Organ Crosstalk in Acute Kidney Injury

Carlos Guido Musso • Adrian Covic

Editors

Organ Crosstalk in Acute Kidney Injury

Basic Concepts and Clinical Practices

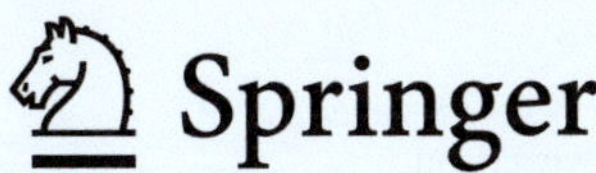 Springer

Editors
Carlos Guido Musso
Nephrology Division
Hospital Italiano de Buenos Aires
Buenos Aires, Argentina

Adrian Covic
Grigore T. Popa University of Medicine
Iasi, Romania

ISBN 978-3-031-36791-5   ISBN 978-3-031-36789-2   (eBook)
https://doi.org/10.1007/978-3-031-36789-2

This Springer imprint is published by the registered company Springer Nature Switzerland AG
The registered company address is: Gewerbestrasse 11, 6330 Cham, Switzerland

To Dr Anita Amalia Rossi, Dr Carlos Adolfo Félix Musso, Doña Juana del Rosario Caballero (Tata), and Don Santiago Castellane (Alo), for their immense love. Carlos G. Musso, MD, PhD.

To my wife. A. Covic, MD, PhD, FRCP, FERA, FESC.

Foreword

The ancient approach to medicine promoted by Hippocrates claimed that "the health of the body depends by the equilibrium of the different components that contribute to the continuum of organs and spirit." Subsequently, Claude Bernard described the concept of the "internal milieu," i.e., the internal environment where cells and tissues can live in optimal conditions only when a stable composition of the fluids is achieved and maintained. Homer Smith added to these concepts the important contribution of the kidneys in his book "from fish to philosopher" confirming that life as we know is made possible by the homeostatic capacity of the kidneys. In Greek, the term "oλoσ" means "whole" and it is normally utilized to describe something whose entire structure is made by the contribution of different parts. In spite of the bad reputation of the term "holistic medicine," normally representing an alternative non-orthodox approach to patient management, we should not neglect the fact that our body is a living organism owing its survival to the contribution of different equally important organs and apparatus. If we agree on this simple concept, it becomes clear that we cannot cure a patient focusing on one single organ, but we must consider the body as a complex entity where various organs are in continuous interaction and exchange of signals and information. While this is known in classic physiology, it tends to be neglected during pathological processes and diseases. Among these conditions, critical illness represents a situation where physicians and specialists tend to focus their attention on one specific organ or apparatus while overlooking important signals coming from the whole body or other organs. This concept has been recently highlighted with the term "organ cross-talk," i.e., the continuous interaction among different organs. Due to this cross-talk, one dysfunctioning organ may affect another organ or multiple organs at the same time. Often this interaction is mediated by physical (pressures and flows), chemical (acid-base and electrolytes), and biological (cytokines, chemokines) signals. In this view, special pathological conditions have been studied, defined, and classified as multidirectional and temporally regulated. This is the case of cardio-renal syndromes, hepato-renal syndromes, cardio-metabolic syndromes, brain-kidney and lung-kidney interactions. Different organs have in common two important components: the vascular endothelium and the circulating blood. Both components can be significantly affected by a dysregulation of the immune system, and this is what typically occurs in sepsis where the inevitable consequence is a multiple organ dysfunction syndrome mediated by a significant yet altered organ cross-talk. What happens to other organs during a physiological event such as pregnancy? What is the effect of a drug designed to heal one organ on other remote organ systems? In recent years, we had to learn about physiological and pathological interactions between native organs, but now we face other challenges. Advancements in technology and application or extracorporeal therapies impose today to learn about another type of interaction: the artificial organ cross-talk. We must be aware of the effects of different extracorporeal organ support systems (ECOS) on various organs, on their function, and on their processes of healing and recovery. It is not uncommon to see a patient with different ECOS such as CRRT + ECMO, CVVHD + ECCO2R, and hemoperfusion + hemodialysis. In all these cases, we should further expand our understanding of the mechanisms of different artificial organs studying possible interactions between them and a fully artificial organ cross-talk.

In my life, I spent a lot of time to bring it to the attention of the scientific community what we call the "Vicenza Model." For years, instead of sending the patient to departments and units, we have made clear that specialists of different disciplines should come to the bedside to discuss together patient's conditions. This multidisciplinary approach led to new specialties such as critical care nephrology and cardio-renal medicine. Organ interaction required physician interaction.

This book is unique in its kind, providing information about various forms of organ cross-talk and suggesting moving beyond single organ or disease, taking care of the patient in his/her whole structure. This is a very important message for young investigators and physicians, but the message can be expanded further. The perfect approach and support for the patient includes the care of the spirit and the psychological mechanisms that may influence the severity of illness, the immune response, and the capacity to fight the disease and the adverse events of life.

DIMED - University of Padova   Claudio Ronco
Padova, Italy

Department of Nephrology Dialysis and Transplantation
International Renal Research Institute of Vicenza (IRRIV)
AULSS8 Regione Veneto, San Bortolo Hospital
Vicenza, Italy

Contents

Chapter 1
Nosology and Semiotics

Morten Tønnessen

1.1 Introduction

The central medical terms 'sign' and 'symptom' are semiotic concepts, with symptoms being a class of signs. There are both natural signs, which are typically exchanged within or between bodies, and conventional (human-made) ones, such as words and cultural imagery. In this chapter, I explain how semiotics, the theory of signs, is relevant for medicine and health studies. I make use of a perspective that draws heavily on biosemiotics, which can be understood as the part of semiotics which is concerned with the study of signs in the realm of the living (biology).

The broad relevance of semiotics for natural science has been emphasized by several scholars [1–3]. In this context, particular attention has been devoted to application of semiotic ideas and models in the study of biological phenomena. However, the acknowledgement of the semiotic nature of the realm of the living is even better established in the context of various human phenomena, ranging from psychological and social to cultural phenomena. An important aim for biosemiotic medicine should be to integrate our knowledge about human biology and medicine with our knowledge about these other human phenomena in so far as they make a difference for disease and health phenomena, within a comprehensive semiotic framework.

Nosology is the theory or study of diseases, or more specifically "the scientific study and classification of diseases and disorders, both mental and physical" [4]. As such, it is related to the concept of *diagnosis* and the practice of *diagnostics*, where making a diagnosis often, and historically, entails recognizing a disease or condition by its signs and symptoms. Classification of diseases has changed considerably over time. Attempts at developing classifications of diseases go all the way back to ancient Greece, but "the first serious attempt to develop a comprehensive approach

M. Tønnessen (✉)
Department of Social Studies, University of Stavanger, Stavanger, Norway

C. G. Musso, A. Covic (eds.), *Organ Crosstalk in Acute Kidney Injury*,
https://doi.org/10.1007/978-3-031-36789-2_1

to the classification of disease" was made in the sixteenth century [5].[1] Since the eighteenth century, it has been recognized that many diseases affect particular organs, and since the middle of the nineteenth century, there have been international classifications of diseases.[2] Even so, there is no general agreement in contemporary philosophy of medicine about what constitutes disease or health [6]. In psychiatric nosology, there is substantial disagreement about if or to what extent classification of diseases should refer to natural kinds, social constructs and/or practical kinds [7].

The condition that today goes under the name acute kidney injury (AKI) has been subjected to numerous different terms throughout history [8]. While competing definitions of AKI have been developed and applied clinically, establishing an ideal, universal definition of AKI has proven challenging, as AKI is a syndrome of many causes [9]. The fact that AKI can result in multi-organ dysfunction or be a first indication of a more complex clinical picture has made scholars study AKI in light of organ crosstalk [10, 11].

'Organ crosstalk' refers to "the complex and mutual biological communication between distant organs mediated by signaling factors" [12].[3] The term has received increasing attention over the last 10 years or so, as several new types of organ crosstalk/interaction have been identified. In the context of nephrology, this includes cardio–pulmonary–renal interactions, hepato-renal (kidney–liver) crosstalk, heart–kidney crosstalk, kidney–brain crosstalk, kidney–gut crosstalk, kidney–lung crosstalk, the cardio–renal axis, kidney–bone crosstalk, and muscle–kidney crosstalk.[4] While under normal circumstances neurons and bloodstream facilitate "interaction between the organs for maintaining an adequate homeostasis," the communication entailed in organ crosstalk can also facilitate "the spread of damage mediators" [10].[5]

As Danesi and Zukowski point out, "despite the fact that the discipline of semiotics traces its roots to the medical domain in the ancient world," medical semiotics "has never really gained a foothold in either semiotics itself or medical science" [13]. They define medical semiotics as "the study of the connection between the biosphere and the semiosphere in all areas of health and disease."[6] Current research which can be categorized as 'medical semiotics' does not systematically cover all major areas of medical research. However, Tredinnick-Rowe and Stanley claim that there are "many areas of clinical practice in which semiotics could be applied," and argue that a semiotic approach in medicine could function "as a qualitative counterpoise to existing bio-statistical approaches in medicine and healthcare" [14].

---

[1] 2011:9.

[2] 2011:9,10.

[3] 2019:825.

[4] 2019:827.

[5] 2019:2203.

[6] 2019:4.

Biosemiotic medicine has been approached from different angles, including body language and interpersonal interaction [15], patient agency and subjective aspects of symptom formation [16], and the interaction of biological and cultural factors of health and illness [13]. The approach of Musso et al. [11] builds on the recognition of a semiotic network which links the whole body and can be conceptualized as a 'biosemiotic plane' that is intimately related to the body's 'structural plane.' In this perspective, diseases should be reconceptualized as disorders on the biosemiotic plane involving pathogenic biosemiosis (i.e. biological sign exchange), since damage on the structural plane is typically preceded by abnormal processes on the biosemiotic plane.

The chapter is structured as follows. I start by outlining a brief historiography of the interrelations between semiotics and studies of health/medicine and also present semiotic aspects of nosology. Next, I introduce fundamental elements of a biosemiotic perspective on human health, focused on the 'Umwelt' notion; a biosemiotic view of the relation between the body and the environment; a biosemiotic view of the relation between physiology, behaviour and perception; and the notion of 'endosemiosis,' encapsulating somatic sign processes. The final section of the chapter comprises contributions to biosemiotic medicine. These include discussing how such an approach can be regarded as process-based medicine, the way in which biosemiotic medicine can bridge studies of human and animal health, and how it can be understood as involving a conception of the human being as a system of interrelated sign systems. In relation to the latter topic, the human microbiome is discussed as a context for the way in which the human organism can be conceived of as an ecosystem. The section concludes by discussing how organ crosstalk can be understood within a biosemiotic framework.

1.2 A Brief Historiography of Semiotics and Health/ Medicine

Through history, semiotic ideas and concepts have been applied in medical literature and contributed to our attempts at providing definitions and explanations of health and disease phenomena and identifying causes of diseases. In this section I outline a historiography of connections between semiotics on the one hand and medicine and health studies on the other.

At its historical beginning, semiotic discourse was indistinguishable from medical discourse. Danesi and Zukowski credit Hippocrates (ca. 460–377 BCE) for being "the founder of both medicine and semiotics,"[7] referring to his coining of the term *semiotiké'* meaning "medicinal diagnosis" [13]. In Greek Antiquity, the art of healing was called *techne semeiotike*, indicating a craft involving the skills to interpret signs [14, 17]. The term 'semiotics' itself is derived from the Greek word

---

[7] 2019:3,5.

for 'sign,' *sēmeion* (σημεῖον). As Deely [18],[8] cited in Tredinnick-Rowe and Stanley [14], observed, semiotics initially referred to "that specific branch of medicine concerned with [...] symptoms, the signs of diseases". More than 500 years after Hippocrates lived, Galen (ca. 129–216) classified semiotics as one of the six principal branches of medicine [19].[9]

Through its central role in Greek Antiquity, semiotic terminology in medicine has also played a role in Roman times and the Middle Ages, as well as in later centuries. Hess outlines medical semiotics in the eighteenth century, as it facilitated combining empirically based rules of instruction with theoretical knowledge drawn from emerging sciences [20]. Traces of the Greeks' mixture of semiotic and medical thinking were still discernible in English language use in the nineteenth century. In *The Imperial Dictionary of the English Language* [21], 'Semeiotics' is said to have two meanings, firstly, "The doctrine or science of signs," and secondly, in pathology, "that branch which teaches how to judge of all the symptoms in the human body, whether healthy or diseased; symtomatology" (cited in Deely [18] and Tredinnick-Rowe and Stanley [14]).

In the early work of the theoretical biologist Jakob von Uexküll (1864–1944), the originator of the Umwelt theory, some views on health and pathology appear in his writings on Umwelt theory [22, 23]. "Die Biologie in ihrer Stellung zur Medizin" [24] reports from a lecture he gave on how biology relates to medicine, in which he does not appear to have addressed specifically medical questions, but argued for the relevance of his biological outlook.

More focused and in-depth work on medicine from a semiotic perspective was done by Jakob's son Thure von Uexküll (1908–2004). Towards the end of his life, Thure von Uexküll played a central role in the establishment of modern biosemiotics [25, 26].[10] Being a physician and professor of psychosomatic medicine, he had throughout his career pioneered and promoted psychosomatic medicine in Germany. In his writings that explicitly address connections between semiotics and medicine [27–29], Thure von Uexküll contrasts a semiotic approach to medicine with a mechanistic approach narrowly based on natural science. His basic premise is that behaviour should be seen as "the response to signs," while physical and chemical processes can serve as vehicles for transportation of meaning or information.[11] All cells in the human body are connected via sign processes.[12] With regard to the Umwelt theory's relevance for medicine, Thure von Uexküll indicated that medicine's inability to integrate physical and psychological aspects of patients' problems could only be overcome by showing interest "in the 'reality' in which the patient lives himself" (i.e. the patient's Umwelt) [30].[13]

---

[8] 2006:76.

[9] 2001:75.

[10] The latter includes a selected bibliography.

[11] 1999:649.

[12] 1986:204.

[13] 2004:374.

According to Thure von Uexküll, the need for sign theory in medicine is most obvious in psychosomatic medicine [27].[14] "The unique position of psychosomatic medicine in Germany" is "largely down to the continuous engagement of Thure von Uexküll" [31]. His legacy in the German context includes the fact that subjects such as psychology, sociology, and psychosomatic medicine are included in the undergraduate medical curriculum, and that several thousand hospital beds are reserved for patients with psychosomatic disorders. In Thure von Uexküll's view, "the progression of a disease depended just as much on the personality, attitude, and the social circumstances of a patient as on his or her medical condition" [31]. Moreover, he regarded "the human being as a system in the environment of other systems" [31], i.e. he contextualized human health in a social and ecological setting.

Tredinnick-Rowe notes that there is currently a "total absence of medical semiotics in the curriculum of medical schools in the English speaking world", and asks whether the works of Thure von Uexküll could "offer a possible step towards a resurrection of medical semiotics in clinical education" [32].[15] In their overview of contemporary research in medical semiotics, Tredinnick-Rowe and Stanley [14] mention work done in gerontology, immunology, psychiatry, psychosomatic medicine and public health. Explicitly semiotic methods are taught in clinical skills courses in psychiatry and neurology in the context of disease identification and categorization in Latin American countries.

While it can be argued that all human thinking and therefore also all psychiatric symptoms are related to the functioning or dysfunction of symbol processes, semiotic approaches to psychopathology have not had any major impact on psychiatry and psychology in recent decades [32]. In this context, Andersch argues that there is an unrealized potential for cooperation between the medical profession and established subfields of semiotics such as biosemiotics and neurosemiotics [33, 34].[16]

1.3   Semiotic Aspects of Nosology

As we saw in the last section, nosology has historically been associated with and made use of semiotic terms. The relevance of semiotics for nosology has also been emphasized by several contemporary scholars. In this section I outline semiotic aspects of nosology.

According to Staiano-Ross, the symptom, as a term, refers to a clinical, objective sign as well as the patient's subjective experience and interpretation of their own health [35]. It can thus be seen as a natural sign at the same time as it has cultural aspects. Rather than understanding symptoms merely as biologically coded events,

---

[14] 1982:212.

[15] 2017:1.

[16] The latter offers a biosemiotic take on neurosemiotics.

she suggests looking at symptoms as indicative of the misadventures of a body and the condition of its associated Umwelt, and therefore as biocultural events. In a similar vein, Danesi and Zukowski, while acknowledging that all "species have a species-specific bodily warning system that alerts them to dangerous changes in the bodily states," stress that "in the human species bodily states are also representable and thus interpretable in culture-specific ways" [13].[17] This implies that both the definition of and the experience of diseases have a cultural aspect, and are related to cultural norms about what is regarded as healthy and sick. Relatedly, Kirmayer points out that "diagnoses serve to position individuals by assigning the sick role," which has personal as well as societal consequences [36].[18]

As Nessa notes, a medical consultation "often starts with the patient presenting a symptom, a bodily sensation of some kind" [37].[19] He portrays the clinical model at work in situations in which diagnoses are being made as involving the triadic relation Symptom–Disease–Diagnosis, corresponding to the semiotic structure Sign–Reference–Meaning).[20] According to Tredinnick-Rowe and Stanley, the physician must "link together signs, history and symptoms that are indicative of a particular pathology" by "weaving together facts into a strong inferential chain" [14]. Thure von Uexküll stresses that the physician is a meta-interpreter of the patient's symptoms, and that the physician and the patient must establish a common reality [29].[21] He sees symptoms as originating from "a disrupted flow of information in which objective and subjective evidences of an illness (signs and symptoms) appear" [28].[22] Burnum emphasizes that medical diagnosis always relies on interpretation of signs, and that getting it right requires recognition of relevant contexts [38]. As he notes, since "interpretation is subjective, it is subject to bias and to the constraints of personal experience" [38].[23] Soldati et al. emphasize doctors' use of abduction and various manipulative actions aiming at eliciting signs in the diagnosing process [39]. Thure von Uexküll cautions that such machine-supported capabilities, although they facilitate progress in medicine, do not eliminate the need for interpreting the patient's subjective signs [28].[24] An important task for the physician in his view is to carry out "the semiotic analysis of the subjective meaning which objective evidences of illness imply" [28].[25]

In their overview of contemporary research in medical semiotics, Tredinnick-Rowe and Stanley mention work done on aphasia, Alzheimer's, anorexia, autism, chronic pain, depression, dementia, fibromyalgia, HIV, obesity and schizophrenia

---

[17] 2019:86.

[18] 2005:193.

[19] 1996:364.

[20] 1996:368.

[21] 1999:653.

[22] 1986:215.

[23] 1993:942.

[24] 1986:205.

[25] 1986:215.

[14]. As this rather limited selection of medical conditions shows, research in medical semiotics does not to date cover all major diseases in any systematic and comprehensive manner, as a full-fledged research paradigm should. Tredinnick-Rowe and Stanley call for "a more comprehensive dialogue between biosemiotics and the use of semiotics in medicine," which may alleviate the situation [14].

1.4 Fundamental Elements of a Biosemiotic Perspective on Human Health

So far in this chapter, we have looked at interrelations between semiotics and medicine, and semiotic aspects of nosology. In so far as what we aim for is comprehension of bodily processes, within semiotics, biosemiotics is particularly relevant. In this section, I present fundamental elements of a biosemiotic perspective on human health, starting with the human Umwelt, i.e. the subjectively experienced lifeworld of human beings, and ending with endosemiosis, the most relevant category of signs in the context of bodily processes.

1.4.1 The Umwelt

A natural starting point for a biosemiotic perspective on human health is the notion of Umwelt. The Umwelt theory in its classical version was developed by Jakob von Uexküll, with major works appearing between 1909 and 1940 [22, 23, 40, 41]. In its updated version, Umwelt theory is a central part of the foundation of contemporary biosemiotics.

According to Uexküll, any animal is endowed with an Umwelt, i.e. a subjectively experienced lifeworld. In terms of biology, this includes the human being. The Umwelt is constituted by signs that are perceived as meaningful by the organism as a whole. What all creatures endowed with an Umwelt have in common is that anything that appears to the organism as meaningful does so within the framework of the Umwelt.

The Umwelt is the realm of our experiences as well as the realm in which our behaviour takes place. In Uexküll's view, behaviour is best understood as continuous response to what we experience. This is expressed by Uexküll's most famous figure, the so-called functional cycle (also called functional circle), where an act is depicted as the functionally justified response to some perceived object [41]. In Uexküll's view, the goal of any action is to make the perceived object disappear from the perceptual field by handling it appropriately. The most fundamental acts of animals include relating to some perceived objects as potential food, enemies or a sexual partner, and relating to the physical medium that the organism navigates within. The disappearance of perceived objects may imply, e.g., that a prey animal has been caught and consumed, that a predator has been avoided, that a sexual partner has been approached, or that the animal has passed through a particular physical medium.

The Umwelt is constituted by the *Merkwelt* (perceptual world) and the *Wirkwelt* (operational world). At a lower level of biological organization these are in turn constituted by *Merkzeichen* (perceptual signs) and *Wirkzeichen* (operational signs). Operating at a cellular level, according to Uexküll such signs represent the biosemiosis which is the foundation of consciously experienced phenomena.

The human Umwelt share basic features, such as the ones described so far, with the Umwelt of other animals, but is distinguished, first, by the way we humans make use of language and abstract thinking [42].[26] This in turn colours our perception even of tangible objects. No matter how distinct the human lifeworld may appear in comparison with the lifeworlds of other animals, we should not forget that when in crisis, human beings also tend to revert to more basic perceptions and actions. The logical starting point for any sound health care philosophy is thus to take care of fundamental bodily needs first.

When human beings relate to their own diseases, exactly what actions are required is not as straightforward as in the simpler cases of satisfying, e.g., hunger or sexual needs. The 'perceived object' may be complex, and it may not be possible to perceive it momentarily. Furthermore, the individual human being itself is not necessarily capable of perceiving the object satisfactorily. Appropriate actions may require the guidance of trained specialists.

This has several implications. First, a human being needs perceptual assistance, as it were, in figuring out the meaning of the 'perceived object' which indicates the incidence of a disease. Within a psychosomatic framework, the patient's own experience nevertheless remains significant [35]. Second, the perception of the disease-related object thus turns into a group task. And third, the appropriate actions that follow from correct identification of a disease may or may not be carried out by the patient him- or herself; they may have to be carried out by an external party (e.g. a doctor or a nurse).

In line with Uexküll's model of the functional cycle [41], successful action against the perception of a disease should result in the disappearance of the perceived object, i.e. the perceived disease. In a psychosomatic perspective, the subsequent perception of the patient's condition following recovery may also be a group task.

---

[26] The latter includes discussion of different views on humans' capabilities and place in nature.

1.4.2   Body and Environment

In the time of von Uexküll's most intense theory development, many theories about biological holism were presented. Many of these theorists "used the model of an organism as a unifying explanatory tool for all levels of reality" [43].[27] To von Uexküll, the organism rather represented the centre of subjectivity and sentience.

By way of the functional cycle, the Umwelt theory aims to say something about the relation between an organism's body and the environment [41]. More specifically, the Umwelt theory stresses that what an organism perceives in its environment, and what it acts upon in its environment, contributes to the constitution of what we could call *the extended organism* (the organism-in-its-environment as a whole). Phrased differently: If you want to understand the perception and behaviour of an organism, you must study its perception and behaviour in its proper context, namely from the perspective of the extended organism. Physiological studies alone are not telling of behaviour; behavioural studies require an environmental perspective that goes beyond the physical organism itself. Hoffmeyer, referring to the fact that a human body has "perhaps as much as 30 km^2 of membrane structure," stresses "how the skin, on the one hand, makes us belong in the world, and on the other hand, is part of the huge landscape of membranes across which the semiotic self incessantly must be reconstituted" [44].[28]

Applied to the study of diseases, a biosemiotic perspective entails that a first step should be to identify the relevant environmental context of a disease. For complex diseases or disorders, this might have to involve the entire environmental context of a human individual.

Given the ubiquity of signs and sign processes, applying a semiotic perspective may be appropriate for the study of complex wholes in the realm of the living [16, 29]. Giorgi et al. thus suggest that the biopsychosocial model can be better understood if approached biosemiotically [45].[29] Relatedly, Grzybek (1993) suggests that empirical semiotics "may [...] offer our first hope of a unifying methodology for the cognitive sciences" [46].[30]

1.4.3   Physiology, Behaviour and Perception

In a biosemiotic perspective, physiology, behaviour and perception should be studied in conjunction, since these phenomena are interrelated. Umwelt theory is founded on the combination of physiological and behavioural studies.

---

[27] 2008:379.

[28] 2008:175,169.

[29] 2020:369.

[30] 1993:1.

A central notion in Uexküll's work is that of the 'Bauplan' (literally: blueprint or construction plan), which is the organism's physiological and functional organization. Early on in his first major work, *Umwelt und Innenwelt der Tiere*, von Uexküll states that it is the Bauplan, depicted as a spatial scheme, that shows us how different parts of the organism, and different processes that take place within the organism, are connected [22].[31] This, however, does not establish the physical organism alone as a functional unit. But the Bauplan furthermore largely determines the exact nature of the Umwelt of an organism and directs it towards seeking out that in its physical environment which suits it given the way the organism itself is built.[32] And this is the proper context for organismic functionality—a functioning organism is an organism that is active in a suitable environment, and the organism as a functional unit is constituted by the organism and the environment in liaison.

As Brentari remarks, the Bauplan can in some cases be understood as "a structure which actually exists in the organism"—i.e. an ontological reality, but in other cases von Uexküll appears instead to refer to a scientific model reconstructed for the purpose of understanding an organism—i.e. an epistemological tool [47].[33] In his case-specific scientific work, von Uexküll often used the term "to refer to the structure and the organization of the animal itself" [47].[34]

Musso et al.'s conception of the organism's structural plane and biosemiotic plane [11] could be understood in light of von Uexküll's notion of Bauplan. In their understanding, not only the structural plane but also the biosemiotic plane should be understood in material terms, since the vital information flow on the biosemiotic plane typically involves exchange of signalling molecules such as hormones and neurotransmitters, cytokines and autacoids. Various flows of organic substances thus mediate sign exchange, with the sign processes having obvious material aspects. The vital information flow on the biosemiotic plane sustains and has an impact on the structural plane over time. Like von Uexküll's Bauplan notion, Musso et al.'s conception of the organism as having a structural plane which is integrated with a biosemiotic plane [11] also has both a material and a functional aspect, and explains functionality in terms of biosemiosis.

1.4.4   Endosemiosis

With signs permeating the realm of the living, we have good use of a distinction between sign processes that are internal to the body and those that are not. This is found in the distinction between 'exosemiosis' and 'endosemiosis,' where the suffix '-semiosis' means sign exchange or sign action [48]. Exo- and endosemiosis refer

---

[31] 1909:12.

[32] 1909:5.

[33] 2015:60.

[34] 2015:77.

to semiosis that is external and internal to the body respectively. Specifically, von Uexküll T and Geigges define endosemiosis as referring to "processes of sign transmission inside the organism".[35] They describe the cell as the "most elementary integrating unit" of biosemiosis, and observe that "all sign processes occurring in multicellular organisms are 'endosemiotic,' no matter whether we look at fungi, plants, animals, or humans".[36] The authors operate with a hierarchical system of different integration levels, starting with microsemiosis (sign exchange within cells) and proceeding to cytosemioses (sign exchange between cells) and organ semiosis. A fourth integration level involves the immune system and the nervous system, which envelop the whole body and together constitute the inner world of the organism.[37] In the context of the immune system, they remark that as "a transport system for sign vehicles, the bloodstream is considerably slower" than the nervous system.[38]

"All endosemiotic sign processes" are said to be "indirectly linked to phenomena in the organism's environment," with the link between the nervous system and the locomotor apparatus exemplifying how the inner world of the organism (the 'Innenwelt' in Jakob von Uexküll's terminology) reflects its Umwelt [48].[39] Von Uexküll T and Geigges support the pragmatic idea that signs are generally "for somebody."[40] On the most basic level, this implies that the cell is the interpreting unit in the case of microsemiosis. They are somewhat reluctant, however, to attribute subjecthood at levels in-between the cell and the organism, stating that "[d]ifficulties arise […] if it has to be decided whether a cell aggregation, a tissue, or an organ should be regarded, in an endosemiotic sense, as the addressee "for whom" certain sign processes may possess a pragmatic meaning."[41] There is in their view no "one-dimensional hierarchical order" for endosemiotic processes, "but several ramified orders and numerous feedback loops between them" [48].[42]

This foundational understanding of endosemiosis is supplemented by Sebeok, who states that various biological codes, characterized by Sebeok as "syntax-controlled semiotic systems," play an important role in regulating and directing several forms of endosemiosis [49].[43] He specifically mentions the genetic code, neural code, immune code and metabolic code.

A contemporary contribution to biosemiotic medicine which may inform our understanding of endosemiosis is provided by Nowlin, who investigates the role of dysfunctional signalling processes in human pathology within a biosemiotic

---

[35] 1993:283.
[36] 1993:283.
[37] 1993:286.
[38] 1993:302.
[39] 1993:283.
[40] 1993:299.
[41] 1993: 299.
[42] 1993:300.
[43] 1996:107–108.

framework [50]. In immunology, it is well established that allergies are related to inappropriate defence reactions of the immune system. Nowlin's core hypothesis is that *errant defense*, far from being limited to immunology, "is a universal physiological phenomenon that can occur with any system in the body," and "results from dysfunctional signaling processes which alter stimulus interpretation, leading to erroneous perception of threat."[44] She argues that identification of threats is a primitive function that occurs in all animals, and that "living systems in the body have evolved with defense mechanisms" to protect the integrity of cells and organs.[45] Defining errant defence as "any negative, pathological or abnormal physiological reaction to a benign stimulus," she explains such reactions as the response to a system's negative valuation of a stimulus, with the purpose of the defence reaction being to "preserve the 'self'" of the system [50].[46]

1.5   Contributions to Biosemiotic Medicine

After having presented the fundamental elements of a biosemiotic perspective on human health in the previous section, I now proceed to make a few more explicit contributions to biosemiotic medicine. This will include approaching biosemiotic medicine from different angles, namely in its character of being process-based medicine, and in providing a bridge between human and animal health studies. It will further include presenting a conception of the human being as a system of interrelated sign systems, and a framing of the human organism as an ecosystem in the context of the human microbiome. To draw the chapter to a close, some remarks are made on how organ crosstalk can be understood within a biosemiotic framework.

1.5.1   *Process-Based Medicine in Light of the Ontogeny of the Human Being*

According to Musso et al., modern medicine suffers from an overreliance on physiological and physiopathological points of view and neglect of processual perspectives [11]. In their view, both the structural plane and the biosemiotic plane of an organism can be regarded as temporal, developing entities, with the structural plane having a slow pace (slow and in some cases permanent changes) and the biosemiotic plane a fast pace (rapid and more dynamic changes). Instead of basing diagnoses on identification of damaged organs, we should in this view aim for earlier diagnoses based on early detection of pathogenic crosstalk. They call this

---

[44] 2021:155.

[45] 2021:158.

[46] 2021:158,157.

'biosemiotic process medicine' [11, 51]. In a somewhat similar manner, von Uexküll T and Geigges refer to 'semiotic anatomy,' with 'anatomy' denoting "dynamic structures being constantly constructed and transformed," and "the vital relations between the organism's cells and organs [...] established and maintained by information transmission through signs" [48].[47]

It is an established fact that any organism's body takes shape gradually in the course of the organism's development until it reaches the stage of the adult organism [52].[48] This is naturally the case for the human body as well—including organ systems, such as the urinary system. The coming to be of a body clearly demonstrates that physiology has processual aspects. However, conceiving of an organism's body as a mature body *only* simplifies the understanding of the body to an unwarranted extent. Neither is the perspective of the origination of adult organisms always sufficient to understand the health condition of adult organisms.

In the context of process-based medicine, it is worth noting that the term 'ontogeny' can be applied to two different temporal perspectives: either the development of an organism from an egg to an adult organism, or the development of an organism throughout its lifespan. In the latter sense, ontogeny covers any organismic development whatsoever, and in this perspective, it becomes clear that organisms are subject to processes of change throughout their lives, and not only in their initial, forming, developmental stages. For instance, normal development of the urinary system involves the emergence of voluntary control of urination. But in some cases, humans lose this function at some later life stage. As all individuals who are fortunate enough to die of old age demonstrate, processes of change, including physiological ones, occur at all life stages.

The idea that physiology, behaviour and perception should be studied in conjunction—an idea which is prominent in biosemiotic thinking, among other strains of thought—has implications for the understanding of process-based medicine. In the same vein, it also has implications for our understanding of biosemiotic medicine as process-based medicine. Beyond the processual aspects of human ontogeny, which have already been mentioned, there are further processual aspects to physiology as well, related to the integration of physiology with behaviour and perception. The functioning of a living body is intimately related to the perceptual and behavioural repertoire its physiological makeup enables at any point in time. This functioning is not static, but subject to change throughout the lifespan—potentially at any given moment. Whenever diseases or disorders affect the functioning of specific organs, they tend to affect the functioning of the body as a whole as well. When physiological malfunctioning occurs, the patient's perception and behaviour are often immediately affected.

---

[47] 1993:284.

[48] The latter offers a portrayal of human ontogeny in an Umwelt perspective.

1.5.2 Biosemiotic Medicine Within and Beyond Human Health Studies

Over the last few years, the One Health agenda has increasingly been recognized, for instance by the World Health Organization. The core idea of the agenda is that human and animal health should be seen in context, and that professionals in human medicine and veterinary medicine should interact and learn from each other. As Day points out, the contemporary One Health agenda has deep historical roots in comparative medicine and comparative anatomy through centuries of work, including that of classics within infectious disease research [53]. Zinsstag et al. refer to developments over the second half of the twentieth century and 'One Medicine' as a precursor to One Health [54]. Since the 1980s, an increasing international focus on sustainable development has stimulated interest in relations between human and animal health and ecosystems.

A key issue related to connections between human and animal health is zoonotic diseases, which often involves a "transmission chain from wildlife to livestock and to people" [54].[49] Zinsstag et al. call for simultaneous studies of zoonoses in people and animals and an integrated health system addressing health issues across species [54]. Wondwossen et al. address how a 'global One Health paradigm' can improve the tackling of infectious diseases, especially in low-resource settings in poorer countries [55]. Writing 5 years before the Covid-19 pandemic, they state that 75% of newly emerging infectious diseases are zoonoses, and that the top 56 zoonoses cause 2.5 billion cases of human illness and 2.7 million deaths per year. Wondwossen et al. argue that an integrated surveillance system drawing on reports from environmental monitoring as well as human and animal health diagnostic systems is required to better tackle infectious diseases [55].

In extension of the One Health agenda, Pinillos et al. have suggested a One Welfare agenda where human and animal welfare are studied in conjunction [56]. They argue that interdisciplinary collaboration would deepen our understanding of the interconnections of human, animal and environmental factors, and benefit both animal welfare and human wellbeing. In the context of diseases, Pinillos et al. point out that "poor animal welfare result[s] in increased release and virulence of a number of zoonotic diseases" [56].[50]

With its foundation in biosemiotics, which involves a semiotic perspective on issues in biology at large, biosemiotic medicine is well positioned to contribute to comparative studies of health issues in humans and animals. If developed further, it even has the potential for contributing to establishing a more comprehensive theoretical framework for the One Health agenda. Similar claims could be made with regard to the One Welfare agenda. As Danesi and Zukowski indicate, medical semiotics can draw on Jakob von Uexküll's idea that "organisms are distinguished by semiosis," implying that "a species interprets symptoms, and reacts to them, in

---

[49] 2005:2143.

[50] 2016:413.

its own peculiar biologically-programmed way," in accordance with its exact anatomy [13].[51] There is thus a potential for comparative studies with animal health issues whenever human anatomy resembles animal anatomy.

This applies to acute kidney injury as well as to any other disease or health issue that is rooted in anatomical factors which can be studied in a comparative perspective. Given that all vertebrate animals—i.e. all mammals, birds, reptiles, amphibians, and fish—have kidneys, the potential for comparative studies of AKI and similar health issues across species is considerable. Rather than limiting such studies to applying animal models to human cases of AKI, a One Health approach implies that learning should go both ways in-between human and animal medicine [54].

1.5.3   The Human Being Conceived of as a System of Interrelated Sign Systems

In biosemiotics, it is commonplace to frame the operation of signs in terms of sign processes and sign systems. As stressed by Sharov and Tønnessen, semiosis, or the use of signs, should always be associated with, and understood in light of, the semiotic agents that control or perform the semiosis [2]. The human being as an individual organism is one such semiotic agent which is endowed with what we can call 'semiotic agency,' i.e. the ability to make use of signs. In addition to being a semiotic agent at the organismic level, any organism incorporates a number of subagents, which can be understood as involving autonomous sign systems operating at sub-organismic levels of biological organization. We can therefore understand the human organism—and any other organism—as a system of interrelated sign systems [2].

This perspective on the human organism stresses the importance of a semiotic approach to health issues, and the systemic and organized nature of most sign processes. In the context of biosemiotic medicine, the conception of the human being as a system of interrelated sign systems provides a theoretical framework for studying the interrelation between different somatic sign processes. As Thure von Uexküll writes, "for the introduction of semiotics into the science of medicine, it is essential to describe the connections that exist between the different levels and their sign processes" [28].[52] This is relevant for the study of organ crosstalk on one condition, namely that we can conceive of human organs, or at least organs involved in organ crosstalk, as subagents of the organism-level semiotic agent, and therefore as involving their own organ-specific autonomous sign system. More specifically, organs are subagents that partake in an organ system, which can likewise be understood as a subagent of the organism-level semiotic agent. For clarity, we may distinguish between the different organizational levels of subagents in this context

---

[51] 2019:30.
[52] 1986:211.

by referring to first-order and second-order subagents, with first-order subagents representing the highest level of organization. In this view of the human body approached as an organism endowed with semiotic agency, the kidneys constitute a second-order subagent partaking in the urinary system as a first-order subagent of the human organism.

An organ is commonly defined as a collection of tissues that are joined in a structural unit to serve a common function. The study of organ crosstalk is particularly relevant for understanding the function and dysfunction of organs that can be explained by reference to endosemiosis occurring between organs. In the conception of Musso et al., the organism is formed by the combination of a structural plane and a biosemiotic plane [11]. In this view, flows of various signalling molecules that act as biosigns functionally connect vital organs, and organs may be seen as both anatomical structures that produce crosstalk and as products of such crosstalk [11]. This is also in line with von Uexküll T and Geigges' conception of "semiotic anatomy" [48].

Drawing on "the biosemiotic position which recognizes cells and organs as semiotic systems," Nowlin portrays the body as "a community of living systems within living systems, or selves within selves, each with their own boundary and need to interpret and respond to the surrounding environment" [50].[53] Organs are living systems in this sense [2, 50]. Each system "must be able to respond to a quasi-negative environment that includes increasingly complex and every-changing stimuli," and given that "interpretive systems are not always accurate" and that "fallibility is a basic feature of semiosis," any "system in the body is capable of reacting inappropriately to a harmless stimulus, exogenous or endogenous," and thus of enacting what Nowlin calls errant defence [50].[54]

While some of the functions of an organ system are performed locally, others may require coordinated whole-body action performed at the level of the organism. In the context of the urinary system, urination is an example of a function that requires organism-level action. Urination occurs as a reflex in infants, but by voluntary action in healthy children and adults. In the perspective of Umwelt theory, it is worth recalling that the 'functional cycle' applies to any act performed by the organism as a whole [41]. Within this framework, the act of urinating can be understood as an act that is tailored to neutralize the individual human being's sensation that the urinary bladder is full.[55] After emptying the bladder and thus disposing of waste from the body, the sensation vanishes, and the individual can proceed to focus on other tasks. While the cognitive mechanism involved is likely quite straightforward, the act of urinating nevertheless requires the participation of the brain, the nervous system and muscles, and thus coordinated whole-body action.

---

[53] 2021:158.

[54] 2021:176,158.

[55] Urination is also performed by voluntary control in many animals. In some species, such as wolves, dogs, rats and mice, urination has additional functions beyond disposal of waste material, in that urine is left at specific locations as a sign with social or practical significance, for their own perusal or that of fellow specimen.

As this fact illustrates, even though the urinary system for the most part functions as an autonomous subsystem of the organism as a whole—encompassing a first-order subagent of the human organism—the urinary system regularly involves the organism as a whole in its functioning as well. This involvement is induced by way of signals communicated via the nervous system. From a semiotic point of view, we can observe that the body, as a system of interrelated sign systems, relies on coordinated dynamic interaction between different levels of semiotic agency.

1.5.4 The Human Microbiome: The Human Organism Conceived of as an Ecosystem

In the previous subsection we discussed how the human organism can be conceived of as a system of interrelated sign systems, with organ systems and organs acting as first-order and second-order subagents of the human organism as a whole. In this subsection, the human microbiome—involving microorganisms that utilize various body sites in the human organism as habitat—is approached as exemplifying that the human organism can in some contexts serve as an ecosystem for other species.[56] Despite the radical difference between conceiving of the human organism as an agent and individual and conceiving of it as an ecosystem, the two perspectives are compatible and are in effect in operation simultaneously.

As noted in Sect. 1.4.2, "Body and Environment," rather than an isolated organism, a functioning organism is a whole constituted by the organism-and-its-environment. Recent investigations into the nature of the human microbiome, which involve bacteria, archaea, fungi, protists and viruses that permanently live in a human body, are informative in this regard [57]. As Knight et al. recount, improved methods for DNA analysis have in recent years made microbiome research possible that is now reshaping our understanding of human biology. This includes "rapid discovery of new links between diseases and the microbiome," e.g. on the gut–brain axis, and investigations of "crosstalk between the microbiome and epigenetic regulation" which "may also modulate disease susceptibility" [57].[57]

It is by now well established that the development of human infants and children relies on the maturation of the infant's microbiome, which is significantly affected by whether birth occurs vaginally or by cesarean section [57].[58] It is likewise well established that antibiotics usage can have a long-term detrimental effect on the gut microbiome [57].[59] However, only a fraction of the 2 kg of microbial biomass in a typical adult, which likely has a gene content "exceeding the ~20,000 human genes

---

[56] Parasites are another example of organisms that can take up residence in the human body.

[57] 2017:75,78.

[58] 2017:72–73.

[59] 2017:73.

by at least a factor of 100," and which includes an estimated 39 trillion microorganisms in the gut alone, has been studied [57].[60]

The existence of the microbiome implies that the human organism as a coordinated whole has to relate not only to its own bodily subsystems, but also to a number of other internal agentive powers in the form of microbes. The human microbiome can be regarded as an interface between the human organism as conceived of in species-specific terms and our actual ecology, where we as humans co-exist with several other species, some of which we depend on for our normal functioning. More specifically, the human microbiome can be seen as the microbic ecology we carry with us, in us or on us, as organisms. This perspective shows us that a living human body is in fact a multi-species entity, that the human species is not self-contained, and that no sharp distinction can be drawn between the human body or organism and the environment in which we live. The human microbiome supplements the human organism's own complexity in intricate ways and contributes to making the study of health and diseases even more challenging.

1.5.5   A Biosemiotic Understanding of Organ Crosstalk

A biosemiotic view on organ crosstalk can build on conceiving of organs and organ systems as semiotic subagents that operate within the biological context of the human organism and that each involves sign systems that are specific to organs and organ systems. Combined with a conception of the human organism as a system of interrelated sign systems, this opens a research avenue in which the interrelation of various somatic sign systems can be studied, including in the context of organ crosstalk.

In this view, each organ engages in two kinds of endosemiosis, with one occurring internally within the tissues of the organ itself, and the other occurring in-between the organ and other organs within the organism. We can call these two kinds of endosemiosis 'intra-organ endosemiosis' and 'inter-organ endosemiosis' respectively. The latter is particularly relevant for the study of organ crosstalk. Intra-organ endosemiosis is most relevant for understanding functions that organs can perform locally, and may relate, e.g., to signalling within the tissues of an organ. Any organ system relies on some inter-organ endosemiosis occurring between the organs involved in the organ system. Furthermore, inter-organ endosemiosis should always be taken into account when studying organ functioning that requires involvement of the organism as a whole. In humans (and all sentient animals) this often involves signalling via the nervous system. In cases where inter-organ endosemiosis interferes with functioning that is normally performed locally within an organ, it becomes relevant in studies of such functions as well.

---

[60] 2017:66,78.

Table 1.1 Typology of biosemiosis in relation to organs

Level of organization	Semiosis internal to unit	Which may be equal to …	Semiosis between units	Which may be equal to …
Cell	Intra-cellular endosemiosis		Inter-cellular endosemiosis	Intra-tissue endosemiosis Intra-organ endosemiosis **Intra-organ system endosemiosis** Organismic endosemiosis
Tissue	Intra-tissue endosemiosis	Inter-cellular endosemiosis	Inter-tissue endosemiosis	Intra-organ endosemiosis **Intra-organ system endosemiosis** Organismic endosemiosis
Organ	Intra-organ endosemiosis	Inter-cellular endosemiosis Inter-tissue endosemiosis	**Inter-organ endosemiosis**	**Intra-organ system endosemiosis** **Organismic endosemiosis**
Organ system	**Intra-organ system endosemiosis**	**Inter-cellular endosemiosis** **Inter-tissue endosemiosis** **Inter-organ endosemiosis**	**Inter-organ system endosemiosis**	**Organismic endosemiosis**
Organism	Organismic endosemiosis	Inter-cellular endosemiosis Inter-tissue endosemiosis **Inter-organ endosemiosis** **Inter-organ system endosemiosis**	Exosemiosis	Ecological semiosis Social semiosis

As shown in Table 1.1, a typology of biosemiosis can be built on the commonly held conception that an organism is constituted by cells that make up tissues, that in turn make up organs, that in turn make up organ systems, that in turn make up the organism. In the table, types of semiosis that are particularly relevant for organ crosstalk are highlighted using bold font. The dynamic interaction between different levels of agency at different levels of organization is accentuated by indications of how semiosis internal to a unit at one level may be equal to semiosis between units at lower levels of organization (third column). Likewise, it is also indicated how semiosis between units at one level may be equal to semiosis internal to a unit at higher levels of organization (fifth column). In many cases, one and the same sign process can be approached from different perspectives, depending on the level of organization that is emphasized. The two most relevant types of biosemiosis in the context of organ crosstalk are inter-organ endosemiosis and intra-organ system endosemiosis. However, considering the dynamic interaction between different levels of agency, such endosemiosis may involve sign exchange within an organ system or within the organism as a whole (in the case of inter-organ endosemiosis), as well as sign exchange between cells, between tissues and between organs (in the case of intra-organ system endosemiosis).

Endosemiotic sign exchange often takes the form of cell signalling. This may involve, e.g., autocrine signalling in an intracellular context, and paracrine signalling or juxtacrine signalling in a local intercellular context. Longer-distance sign exchange typically involves endocrine signalling via the endocrine system or neurocrine signalling via the nervous system. Also relevant in the context of cell signalling is signal transduction, which concerns cells' utilization of signals originating from outside the cell.

Most of the human body's organs are engaged in endosemiosis only—in other words, the sign processes they are involved in are limited to occur within the physical organism. In contrast, the sense organs related to the external senses— namely the skin, eyes, ears, nose, mouth and vestibular system—are primarily engaged with exosemiosis. The sign processes they are involved in generally play a role in receiving and interpreting external signals from other organisms or from the external environment. Moreover, organs involved in whole-body expressive actions, such as the larynx and voluntary muscles involved in the musculoskeletal system/ human locomotor system, may also play a part in exosemiosis, by contributing to communicative acts. The sense organs that are related to the internal senses are engaged in endosemiosis on par with most of the other organs.

With regard to the term 'acute kidney injury,' George [8] raises the question of whether 'injury' is really "a preferable term by which to describe acute impairment of renal function?"[61] As he points out, 'injury' typically refers to physical damage, and using this term therefore in effect "poses a structural term to convey the meaning of a syndrome of malfunction."[62] In doing so, we are "describing a physiological *process* in anatomical words" [8].[63] This is a pertinent point to make in light of our earlier discussion of biosemiotic medicine in its aspect of being process-based medicine (cf. Sect. 1.5.1). As stressed there, the functioning of a living body is not static, but subject to change throughout the lifespan. If diseases or disorders affecting specific organs can be explained by organ crosstalk, malfunction will be best understood in a processual perspective. Understanding organ crosstalk within a biosemiotic framework likewise aligns with a processual perspective on organ

---

[61] 2018:5.

[62] 2018:5.

[63] 2018:5, emphasis added.

functioning and malfunction, since it involves what we can understand as a flow of semiosis which may change over time.

Whether the context is AKI or health care more generally, proper patient care requires that attention is paid to the first-person experimental perspective that is encapsulated in the Umwelt notion, and the implied change in Umwelt experience [58].[64] While AKI has multiple features, many of which are not experienced directly by the patient, a key measure of successful treatment of AKI must be an improvement in the patient's experience of health and disease before vs. after the treatment. Given a biosemiotic perspective on organ crosstalk, this requires seeing connections between the endosemiosis occurring in the kidneys and the kidneys' interrelation with the human organism as a whole. Such connections may become discernable in the disturbance of a regular function, such as urination, or in various AKI-related symptoms (e.g. nausea, fatigue, irregular heartbeat, shortness of breath) that trigger the patient to perform perceptible whole-body actions and responses. What disturbance in functions that are performed voluntarily and symptoms that affect the perception of the body as a whole have in common is that they significantly impact the patient's experience of his or her life, and thus the patient's experienced quality of life. While the problems may in a sense be 'located' in the kidneys, they may be caused by dysfunctional organ crosstalk involving other parts of the body. When the health issues are severe enough, there is a risk that one dysfunctional organ can dominate the patient's attention and experience, thus further distressing the human organism as a whole.

Nowlin's theorizing on the errant defence reactions of various systems in the body [50] is informative in the context of organ crosstalk. As she points out, in some cases where errant defence reactions occur, "medical tests are unable to detect a physical cause," but this may be because "the cause is semiotic: the reacting system is 'perceiving' a harmless stimulus as a threat and responding inappropriately."[65] A better understanding of what occurs at what Musso et al. call the biosemiotic plane [11] is then required. Nowlin speculates that "endogenous signals from the body's various systems can become associated with unconditioned stimuli," and indicates a need for research on the role of the Sympathetic Nervous System "in the defensive reaction of specific organs or systems" [50].[66]

The main pillars of a biosemiotic theoretical framework for understanding organic crosstalk are already in place. More empirically oriented research is needed on several fronts, ranging from endosemiotic sign exchange, the connections between different somatic sign systems, and organ-related defence reactions, to patients' Umwelt experience and sign-based doctor–patient interaction. Further theoretical refinement is also needed, to improve our understanding of how various sign processes are at work in the context of medicine.

---

[64] The latter addresses 'Umwelt transitions.'

[65] 2021:160.

[66] 2021:168,174.

References

1. Anderson M, Deely J, Krampen M, Ransdell J, Sebeok TA, von Uexküll T. A semiotic perspective on the sciences: steps toward a new paradigm. Semiotica. 1984;52(1/2):7–47.
2. Sharov A, Tønnessen M. Semiotic agency: science beyond mechanism. Cham: Springer Nature; 2021.
3. Pelkey J, Walsh Matthews S. Semiotics in the natural and technical sciences (Bloomsbury semiotics volume 2). London: Bloomsbury Academic; 2022.
4. APA dictionary of psychology. Nosology. American Psychological Association, 2021. https://dictionary.apa.org/nosology.
5. Moriyama IM, Loy RM, Robb-Smith AHT. Development of the classification of diseases. In: Rosenberg HM, Hoyert DL, editors. History of the statistical classification of diseases and causes of death. Hyattsville, MD: National Center for Health Statistics; 2011. p. 9–22.
6. Reiss J, Ankeny RA. Philosophy of medicine. In: Zalta EN, editor. The Stanford encyclopedia of philosophy; 2016. https://plato.stanford.edu/archives/sum2016/entries/medicine. Accessed 05 Dec 2021.
7. Zachar P, Kendler KS. The philosophy of nosology. Annu Rev Clin Psychol. 2017;13:49–71. https://doi.org/10.1146/annurev-clinpsy-032816-045020.
8. George CRP. The rise and fall of acute tubular necrosis – an exercise in medical semiotics. Giornal italiano di nefrologia. 2018;35(Supplement 70):138–42.
9. Thomas ME, Blaine C, Dawnay A, Devonald MAJ, Ftouh S, Laing C, et al. The definition of acute kidney injury and its use in practice. Kidney Int. 2015;87:62–73.
10. Capalbo O, Giuliani S, Ferrero-Fernández A, Casciato P, Musso CG. Kidney–liver pathophysiological crosstalk: its characteristics and importance. Int Urol Nephrol. 2019;51:2203–7. https://doi.org/10.1007/s11255-019-02288-x.
11. Musso CG, Musso-Enz VP, Musso-Enz GM, Capalbo MO, Porrini S. Organic crosstalk: a new perspective in medicine. Biosemiotics. 2022;14:829–37. https://doi.org/10.1007/s12304-021-09459-3.
12. Armutcu F. Organ crosstalk: the potent roles of inflammation and fibrotic changes in the course of organ interactions. Inflamm Res. 2019;68:825–39. https://doi.org/10.1007/s00011-019-01271-7.
13. Danesi M, Zukowski N. Medical semiotics: medicine and cultural meaning. München: Lincom; 2019.
14. Tredinnick-Rowe J, Stanley DE. Semiotics in health and medicine. In: Pelkey J, Walsh Matthews S, editors. Semiotics in the natural and technical sciences (Bloomsbury semiotics volume 2). London: Bloomsbury Academic; 2022.
15. Cowley S, Major JC, Steffensen SV, Dinis A. Signifying bodies: biosemiosis, interaction and health. Braga: Portuguese Catholic University; 2010.
16. Goli F, editor. Biosemiotic medicine: healing in the world of meaning (studies in neuroscience, consciousness and spirituality 5). Cham: Springer; 2016.
17. Baer E. Medical semiotics. Lanham: University Press of America; 1988.
18. Deely J. On 'semiotics' as naming the doctrine of signs. Semiotica. 2006;158:1–33.
19. Sebeok TA. Signs: an introduction to semiotics. 2nd ed. London: University of Toronto Press; 2001.
20. Hess V. Medical semiotics in the 18th century: a theory of practice? Theor Med Bioeth. 1998;19:203–13. https://doi.org/10.1023/a:1009957730860.
21. Annandale C. The Imperial dictionary of the English language. London: London Blackie & Son; 1883.
22. von Uexküll J. Umwelt und Innenwelt der Tiere. Berlin: Verlag von Julius Springer; 1909.
23. von Uexküll J. Umwelt und Innenwelt der Tiere. 2nd ed. Berlin: Verlag von Julius Springer; 1921.
24. von Uexküll J. Die Biologie in ihrer Stellung zur Medizin. Written by Kowitz Klin Wochenschr. 1927;6(24):1164–5.

25. Kull K, Hoffmeyer J. Thure von Uexküll 1908–2004. Sign Syst Stud. 2005;33(2):487–94.
26. Tiivel T, Kull K. Thure von Uexküll: Symbiosis of biology, medicine, and semiotics. In: Wagner E, et al., editors. From symbiosis to eukaryotism. Geneva: University of Geneva; 1999. p. 657–61.
27. von Uexküll T. Semiotics and medicine. Semiotica. 1982;38(3/4):205–15.
28. von Uexküll T. Medicine and semiotics. Semiotica. 1986;61:201–17.
29. von Uexküll T. The relationship between semiotics and mechanical models of explanation in the life sciences. Semiotica. 1999;127(1/4):647–55.
30. von Uexküll T. Eye witnessing Jakob von Uexküll's umwelt theory. Sign Syst Stud. 2004;32(1/2):374–5.
31. Tuffs A. Thure von Uexküll: a pioneer of psychosomatic medicine. Obituary BMJ. 2004;329(7473):1047.
32. Tredinnick-Rowe J. The (re)-introduction of semiotics into medical education: on the works of Thure von Uexküll. Med Humanit. 2017;43:1–8.
33. Andersch N. Semiotics in psychiatry and psychology. In: Pelkey J, Walsh Matthews S, editors. Semiotics in the natural and technical sciences (Bloomsbury semiotics volume 2). London: Bloomsbury Academic; 2022.
34. Tønnessen M. Beyond the human animal: Towards a cross-species neurosemiotics. In: García A, Ibanez A, editors. The Routledge Handbook of Semiosis and the Brain, 82–96. Routledge; 2022.
35. Staiano-Ross K. The symptom. Biosemiotics. 2012;5:33–45. https://doi.org/10.1007/s12304-011-9112-6.
36. Kirmayer LJ. Culture, context and experience in psychiatric diagnosis. Psychopathology. 2005;38:192–6. https://doi.org/10.1159/000086090.
37. Nessa J. About signs and symptoms: can semiotics expand the view of clinical medicine? Theor Med Bioeth. 1996;17(4):363–77.
38. Burnum JF. Medical diagnosis through semiotics: giving meaning to the sign. Ann Intern Med. 1993;119:939–43.
39. Soldati G, Smargiassi A, Mariani AA, Inchingolo R. Novel aspects in diagnostic approach to respiratory patients: is it the time for a new semiotics? Multidiscip Respir Med. 2017;12:15. https://doi.org/10.1186/s40248-017-0098-z.
40. von Uexküll J. Bedeutungslehre (Bios. Abhandlungen zur theoretischen Biologie und ihrer geschichte sowie zur Philosophie der organischen Naturwissenschaften Bd. 10). Verlag von J. A. Barth; 1940.
41. von Uexküll J. A foray into the worlds of animals and humans with a theory of meaning. In: O'Neil JD, editor. Minneapolis, MN: University of Minneapolis Press; 2010.
42. Jaroš F, Maran T. Humans on top, humans among the other animals: narratives of anthropological difference. Biosemiotics. 2019;12(3):381–403.
43. Magnus R. Biosemiotics within and without biological holism: a semio-historical analysis. Biosemiotics. 2008;1(3):379–96. https://doi.org/10.1007/s12304-008-9021-5.
44. Hoffmeyer J. The semiotic body. Biosemiotics. 2008;1(2):169–90. https://doi.org/10.1007/s12304-008-9015-3.
45. Giorgi F, Tramonti F, Fanali A. A biosemiotic approach to the biopsychosocial understanding of disease adjustment. Biosemiotics. Universitätsverlag Dr. Norbert Brockmeyer. 2020;13(3):369–83.
46. Grzybek P. Psychosemiotics – Neurosemiotics: what could/should it be? In: Grzybek P, editor. Psychosemiotik – Neurosemiotik. Bochum, Universitätsverlag Dr. Norbert Brockmeyer; 1993. p. 1–14.
47. Brentari C. Jakob von Uexküll: the discovery of the umwelt between biosemiotics and theoretical biology (biosemiotics 9). Dordrecht: Springer; 2015.
48. von Uexküll T, Geigges W, Herrmann J. Endosemiosis. In: Favareau D, editor. Essential readings in biosemiotics – anthology and commentary (biosemiotics 3). Springer; 2010. p. 283–321. First published in Semiotica 1993;96(1/2):5–51.

49. Sebeok TA. Signs, bridges, origins. In: Trabant J, editor. Origins of language. Budapest: Collegium Budapest; 1996. p. 89–115.
50. Nowlin DM. The role of biosemiosis and dysfunctional signaling processes in human pathology. In: Hendlin YH, Hope J, editors. Food and medicine: a biosemiotic perspective (biosemiotics 22). Springer; 2021. p. 155–82.
51. Musso CG. Biosemiotic medicine: from an effect-based medicine to a process-based medicine. Arch Argent Pediatr. 2020;118(5):e449–53. https://doi.org/10.5546/aap.2020.eng.e44.
52. Tønnessen M. The ontogeny of the embryonic, foetal and infant human umwelt. Sign Syst Stud. 2014;42(2/3):281–307.
53. Day MJ. One health: the importance of companion animal vector-borne diseases. Parasites Vectors. 2011;4:49.
54. Zinsstag J, Schelling E, Wyss K, Mahamat MB. Potential of cooperation between human and animal health to strengthen health systems. Lancet. 2005;366:2142–5.
55. Wondwossen A, et al. The global one health paradigm: challenges and opportunities for tackling infectious diseases at the human, animal, and environment interface in low-resource settings. PLoS Neglected Trop Dis. 2014;8(11):e3257.
56. Pinillos RG, Appleby M, Manteca X, Scott-Park F, Smith C, Velarde A. One welfare – a platform for improving human and animal welfare. Vet Rec. 2016;179:412–3.
57. Knight R, Callewaert C, Marotz C, Hyde ER, Debelius JW, McDonald D, et al. The microbiome and human biology. Annu Rev Genomics Hum Genet. 2017;18:65–86.
58. Tønnessen M. Umwelt transitions: Uexküll and environmental change. Biosemiotics. 2009;2(1):47–64.

Chapter 2
Acute Kidney Injury: Definition and Generalities

Lucas Petraglia, Carlos Guido Musso, and Adrian Covic

2.1 Introduction

The concept of acute kidney injury (AKI) describes a state of reduction of glomerular filtration rate (GFR) in a relatively short period of time that most frequently leads to the accumulation of nitrogenous-waste substances in the blood.

Shaping the definition of AKI has been a long-term discussion but by 2012 KDIGO guidelines agreed that the clinical diagnosis criteria would include having a serum creatinine rise of more than 0.3 mg/dl or 1.5–1.9 times baseline value, and/or a urinary output fall to 0.5 mL/kg/h over 6 h, limited to 7 days [1, 2].

In an attempt to gain a better understanding of AKI, the nephrologist community classifies the phenomenon according to the time frame, the severity of the injury, and the physiology of the underlying mechanism. When time is used as the landmark, the term AKI refers to the clinical manifestation of renal injury initiated and lasting less than 7 days, which can be further subdivided into "transient" ($\leq$48 h) or "persistent" (>48 h). Acute renal disease (ARD) encompasses the clinical setting between 7 and 90 days and chronic kidney disease (CKD) the renal injury that remains and surpasses day 90 from the acute event. While these are subjected to the KDIGO diagnostic criteria, subclinical AKI is an allusion to the increased levels of

L. Petraglia
University of Buenos Aires, Buenos Aires, Argentina

C. G. Musso
Nephrology Division, Hospital Italiano de Buenos Aires, Buenos Aires, Argentina

Research Department, Hospital Italiano de Buenos Aires, Buenos Aires, Argentina

A. Covic (✉)
University of Medicine "Grigore T Popa", Iasi, Romania

AOSR, Iasi, Romania

C. G. Musso, A. Covic (eds.), *Organ Crosstalk in Acute Kidney Injury*,
https://doi.org/10.1007/978-3-031-36789-2_2

renal injury biomarkers preceding any clinical manifestation (creatinemia or oliguria) [3–5].

If severity is considered the axis, then KDIGO 2012 uses the AKIN classification to define three consecutive stages: stage 1: increase in serum creatinine levels >0.3 mg/dL or 1.5–1.9 times the baseline creatinine value, and/or decreased urine output to 0.5 mL/kg/h for 6 h; stage 2: increase in serum creatinine levels 2–2.9 times the baseline creatinine value, and/or decreased urine output to 0.5 mL/kg/h for 12 h.; and finally, stage 3: increase in serum creatinine levels 3 times the baseline creatinine value, increase of serum creatinine >4 mg/dL, initiation of Renal Replacement Therapy (RRT), and/or decreased urine output to 0.3 mL/kg/h for 24 h or anuria for 12 h. This grading has real-life clinical implications as it correlates with mortality even 12 months after the insult [6, 7].

According to the pathophysiology of the insult, we may divide AKI into three different groups: prerenal (accounting for 35% of cases), renal or intrinsic (causing 40% of AKI), and postrenal or obstructive (responsible for the remaining 25%). We will focus on this classification in this chapter [8].

2.2 Prerenal AKI

This comes as a consequence of a fall in renal perfusion that exceeds the capacity of the counter-regulatory response to sustain a near-normal GFR. The most frequent insults can be grouped under volume depletion, systemic vasodilation, increased vascular resistance and diminished effective arterial renal blood flow.

Regarding the depleted intravascular states, free water loss from gastrointestinal tract (diarrhea), kidneys (e.g., poliuria secondary to diuretics or hypercalcemia), and skin and respiratory airway should be considered, as well as hemorrhage or third spacing (burns, peritonitis, muscle trauma). Older patients are especially susceptible to dehydration, and the fact that they show a decreased adaptive ability to maintain renal blood flow and GFR results in AKI. Drugs prescription must be periodically reviewed in older patients, as 25–40% of AKI are related to diuretics, and non-steroidal anti-inflammatory (NSAIDs) can augment the absolute risk of developing the condition [9–11].

Systemic vasodilation is an expected condition in sepsis, anaphylaxis, and the use of certain drugs requiring a prompt removal or treatment of the insult. On the other hand, increased vascular resistance secondary to hepatorenal syndrome or drugs (like cocaine) can be similarly harmful [9–11].

Congestive heart failure, nephrotic syndrome, cirrhosis, perioperative hypotension and renal artery stenosis are responsible for diminished effective arterial blood volume states, and may result in AKI [2, 9–11].

Volume depletion and limited renal perfusion trigger the activation of the renin-angiotensin aldosterone axis, the upregulation of the sympathetic nervous system, and the stimulation of vasopressin secretion. Angiotensin II is a potent vasoconstrictor that acts simultaneously over the afferent and efferent renal arteriole, but its effects are opposed by vasodilator prostaglandins. Although there is a reduction in renal blood flow, the post-glomerular (or efferent) vasoconstriction predominates, making it possible to maintain a close to normal intraglomerular pressure and GFR, augmenting at the same time the filtration fraction (the ratio between GFR and renal plasma flow). AKI will occur when the reduction in renal perfusion exceeds the physiological capacity to preserve GFR [12].

The above-mentioned hormones, together with aldosterone, vasopressin and the sympathetic response, will act over renal tubular cells to increase sodium, water, and urea conservation, which will lower diuresis and urinary sodium concentration (UNa <20 mmol/L) and elevate urine osmolality (UOsm >500 mosm/kg), reduce fractional excretion of sodium (FENa <1%) and fractional excretion of urea (FEUrea <35%), and increase blood urea nitrogen (BUN):serum creatinine ratio (>20:1). These parameters will be seen as long as there is no significant tubule-interstitial damage either from acute injury (acute tubular necrosis) or chronic kidney disease or age-associated defects in sodium, urea, and water conservation [13, 14].

It should be noted that angiotensin converting enzyme inhibitors, angiotensin receptor blockers, and NSAIDs may change renal hemodynamics, leading to AKI when mixed with volume depletion, preexisting CKD, bilateral renal artery stenosis (or unilateral renal artery stenosis with a solitary kidney), chronic heart failure, and diuretic administration [9].

2.3 Renal or Intrinsic AKI

Acute tubular necrosis (ATN) is the most frequent form of renal AKI, and almost 50% of AKI episodes in the hospital setting are related to ATN. When looking at causative insults we may divide them into ischemic or nephrotoxic, but sometimes both can overlap [2].

Contrast media, heavy metals, anaesthetics, organic solvents, antibiotics (e.g., aminoglycosides), antifungal (e.g., amphotericin) antineoplastic drugs (e.g., cis-platinum), and endogenous toxins (myoglobin, haemoglobin, uric acid) are just some of the substances associated with nephrotoxicity [2].

Ischemic ATN is seen in sustained volume depletion and septic states, and the pathophysiology involves altered microvascular flow associated with endothelial damage, ischemia-reperfusion injury to the renal tubular cells, and a cascade of inflammatory reactions. The evolution of ischemic ATN can be summarized in four phases: initiation, extension, maintenance, and recovery. In the first stage, after the insult, renal tubular cells will lose polarity followed by their separation from the neighbor cells and basal membrane, resulting in apoptosis and necrosis. The ongoing vasoconstriction, the intratubular obstruction due to dead cells, and the backleak phenomenon through the damaged epithelium will cause AKI, manifested as an elevation in serum urea and creatinine levels, and in some cases diminished diuresis (oliguria) [2, 11].

The damaged microvascular endothelium and the inflammatory cascade are key factors in the extension stage, where cellular hypoxia and ischemia persist even though the insult has ceased to exist. During the maintenance phase, tubular and endothelial cells will regenerate and repair epithelium if there is no additional aggression, but there will not be a recovery of renal function yet. Finally, during the recovery stage, the kidneys will regain GFR and diuresis (usually poliuria) but tubular function will remain impaired, provoking abnormalities in salt, water, and electrolytes balance. AKI in sepsis has been historically considered to be due to ischemic ATN (as endotoxins provoke renal vasoconstriction) but we now know there is a much more intricate pathway involving inflammatory mediators and endothelial injury. Other possible scenarios where ischemic ATN can be found are small vessels compromise (as in thrombotic thrombocytopenic purpura, haemolytic uraemic syndrome, vasculitis, or malignant hypertension), renal artery dissection, renal vein thrombosis, cholesterol atheroemboli, surgical interventions (cardiac and aortic artery surgery), and contrast-induced nephropathy. Certain conditions like CKD, diabetes, older age, atherosclerosis, hypoalbuminemia, and malignancies predispose to ischemic ATN. As there is no specific treatment to improve renal function, supportive therapy and avoiding further insult is the gold standard. The use of diuretics to transform an oliguric ATN into a non-oliguric one is somehow controversial. Although maintaining diuresis during ATN is a marker of better prognosis, diuretics may only work as a stress test (with better response in those with preserved tubular function) rather than a form of treatment. These drugs can be useful to avoid volume overload, but when there is no diuretic response RRT should be considered [4, 15–22].

Another form of intrinsic AKI is that related to acute interstitial nephritis (AIN) which may be seen in 5–30% of patients. Its histopathological hallmark is an infiltrated tubule-interstitium with lymphocytes and eosinophils. Clinically it can be manifested with the triad fever, rash, and eosinophilia but only 15% of cases evidence the three signs and symptoms. Urine may show sterile pyuria, isomorphic hematuria, casts of white blood cells, and low-grade proteinuria. Eosinophiluria is not a specific finding as it is shared by atheroembolic disease, pyelonephritis, prostatitis, and cystitis. When looking at the most frequent cause of AIN, hypersensitivity to drugs takes the lead as it is involved in 60–70% of AKI episodes. Sulfonamides, penicillin-based antibiotics, cephalosporins, proton-pump inhibitors, and NSAIDs are the main medications to be aware of, and older people may be at higher risk due to polypharmacy. AIN will be evident within 3 weeks of introducing the causative drug, but this timeline is not very accurate and it should be noted that systemic collagen vascular diseases and infections can also be responsible for AIN [8, 11, 15].

Again, there is no specific treatment aside from stopping the responsible drug or resolving the underlying cause. Corticosteroides have been used in small controlled trials but the results are not conclusive. Kidney function is expected to return to baseline within days or weeks, taking longer in older individuals [11, 15].

The glomeruli per se can be involved in the pathway of intrinsic AKI in the setting of acute or rapidly progressive glomerulonephritis. Certain infectious diseases like acute post-infectious glomerulonephritis and infective endocarditis are associated with diffuse proliferative forms. Rapidly progressive (crescentic) glomerulonephritis, which may be secondary to a number of glomerulopathies, such as extracapillary glomerulonephritis, lupus nephritis, and IgA glomerulonephritis, has an aggressive debut and evolves to end stage renal disease within days or weeks if not treated promptly. The clinical presentation is generally that of a nephritic syndrome, with hypertension, hematuria, and proteinuria, and associated AKI. The initial diagnostic workflow must include blood tests with complement levels, antinuclear antibodies, anti-neutrophil cytoplasmic antibodies, and hepatitis B and C antibodies, and in certain cases anti-glomerular basement membrane antibodies and cryoglobulin levels. In most patients the renal biopsy will be mandatory and immunosuppressive treatment will be oriented to the underlying pathology [10, 16].

Both ATN and AIN involve a damaged tubule-interstitium which will condition the diminished reabsorption of sodium, water, and urea. Urine parameters will usually exhibit high urinary sodium concentration (UNa >40 mmol/L), high fractional excretion of sodium (FENa >1%), and high fractional excretion of urea (FEUrea >65%) with a low urinary osmolality (UOsm <350 mosm/kg). It should be noted that older individuals, CKD patients, and those with impaired tubular function may falsely exhibit intrinsic AKI urinary patterns in pre-renal AKI (intermediate syndrome) [11, 13].

2.4 Obstructive AKI

This group represents between 9 and 30% of all AKI. It can be divided according to the anatomy of the obstruction in intrarenal (tubular obstruction due to crystals, blood clots, papillary necrosis) or extrarenal AKI. This latter one can be further classified as upper or lower considering proximal or distal obstruction from the bladder. In upper obstructions with unilateral compromise, AKI will only occur if the contralateral kidney lacks the capacity to compensate for the decrease of GFR. The main associated causes are radiation therapy, retroperitoneal fibrosis, renal lithiasis, and malignancy. Bilateral hydronephrosis is more typical of lower obstructions and can be due to pelvic cancer in women and prostatic pathology in men, but there are also less common causes such as blood clots, ureteral stenosis, and neurologic alterations affecting the urethral sphincter [2, 21].

2.5 AKI Implications

It is difficult to quantify the true magnitude of the prevalence and incidence of AKI as the majority of the large cohorts use different criteria to define it. Still, we know that US registries were reporting an incidence of hospital-acquired AKI of 7.2% by the mid-1990s [16], while Australians described an incidence of 18% [17]. This can be substantially higher in intensive care units where 64% of patients admitted with septic shock may develop AKI in the first 24 h [18] and AKI itself is the reason for 1–7% of general hospital admissions, reaching 30–50% for intensive care units.

AKI has short- and long-term consequences. In the immediate setting it raises mortality, and costs, prolonging assisted respiratory ventilation and also hospital stay. In the more remote follow-up it increases the risk of developing end stage renal disease, increases mortality (particularly from cardiovascular causes), as well as the possibility of a recurrent AKI [19, 20].

Neither markers for early prediction nor direct effective treatments for AKI have yet been found, so the best strategy to preserve kidney function is prevention. In this way sticking to KDIGO guidelines have proved to reduce the incidence and severity of AKI related to cardiovascular surgery. Hopefully, novel biomarkers and predictive models will shape the approach of AKI in the near future [21–25].

2.6 Conclusion

Acute kidney injury is a highly prevalent condition in critically ill patients and hospital settings and it has short- and long-term clinical consequences. Each of the various AKI definitions and classifications described seeks to achieve an effective diagnostic and therapeutic approach to this condition.

References

1. KDIGO clinical practice guideline for acute kidney injury. Kidney Int Suppl. 2012;2:1–38.
2. Musso CG, Rosell C, Gonzalez-Torres H, Ordonez JD, Aroca-Martinez G. Primary prevention for acute kidney injury in ambulatory patients. Postgrad Med. 2020;132:1–3. https://doi.org/1 0.1080/00325481.2020.1795484.
3. Beker BM, Corleto MG, Fieiras C, Musso CG. Novel acute kidney injury biomarkers: their characteristics, utility and concerns. Int Urol Nephrol. 2018;50:705–13.
4. Musso CG, Silva D, Propato F, Molin AY, Velez-Verbel M, Lopez N, Terrasa S, Gonzalez-Torres H, Aroca-Martinez G. Daily urinary sodium excretion monitoring in critical care setting: a simple method for an early detection of acute kidney injury. Indian J Nephrol. 2021;31(3):266–70.
5. Koyner JL, Thakar CV, Hladik G, et al. Nephrology self-assessment. Program. 2017;16(2):1–88.
6. Siew ED, Parr SK, Abdel-Kader K, Eden SK, Peterson JF, Bansal N, Hung AM, Fly J, Speroff T, Ikizler TA, Matheny ME. Predictors of recurrent AKI. J Am Soc Nephrol. 2016;27(4):1190–200.
7. Palevsky PM, Liu KD, Brophy PD, Chawla LR, Parikh CR, Thakar CV, Tolwani AJ, Waikar SS, Weisbord SD. KDOQI US commentary on the 2012 KDIGO clinical practice guideline for acute kidney injury. Am J Kidney Dis. 2013;61(5):649–72.
8. Coca SG. Acute kidney injury in elderly persons. Am J Kidney Dis. 2010;56:122–31.
9. Abdel-Kader K, Palevsky P. Acute kidney injury in the elderly. Clin Geriatr Med. 2009;25(3):331–58. https://doi.org/10.1016/j.cger.2009.04.0.

10. Giannopoulou, M, Roumeliotis S, Eleftheriadis T, and Liakopoulos V. Acute kidney injury in the elderly. In Musso, Carlos Guido; Jauregui, José Ricardo; Macías-Núñez, Juan Florencio; and Covic, Adrian (Eds.): Clinical nephrogeriatrics: an evidence-based guide. Cham. Springer. 2019: 123–131.
11. Musso CG, Liakopoulos V, Ioannidis I, et al. Acute renal failure in the elderly: particular characteristics. Int Urol Nephrol. 2006;38:787–93.
12. Musso CG, Jauregui J. Renin-angiotensin-aldosterone system and the ageing kidney. Expert Rev Endocrinol Metab. 2014;(9):1–4.
13. Benozzi P, Vallecillo B, Musso CG. Urinary indices: their diagnostic value in current nephrology. Front Med Health Res. 2017;1(1):1–5.
14. Makris K, Spanou L. Acute kidney injury: definition, pathophysiology and clinical phenotypes. Clin Biochem Rev. 2016;37(2):85–98.
15. Praga M, Gonzalez E. Acute interstitial nephritis. Kidney Int. 2010;77:956–61.
16. Sethi S, De Vriese A, Fervenza F. Acute glomerulonephritis. Lancet. 2022;399(10335):1646–63. https://doi.org/10.1016/S0140-6736(22)00461-5.
17. Nash K, Hafeez A, Hou S. Hospital-acquired renal insufficiency. Am J Kidney Dis. 2002;39:930–6.
18. Uchino S, Bellomo R, Goldsmith D, Bates S, Ronco C. An assessment of the RIFLE criteria for acute renal failure in hospitalized patients. Crit Care Med. 2006;34:1913–7.
19. Rewa O, Bagshaw S. Acute kidney injury—epidemiology, outcomes and economics. Nat Rev Nephrol. 2014;10:193–207.
20. Liaño F, Felipe C, Tenorio MT, Rivera M, Abraira V, Sáez-de-Urturi JM, Ocaña J, Fuentes C, Severiano S. Long-term outcome of acute tubular necrosis: a contribution to its natural history. Kidney Int. 2007;71(7):679–86.
21. Odutayo A, Wong CX, Farkouh M, Altman DG, Hopewell S, Emdin CA, Hunn BH. AKI and long-term risk for cardiovascular events and mortality. J Am Soc Nephrol. 2017;28(1):377–87.
22. Rennke HG, Denker BM. Renal pathophysiology: the essentials. Baltimore, MD: Lippincott Williams & Wilkins; 2007.
23. Musso C, Aguilera J, Otero C, et al. Informatic nephrology. Int Urol Nephrol. 2013;45(4):1033–8.
24. Negi S, Koreeda D, Kobayashi S, et al. Acute kidney injury: epidemiology, outcomes, complications, and therapeutic strategies. Semin Dial. 2018;31(5):519–27.
25. Malhotra R, Siew E. Biomarkers for the early detection and prognosis of acute kidney injury. Clin J Am Soc Nephrol. 2017;12(1):149–73.

Chapter 3
Hormones

Maria Fabiana Russo-Picasso and Erica Springer

3.1 General Principles of the Endocrine System

3.1.1 Structure, Organization, and Function of the Endocrine System

The endocrine system is one of the systems, like the nervous and immunologic systems, that are involved trans-sectionally in the regulation and maintenance of homeostasis throughout the organism.

The endocrine system entails the production of chemical mediators (hormones) that circulate in the bloodstream and act on target organs away from the endocrine gland that produces them. To that end, the endocrine gland secretes the hormones into the extracellular fluid (ECF), lymph, or bloodstream.

On the other hand, non-traditional cells or tissues with endocrine function within other systems have been described. For example, adipocytes secrete chemical mediators like adiponectin that act upon distant organs or tissues. Likewise, the small intestine secretes glucagon-analogues into the general circulation. Recently, the concepts of hormone and endocrine regulation have been expanded to include chemical mediators that act upon a target organ close to the endocrine gland (paracrine regulation) and even when the chemical mediator acts upon the endocrine gland that produces it (autocrine regulation) [1].

Hormones are classified according to their chemical structure and composition: proteins and peptides (including modified amino acids, short peptides, and large proteins) or steroid hormones (Table 3.1) [1–3].

M. F. Russo-Picasso (✉) · E. Springer
Endocrinology Division, Department of Medicine, Hospital Italiano de Buenos Aires, Buenos Aires, Argentina
e-mail: maria.russopicasso@hospitalitaliano.org.ar

C. G. Musso, A. Covic (eds.), *Organ Crosstalk in Acute Kidney Injury*,
https://doi.org/10.1007/978-3-031-36789-2_3

Table 3.1 Hormone classification

Hormone type	Hormone subtype	Structure	Hormone example	Gland
Peptides and proteins	Amines	Modified amino acids	Thyroxine: a molecule of tyrosine coupled to four atoms of iodine	Thyroid
	Peptides	Short chain of amino acids	Thyrotropin-releasing hormone: a tripeptide consisting of glutamate, histidine and proline	Hypothalamus
	Proteins	Long chains of amino acids, sometimes more than one bound together by disulfide bridges	Insulin: Two chains of 21 and 30 amino acids each bound by disulfide bridges	Pancreatic islet beta cells
Steroids		Derived from cholesterol	Testosterone, estrogen, and progesterone (sex hormones) Modified cholesterol ring with 17beta-hydroxy and 3-oxo groups, together with an unsaturated double bond at C-4-C-5	Testicles and ovaries (gonads)

3.2 Hormone Synthesis: Basic Concepts

Protein and peptide hormones are the most abundant in the organism, and are synthesized following the steps of other secretory products in the endoplasmic reticulum. The first product of synthesis is a precursor molecule of comparatively larger size but without biological activity, or "prohormone." This precursor is then cleaved to originate smaller molecules, with biological activity, that are then stored in secretory vesicles; these vesicles are a reservoir of hormones that are released upon stimulation. Many of the protein and peptide hormones are glycoproteins that contain oligosaccharide chains (glycans) covalently attached to amino acid side-chains. These side-chains determine their biological activity and metabolic clearance, for example, thyroid-stimulating hormone (TSH), follicle-stimulating hormone (FSH), and chorionic gonadotropin.

Steroid hormones are synthesized from cholesterol in circulating lipoproteins, or synthesis "de novo." Production of these hormones is widely distributed, in such a way that several tissues can synthesize them from available precursors (e.g., neurosteroids produced in the brain). In contrast to protein and peptide hormones, steroid hormones are not stored in secretory vesicles before the stimuli by a secretagogue [1, 2].

3.2.1 Transport

Hormones are released to the bloodstream unbound or "free" or bound to carrier proteins. Free hormones can diffuse from the intravascular space to the interstitial fluid around the target organ, and interact with its receptor, be it on the membrane or after going through the plasma membrane, in the cytoplasm; it is the "active" form of the hormone. Hormones bound to carrier proteins act as a reservoir in the circulation, and they must be released from the carrier before they can bind to their receptor. Bound hormones circulate in equilibrium with the free hormones, and act as buffers of changes in the concentration, bioavailability, and actions of free hormones at the target organs: about 1–10% of the total hormone mass circulates unbound to proteins.

Most carrier proteins are globulins, and many of them are specific to the hormone they transport (thyroxine binding globulin, sex hormone-binding globulin, etc.). However, there are proteins that bind to several substrates with low specificity and affinity, such as albumin (albumin binds testosterone, thyroxine, and calcium ions). Carrier proteins are synthesized in the liver, and hence liver synthetic dysfunctions affect hormone bioavailability. In general, protein and peptide hormones are hydrophilic and circulate unbound to proteins, with the notable exception of thyroid hormones, whereas steroid hormones are lipophilic and require carrier proteins to circulate [1, 2].

The bioavailability of hormones at the target organs depends on the rate of secretion and the rate of elimination from the bloodstream and ECF, that is, through metabolic modification, internalization of the hormone-receptor complex, and fecal and urinary excretion. Most hormones are degraded or transformed in the liver, while some undergo chemical changes in peripheral target tissues, like the conversion of testosterone to dihydrotestosterone. The metabolic clearance rate (MCR) refers to the volume of plasma that is cleared of a hormone in a unit of time in stable conditions. As binding to proteins makes hormones inaccessible to metabolic degradation and urinary excretion, it also impacts the MCR and prolongs hormone circulating half-time [3].

3.3 Mechanisms of Hormone Action

Hormones elicit a biological effect by binding to specific receptors at target tissues. There are two basic concepts related to hormone action:

- Affinity: Hormones exert their actions at very low plasma concentration; therefore receptors must have a very high affinity for their ligand. Affinity is the strength of the binding of the ligand to its receptor. It is measured as the rate of association and dissociation of the hormone-receptor complex in equilibrium. The equilibrium dissociation constant is defined as the hormone concentration needed to bind 50% of the hormone-union moieties in the available receptors.

- Specificity: This is the capacity of the receptor to bind to a hormone and not to similar molecules. For example, Type 1 receptors for mineralocorticoids also have a high affinity for glucocorticoids.

The responsiveness of target tissues to hormone action can change according to physiological conditions, and is measured in dose/response curves as basal activity (activity in absence of the hormone) and the threshold of response (the concentration of hormone that produces the first detectable effect); the median effective dose (ED50) is the concentration at which 50% of the maximum response is achieved, and maximum response (E_{max}) reflects the functional mass of the target tissue, the number of receptors, and their functional efficiency [3].

The binding of a receptor to its ligand is a saturable process, although most hormones produce E_{max} without binding to 100% of available receptors. On the other hand, exposure to the ligand produces a decrease in the number of functional receptors, by internalization or sequestration of membrane receptors (a process called "downregulation"), or their desensitization by a chemical modification like phosphorylation, a change in the second messenger, or the production of an inhibitor of its signal. Less frequently, there are cases of "upregulation" mediated by an increase in the number of receptors for a hormone that has shown low concentrations, or in response to the binding of another hormone to its receptor: this is the case of FSH and estradiol receptors, whereby the binding of FSH to its receptor upregulates estrogen receptors during the menstrual cycle [3].

3.3.1   Types of Receptors

Hormone receptors are classified according to their location: membrane receptors and intracellular receptors. Protein hormones that are unable to penetrate the cell membrane bind to membrane receptors whereas thyroid and steroid hormones can diffuse through it and bind to intracellular receptors. Recently, thyroid hormone transporters that carry thyroid hormones through the cell membrane in some tissues have also been identified (e.g., MCT8 expressed in the liver and brain).

3.3.2   Membrane Receptors

Membrane receptors are inserted in the cell membrane of cells in the target tissues. The formation of the hormone-receptor complex triggers a cascade of chemical reactions, mainly phosphorylation of "second messengers" that ultimately elicit a biological effect. From the functional point of view, membrane receptors are classified as receptors coupled to guanine-binding proteins (G-proteins), receptor tyrosine kinases, and receptors coupled to ion channels [4].

- G-protein-coupled receptors (GPCR): Hormone receptors coupled to G-proteins are characterized by seven transmembrane domains. G-proteins are heterotrimers composed of Gα, Gβ, and Gγ subunits. Upon binding of the hormone to the GPCR, the Gα subunit exchanges guanosin-diphosphate (GDP) for guanosine-triphosphate (GTP) and dissociates from the Gβγ dimer resulting in two functional subunits (Gα and Gβγ), both of which are involved in intracellular signaling. The type of Gα determines which signaling cascades are stimulated or repressed: stimulator of adenylate cyclase (Gαs), an inhibitor of adenylate cyclase (Gαi), or stimulator of phospholipase C (FLC) (Gαq). For example, the stimulation of adenylate cyclase to produce cyclic AMP (cAMP) from ATP results in the binding of cAMP to the regulatory units of protein kinase A (PKA), and the release of the two catalytic units. The catalytic units phosphorylate other intracellular proteins in serine and threonine moieties, other protein kinases, tubular proteins of the cytoskeleton, transcription factors, and ion channels. On the other hand, several genes have cyclic AMP-response elements (CRE) in their promoters, and some proteins that bind to CREs are themselves substrates of PKA. Alternatively, protein Gαq can stimulate FLC, located in the cell membrane. FLC then cleaves phosphatidylinositol bisphosphate and produces diacylglycerol (DAG) and inositol triphosphate (IP 3). IP3 binds to calcium channels in the endoplasmic reticulum and brings about an increase in intracellular concentrations of calcium that modifies the activity of calcium-sensitive enzymes, sometimes through the action of intermediate proteins that bind calcium, like calmodulin, and processes like the release of neurotransmitters. DAG activates protein kinase C, which phosphorylates different proteins in serine and threonine.

  There are several mechanisms in place to switch off hormonal signals besides the unbinding of the ligand to its receptor. Active receptors can be desensitized by phosphorylation to turn off this response or adapt to a persistent stimulus. G protein-coupled receptor kinases (GRKs) phosphorylate serine and threonine residues in intracellular domains of GPCR, allowing the binding of arrestins that block further G protein-mediated signaling and target receptors for internalization. In the FLC pathway, IP3 is dephosphorylated to inositol, and DAG is converted to phosphoric acid. Calcium cytoplasmic concentrations are decreased by ATP-dependent pumps that carry ions into the endoplasmic reticulum or to the ECF [5, 6].

- Kinase-linked receptors: Receptors with kinase activities are transmembrane proteins with an extracellular, hormone-binding domain, a transmembrane domain, and an intracellular catalytic domain. Most kinase-linked receptors have tyrosine-kinase activity (RTK) and consist of a single peptide chain, but some exist as dimeric complexes or dimerize when the ligand binds to the extracellular domain. RTKs first phosphorylate tyrosine residues in the receptor peptide, which enhances phosphorylation activity, and allows the phosphorylation in tyrosine residues of second messengers. Other kinase-linked receptors have serine/threonine kinase, guanylate-cyclase, phosphatase activity, or do not have intrinsic enzymatic activity but associate to proteins that have kinase activity [7].

- Receptors associated with ion channels: These receptors belong to the family of ligand-activated ion channels. The formation of the hormone-receptor complex opens ion channels in the cell membrane and allows the selective influx of different chemical mediators [4, 5].

3.3.3 *Intracellular Receptors*

Intracellular receptors are lipophilic transcription factors located either in the cytoplasm or in the nucleus of the cell. The main hormones that interact with this type of receptor are steroid hormones (adrenal, testicular, and ovarian hormones) and thyroid hormones. These receptors bind to the DNA of target genes and regulate transcription by interacting with other transcription factors that stimulate or repress gene transcription. Glucocorticoid and mineralocorticoid receptors are mainly cytoplasmic, whereas sex hormone and thyroid receptors are located in the nucleus [8].

The molecular structure of nuclear receptors consists of a highly variable N-terminal domain (NDT), a DNA- binding domain (DBD), a hinge domain, and a ligand-binding domain (LBD). The DBD is characterized by eight cysteine residues connected by two zinc atoms to form a highly conserved structure called "zinc fingers" that binds to the hormone-response-element in the promoter sequence of the DNA. Response elements consist mainly of palindromic sequences or direct repeats, and receptors must dimerize forming hetero- or homodimers to bind to them, and also interact with other transcription factors by protein to protein interaction. The LBD is characterized by a hydrophobic "pocket" that is also ligand-specific. The NTD allows for ligand-independent activation of transcription and recruitment of coactivators. Receptor activity can also be modulated by allosteric modifications and post-translational changes, such as phosphorylation and direct binding of molecules to the LBD [8, 9].

Normal signaling by steroid receptors entails the continuous traffic between cytoplasm and nucleus and the binding to a chaperone complex that includes heat-shock protein (HSP) 90, HSP 70, and other proteins. Binding to the chaperone complex ensures that cytoplasmic receptors are adequately folded to bind stably to their ligands. To translocate to the nucleus, the receptor must bind to its ligand and release the chaperone complex. It has also been suggested that the HSP 90 chaperone complex interacts with structures in the nuclear pore and is involved in the transport of steroid receptors between cytoplasm and nucleus [9, 10].

Intracellular receptor modulation of gene transcription also involves interaction with other coactivators and corepressors. The steroid receptor coactivator family (SRC) includes SRC-1, SRC-2, and SRC-3. The structure of SRC consists of an NTD that allows interaction with other coregulators and transcription factors, a serine- and threonine-rich domain that can be dephosphorylated, and a leucine-rich domain that also interacts with nuclear receptors and transcription factors. There are other families such as BRG1, which is involved in chromatin remodeling essential for the formation of the transcription initiation complex. Steroid receptor coactivators also include other coregulators, protein kinases like Akt, and proteases like small ubiquitin-like modifier (SUMO)-specific protease 1 that catalyzes post-translational changes not only of receptors but also of other coactivators.

There are also corepressors (NCORs) involved in the modulation of nuclear receptor activity. Two have been identified and extensively studied: NCOR1 and NCOR2. NCORs have a common structure that consists of two interaction domains (ID1 and ID2) at the C terminus, a deacetylase activation domain (DAD), and three repression domains (RD1, RD2, and RD3) at the N-terminus. RDs can interact with nuclear receptor modifiers such as epigenome-modifying enzymes and chromatin remodelers, while IDs can interact with different nuclear receptors. The DAD domain binds to histone deacetylases (HDAC3) and produces a conformational change essential for DA activity [11].

Genomic actions of steroid and thyroid receptors follow the sequence of ligand-dependent transcription-factor activity. Gene transcription is modulated by the direct binding of the receptor to its hormone-response-element, by protein–protein interactions with other transcription factors, and the interaction with growth factors. The hormone response element has a highly conserved consensus sequence but it is the cooperation of other transcription factors like AP1 and SP1 that gives specificity to this interaction; likewise, chromatin structure modulates accessibility to the response element. Steroid receptors can repress transcription by displacing other transcription factors from binding sites in the DNA and by protein–protein interactions. Other modifications like methylation of promoter sequences and micro-ARN binding to mRNA can also silence genes [8].

Steroid hormones can also bind to specific membrane receptors and activate a non-genomic pathway. The post-receptor pathway is similar to that of G-protein-bound receptors and activates similar protein kinases producing an increase of cAMP, cGMP, and other second messengers to activate the MAPK pathway and lead to the expression of genes related to proliferation and rapid-response genes [8].

3.4 Regulation of Hormone Levels, Synthesis, and Secretion

Regulation of hormone levels involves the control of their synthesis and secretion. Hormone levels in plasma vary in response to circadian rhythms (e.g., cortisol levels peak in early morning hours), ultradian rhythms (estradiol peaks and troughs during the ovarian cycle), in response to physiological parameters like sleep or body temperature (melatonin), or reflecting their pulsatile pattern of release (luteinizing hormone, parathormone). These oscillations are hormone-specific, and essential for their action in target organs and maintenance of homeostasis [12].

Three systems are involved in the control of hormone levels: central nervous system, endocrine system, and different ions or nutrients. Generally, the secretion of one hormone is regulated by several of these mechanisms. For example, parathormone is regulated by calcium, phosphate, and magnesium concentrations but also by 1, 25-dihydroxycholecalciferol [2].

Neural control involves the release of a neurotransmitter close to its target endocrine gland in response to the propagation of an action potential into the axon terminus. This is a fast and acute type of control, with rapid initiation and cessation of the regulatory action. Neural control of endocrine function is exemplified by the hypothalamic–pituitary axis, whereby hypothalamic-releasing (thyroid-releasing hormones (TRH), corticotropin-releasing hormones, etc.) and inhibiting hormones (somatostatin, dopamine) regulate the synthesis and secretion of pituitary hormones like the thyroid-stimulating hormone. Another example is the neural control of the adrenal medulla, which receives direct stimuli from preganglionic sympathetic nerve terminals and releases epinephrine as an endocrine response [2].

Endocrine control of hormone secretion and release is achieved by "feedback loops," whereby a releasing or "tropic" hormone stimulates or inhibits the release of another hormone by the target endocrine gland. Most feedback loops entail the activity of a hypothalamic-releasing or inhibitory hormone that acts on a specific pituitary group of cells (e.g., thyrotrophs) to stimulate the secretion of a pituitary hormone (e.g., thyroid-stimulating hormone) that reaches the thyroid follicular cell via the circulation and stimulates the synthesis and secretion of thyroxine. The concentrations of thyroxine and triiodothyronine in the extracellular fluid inhibit the secretion of both TRH by the hypothalamic nuclei and TSH by the thyrotrophs, thus closing the negative feedback loop. The pituitary and hypothalamic hormones can also inhibit their secretion in a very short negative feedback loop, and the pituitary can inhibit the release of the hypothalamic hormones in a short feedback loop. A positive feedback loop is that in which the target cells increase the secretion of the original tropic hormone. A well-studied example is the stimulation of the secretion of luteinizing hormone by increasing estradiol concentrations to enable its ovulatory surge during the menstrual cycle.

Nutrient and ion control of endocrine function also involves feedback loops. In these feedback loops, the specific hormone controls the concentration of the nutrient or ion that either stimulates or inhibits its secretion. One such example is the release of insulin brought about by the postprandial increase in glucose plasma concentration [2].

3.5 Water and Electrolyte Balance

The total body content and concentration of water and electrolytes are under the complex regulation of several hormones:

1. Antidiuretic (ADH) or arginine-vasopressin (AVP), which regulates total body water and osmolality in ECF.
2. Aldosterone, and the renin-angiotensin-aldosterone system (RAAS), that regulates total mass of sodium and potassium.

3. Insulin and natriuretic atrial peptide, which control the influx and outflux of potassium from the intracellular fluid, and the excretion of sodium, respectively [13].

3.6 Antidiuretic Hormone and Extracellular Fluid (ECF) Osmolality

ADH/AVP is a cyclic nonapeptide synthesized by magnocellular neurons in the paraventricular and supraoptic nuclei of the hypothalamus as a precursor molecule that also includes a neurophysin (neurophysin II) and a C-terminal peptide (copeptin). ADH is then transported in neurosecretory granules along the unmyelinated axons of the neurons that traverse the median eminence and pituitary stalk and is stored at the axonal terminals in the posterior lobe of the pituitary. The release of ADH/AVP is similar to that of neurotransmitters and occurs in response to an action potential. Once released, ADH/AVP circulates freely without binding to a carrier protein, and its half-life in plasma is between 10 and 30 min [14].

The main targets of ADH/AVP action are the cortical and medullary collecting ducts in the kidneys, where it increases permeability to water and favors the reabsorption of solute-free water. In the terminal regions of the collecting ducts, ADH increases the permeability to urea, favoring its diffusion to the ECF. A secondary function of ADH/AVP is to increase vascular tone by increasing the contraction of vascular smooth muscle.

ADH/AVP exerts its actions through three membrane receptors bound to G-proteins:

- V1aR: This receptor is coupled to a Gq protein and stimulates phospholipase C, which cleaves phosphatidylinositol and opens calcium channels found in vascular smooth muscle, liver, kidney, brain, and adrenal glands. The influx of calcium in peripheral vascular smooth muscle results in peripheral vasoconstriction and an increase in vascular resistance.
- V1bR (or V3R): This receptor is bound to a Gq protein and is mainly expressed in corticotroph cells in the anterior pituitary, pancreas, and kidney.
- V2R: This receptor is coupled to a Gs protein and the union to ADH/AVP results in an increase in cAMP. V2R is mainly expressed in the kidney and is the main transducer for the actions of ADH/AVP regarding water reabsorption [15].

3.7 Endocrine Regulation of Water Balance

Total body water and osmolality are regulated in a negative feedback loop by ADH/AVP and thirst. The main stimulus for ADH/AVP secretion is the increase in osmolality of ECF. Central osmoreceptors located in the *organum vasculosum* of the *lamina terminalis*, which lacks a blood–brain barrier, and adjacent hypothalamus near the anterior wall of the third cerebral ventricle, as well as the magnocellular neurons themselves, sense changes as small as 1% in osmolality above or below the osmotic threshold. When osmolality in the ECF increases, there is a net outflow of water from the intracellular fluid to the ECF, and neuron bodies shrink; magnocellular neurons increase the secretion of ADH/AVP by about 1 pg/mL. The stimulus to increase thirst is comparatively insensitive as it requires changes in osmolality of about 5–10% [13].

ADH/AVP actions in the kidney are mediated through the expression of water channels called aquaporins. There are nine different aquaporins identified in the human kidney, four of which have important roles in water homeostasis:

- Aquaporin 1: This is constitutively expressed in the proximal tubule, the descending limb of Henle's loop, and the endothelial cells in the descending vasa recta, and controls the reabsorption of 90% of the water that is filtered by the nephron, independent of ADH/AVP action.
- Aquaporins 2–4: These are exclusively expressed in the principal cells of the distal and collecting ducts. Aquaporin 2 expression is regulated by ADH/AVP. Whereas water permeability is increased in the proximal tubule and Henle's loop, the collecting duct is practically water-resistant in the absence of ADH/AVP. In response to binding of ADH/AVP to V2R in the basolateral membrane of principal cells, activation of PKA results in the phosphorylation of aquaporin 2 and its translocation to the luminal membrane of collector duct cells. Aquaporins 3 and 4 are constitutively expressed in the basolateral membrane of the collecting duct cells, and they are the pathway by which water reabsorbed through aquaporin 2 reaches the ECF of the renal medulla following an osmotic gradient [16].

Vascular events, such as a fall in blood pressure of 10%, or decreases in blood volume, are sensed by pressure-sensing receptors in the cardiac atrium (low-pressure sensors) and the wall of big vessels such as the aorta (high-pressure sensors). These stretch sensors respond to the decrease in the tension of vessel walls and trigger an increase of sympathetic nervous system signaling that ultimately stimulates the secretion of ADH/AVP by magnocellular cells. The binding of ADH/AVP to V1bR in vascular smooth muscle results in the constriction of small vessels and the increase in vascular resistance; furthermore, the vascular-originated release of ADH/AVP sensitizes osmoreceptors to smaller increases in osmolality. Non-osmotic stimuli also include pain, nausea, exercise, hyperthermia, hypoglycemia, and the effect of pharmaceuticals (opioids, etc.) [13].

3.8 Sodium and Potassium Balance and the Renin-Angiotensin-Aldosterone System (RAAS)

Sodium (Na^+) is the main electrolyte in the ECF, and it is maintained in the ECF by the action of Na^+/K^+-ATPase pump, and the overall mass of Na^+ is under aldosterone control through the regulation of sodium excretion by the kidney. Sodium intake in a regular diet is around 4–6 g of salt (sodium chloride), which greatly exceeds the basal requirements of around 500 mg/d. Na^+ fecal loss is negligible, and thus the major regulation of its balance is renal excretion. Most of the filtered Na^+ load (90–95%) is reabsorbed passively in the proximal tubule and the ascending limb of Henle's loop. Reabsorption of the remaining 5–10% occurs in the distal tubule and collecting duct, which is the site of aldosterone regulation [17].

Potassium (K^+) is the main intracellular cation. The Na^+/K^+ -ATPase maintains the ratio of extracellular to intracellular K^+ (1:10), which is the major determinant of resting membrane potentials. The daily intake of K^+ (80–120 mmol/d) greatly exceeds the minimum dietary potassium requirements of 40–50 mmol/d. As with sodium, the major regulator of potassium balance is renal excretion. Most of the K^+ filtered mass is reabsorbed in the proximal convoluted tubules and thick ascending limb of Henle's loop and only about 10% reaches the distal nephron. Secretion of potassium in the distal convoluted tubules and collecting ducts is the main regulator of potassium balance. Aldosterone tightly regulates potassium secretion in the distal tubule by an epithelial sodium channel (also an amiloride-sensitive channel) that couples potassium secretion to sodium reabsorption [18].

K^+ concentration in ECF can also be regulated by insulin and catecholamines in the short term. β2-adrenergic stimuli increase Na1-K1-ATPase activity through a PK-A pathway whereas insulin does so through an insulin receptor substrate protein (IRS-1)–phosphatidylinositide 3-kinase (PI3-K) interaction that ultimately results in membrane insertion of the Na1-K1-ATPase pump mainly in muscle. These events lead to a quick shift of K^+ from ECF to intracellular fluid (ICF), and a fall of K^+ concentrations in plasma. Changes in osmolality and ECF pH also affect potassium concentrations in ICF: an increase in osmolality in the ECF will produce an efflux of K^+ from the ICF to the ECF together with the water shunt. Metabolic acidosis will also shunt K^+ ions from the ICF to the ECF [18].

3.9 The RAAS and the Regulation of Sodium and Potassium Homeostasis

Aldosterone is a steroid hormone synthesized and released by the adrenal gland, and is under the control of two main secretagogues: angiotensin II, potassium, and a secondary one, adrenocorticotrophic hormone (ACTH). Other factors can directly inhibit aldosterone synthesis, such as somatostatin, atrial natriuretic factor, and dopamine.

Aldosterone is part of the RAAS, in charge of the maintenance of extracellular volume, blood pressure, and potassium homeostasis. The rate-limiting step in the RAAS is the secretion of renin. Baroreceptors in the carotid sinuses and aortic arches sense a decrease in arterial pressure and stimulate the release of norepinephrine that stimulates the secretion of renin by juxtaglomerular cells. Stretch-activated ion channels detect a decrease in blood volume, open calcium channels in the juxtaglomerular smooth muscle cells, and stimulate renin secretion. Decreased perfusion pressure and a decrease of sodium load at the distal convoluted tubules are sensed by the *macula densa* cells, stimulating renin release. Additionally, hypokalemia increases and hyperkalemia decreases renin secretion, and potassium exerts a direct effect on the adrenal cortex to increase aldosterone secretion. Sodium loading, on the other hand, inhibits the RAAS [17].

Angiotensinogen is a globulin synthesized in the liver and is cleaved by renin to form angiotensin I. Angiotensin I is converted to an angiotensin II by angiotensin-converting enzymes in the lung and many other peripheral tissues. The action of angiotensin II on aldosterone involves a negative feedback loop that involves the conservation of sodium mass and blood pressure. Angiotensin II acts through the AT1 receptor, stimulating the constriction of vascular smooth muscle, increasing blood pressure, and reducing renal blood flow. It also increases sympathetic tone by increasing the discharge of norepinephrine by sympathetic terminals and the release of epinephrine and epinephrine by the adrenal medulla. The release of aldosterone and ADH/AVP is also mediated through the AT1 receptor, as well as other "non-traditional" functions, such as the stimulation of thirst and the release of corticotropin by the anterior pituitary. Angiotensin II increases vascular resistance in the kidney by constricting vascular smooth muscle, and decreasing glomerular filtration rate, and by doing so, it also decreases sodium and water excretion. On the other hand, it directly stimulates sodium–proton exchange and activates the sodium bicarbonate cotransporter, increasing sodium bicarbonate reabsorption. It also favors ECF reabsorption into the intravascular compartment by increasing efferent arteriole vasoconstriction. Extra-renal production of angiotensin II has been found in adipose tissue, vascular wall, and brain, and may act as a paracrine modulator in the secretion of prostaglandins [19].

Aldosterone actions are mediated by binding to the mineralocorticoid receptor in the cytosol of epithelial cells, mainly in the renal collecting duct. It is then transported to the nucleus where it binds to specific binding domains on targeted genes that lead to the increased expression of the serum and glucocorticoid regulated kinase 1 (SGK1). Increased SGK1 expression results in an increased expression in and activity of the apical sodium channel and the basolateral Na, K-adenosine triphosphatase (ATPase). In this way, aldosterone promotes the Na + reabsorption and K+ secretion. The negative feedback loop is closed by an increased blood volume that inhibits the secretion of renin and aldosterone [20].

3.10 Natriuretic Factors

Natriuretic factors are a family of peptide hormones that counterbalance the actions of the RAAS. Their structure consists of a single strand of amino acids with an acid loop structure formed by a cysteine disulfide bond essential for receptor binding. The family of natriuretic peptides comprises three members: atrial natriuretic peptide (ANP), B-type natriuretic peptide (BNP), and C-type natriuretic peptide (CNP). ANP and BNP are produced in the atria and bind to natriuretic receptor-A (NPR-A) located in the membrane of target cells. NPR-A has a single transmembrane region and catalyzes the formation of cyclic GMP (cGMP) from guanosine-triphosphate (GTP). Natriuretic peptides (NPs) elicit their biologic actions through three different types of cGMP binding proteins: cGMP-dependent protein kinases (PKG), cGMP-regulated phosphodiesterases, and cyclic nucleotide-gated ion channels. CNP is expressed in the brain and endothelial cells where it acts as a paracrine/autocrine regulator through the natriuretic peptide receptor B (NPR-B). Natriuretic peptide receptor-C (NPR-C) binds to the three NPs; it activates an inhibitory G-protein and controls the local concentrations of NPs by receptor-mediated internalization and degradation [19, 21].

Secretion of ANP is regulated by a negative feedback loop: expansion of intravascular fluid increases atrial filling pressure that is sensed by stretch-activated ion channels that result in ANP secretion. ANP release is also stimulated by water immersion and sympathetic stimulation. ANP reduces arterial blood pressure through the inhibition of sympathetic nervous system activity, with the reduction of cardiac contractility and heart rate, and direct actions on the vascular smooth muscle. The increase in cGMP and activation of PKG open potassium channels and inhibit the influx of calcium through voltage-gated calcium channels, as well as the dephosphorylation of contractile proteins by PKG-dependent phosphatases. ANP also inhibits renin by reducing sympathetic tone and through cGMP-regulated phosphodiesterases that decrease cAMP. Aldosterone synthesis and secretion are also directly inhibited by ANP.

ANP increases salt and water renal excretion. ANP decreases sodium reabsorption by inhibiting sodium bicarbonate reabsorption and increasing glomerular filtration rate. It counters the result of ADH/AVP actions by decreasing the osmotic gradient in the medulla and decreasing sodium and water reabsorption in the collecting ducts. ADH/AVP secretion is inhibited through the hypothalamic neurons inhibition. Thirst and salt intake are also decreased by ANP. Thus ANP secretion reduces effective intravascular volume and closes the feedback loop with ANP secretion at normal levels [21, 22].

3.11 Conclusion

Hormones are chemical mediators that reach their target organs via the bloodstream. They are transported in blood exclusively in their free, unbound state or a combination of free states and bound to transporter proteins to enhance their solubility. Only the free hormones are capable of diffusing from the intravascular compartment into the extracellular compartment, and reach their receptors. Receptors are signal transducers located either in the cellular membrane (receptors of protein and peptide hormones) or in the intracellular compartment (receptors for thyroid and steroid hormones). Regulation of hormone secretion and synthesis is achieved through feedback loops, whereby the product of hormone action inhibits the synthesis and secretion of its stimulatory hormones.

Several hormones are involved in the regulation of the total body content and concentration of water and electrolytes: Antidiuretic or arginine-vasopressin regulates total body water and osmolality in extracellular fluid. The aldosterone and the renin-angiotensin-aldosterone system regulate total mass of sodium and potassium. Insulin and natriuretic atrial peptides control the influx and outflux of potassium from the intracellular fluid, and the excretion of sodium.

Endocrine abnormalities in acute kidney injury result from alterations in active hormone levels, which can be increased mainly by impaired renal clearance or degradation, or disorders of feedback regulation. Active hormone activity can be decreased by reduced synthesis rates or decreased activation of prohormone. Alternatively, hormone levels can be normal but the response of the target organ is impaired by the underlying condition.

References

1. Calandra RS. Introducción a la Endocrinología. In: Calandra RS, Barontini MB, editors. Fisiopatología Molecular y Clínica Endocrinológica. Ciudad Autónoma de Buenos Aires: Elli Lilly Interamérica; 2015. p. 147–51.
2. Molina P. General principles of endocrine physiology In: Endocrine physiology. McGraw Hill Medical; 2013. p. 1–24.
3. Feher J. General principles of endocrinology. In Quantitative Human Physiology: An introduction. Academic Press; 2017. p. 853–69.
4. Riera MF, Meroni SB, Pellizzari EH, Cigorraga SB, Juvenal GJ. Mecanismo de acción de hormonas con receptores en la superficie celular. In. Calandra RS, Barontini MB, editors. Fisiopatología Molecular y Clínica Endocrinológica. Ciudad Autónoma de Buenos Aires. Elli Lilly Interamérica 2015: 173–183.
5. Duc NM, Kim HR, Chung KY. Structural mechanism of G protein activation by G protein-coupled receptor. Eur J Pharmacol. 2015;763(Pt B):214–22. https://doi.org/10.1016/j.ejphar.2015.05.016.
6. Syrovatkina V, Alegre KO, Dey R, Huang XY. Regulation, signaling, and physiological functions of G-proteins. J Mol Biol. 2016;428:3850–68. https://doi.org/10.1016/j.jmb.2016.08.002.
7. Trenker R, Jura N. Receptor tyrosine kinase activation: from the ligand perspective. Curr Opin Cell Biol. 2020;63:174–85. https://doi.org/10.1016/j.ceb.2020.01.016.
8. Lüthy IA. Mecanismo de acción de receptores de esteroides. In: Calandra RS, Barontini MB, editors Fisiopatología Molecular y Clínica Endocrinológica. Ciudad Autónoma de Buenos Aires. Elli Lilly Interamérica 2015: 161–171.
9. Rastinejad F, Huang P, Chandra V, Khorasanizadeh SJ. Understanding nuclear receptor form and function using structural biology. Mol Endocrinol. 2013;51:T1–T21. https://doi.org/10.1530/JME-13-0173.
10. Kimmins S, TH MR. Cell Stress Chaperones. 2000;5:76–86. https://doi.org/10.1379/1466-126 8(2000)005<0076:mosrae>2.0.co;2.
11. Sun Z, Xu Y. Nuclear receptor coactivators (NCOAs) and corepressors (NCORs) in the brain. Endocrinology. 2020;161:bqaa083. https://doi.org/10.1210/endocr/bqaa083.
12. De Lavallaz L, Musso CG. Chronobiology in nephrology: the influence of circadian rhythms on renal handling of drugs and renal disease treatment. Int Urol Nephrol. 2018;50(12):2221–8. https://doi.org/10.1007/s11255-018-2001-z.

13. Molina P. Endocrine integration of energy and electrolyte balance. In: Endocrine physiology. McGraw Hill Medical; 2013. p. 249–80.
14. Sparapani S, Millet-Boureima C, Oliver J, Mu K, Hadavi P, Kalostian T, Ali N, Avelar CM, Bardies M, Barrow B, Benedikt M, Biancardi G, Bindra R, Bui L, Chihab Z, Cossitt A, Costa J, Daigneault T, Dault J, Davidson I, Dias J, Dufour E, El-Khoury S, Farhangdoost N, Forget A, Fox A, Gebrael M, Gentile MC, Geraci O, Gnanapragasam A, Gomah E, Haber E, Hamel C, Iyanker T, Kalantzis C, Kamali S, Kassardjian E, Kontos HK, Le TBU LSD, Low YF, Mac Rae D, Maurer F, Mazhar S, Nguyen A, Nguyen-Duong K, Osborne-Laroche C, Park HW, Parolin E, Paul-Cole K, Peer LS, Philippon M, Plaisir CA, Porras Marroquin J, Prasad S, Ramsarun R, Razzaq S, Rhainds S, Robin D, Scartozzi R, Singh D, Fard SS, Soroko M, Soroori Motlagh N, Stern K, Toro L, Toure MW, Tran-Huynh S, Trépanier-Chicoine S, Waddingham C, Weekes AJ, Wisniewski A, Gamberi C. The biology of vasopressins. Biomedicines. 2021:89. https://doi.org/10.3390/biomedicines9010089.
15.) Bichet DG. Vasopressin receptors in health and disease. Kidney Int. 1996;49:1706–11. https://doi.org/10.1038/ki.1996.252.
16. Su W, Cao R, Zhang XY, Guan Y. Aquaporins in the kidney: physiology and pathophysiology. Am J Physiol Renal Physiol. 2020;318:F193–203. https://doi.org/10.1152/ajprenal.00304.2019.
17. Musso CG, Jauregui JR. Renin-angiotensin-aldosterone system and the aging kidney. Expert Rev Endocrinol Metab. 2014;9(6):543–6.
18. Palmer BF. Regulation of potassium homeostasis. Clin J Am Soc Nephrol. 2015;10:1050–60. https://doi.org/10.2215/CJN.08580813.
19. Holt E, Lupsa B, Lee G, Bassyouni H, Peery H. Regulation of salt and water balance. In: Goodman's basic medical endocrinology. Elsevier; 2021. eBook ISBN: 9780128158456
20. Musso CG. Potassium metabolism in patients with chronic kidney disease (CKD), part I: patients not on dialysis (stages 3-4). Int Urol Nephrol. 2004;36(465–468):7.
21. Potter LR, Yoder AR, Flora DR, Antos LK, Dickey DM. Natriuretic peptides: their structures, receptors, physiologic functions, and therapeutic applications. Handb Exp Pharmacol. 2009;191:341–66. https://doi.org/10.1007/978-3-540-68964-5_15.
22. Emmanouel DS, Lindheimer MD, Ai K. Pathogenesis of endocrine abnormalities in uremia. Endocrine Rev. 1980;1:28–44.

Chapter 4
Neurotransmitters and Autonomous Nervous System

Carlos Guillermo Videla

4.1 Introduction

4.1.1 Autonomic Nervous System (ANS)

The ANS functions in an autonomic way which allows changes in our body without being conscious of them. It is formed by pathways of neurons that control multiple organ systems. For this purpose, it uses chemical signals to maintain a correct homeostasis. It is subdivided into the sympathetic nervous system and the parasympathetic nervous system [1, 2].

The sympathetic component has a catabolic function and prepares the body for stressful events; it is also known as the "fight or flight" system.

In contrast, the parasympathetic system component has an anabolic function, which is also known as "rest and digest" function.

Most of the organs of the body are innervated by both components. For example, sympathetic action on the heart increases inotropism, heart rate, and blood pressure; and parasympathetic action decreases blood pressure, heart rate, and inotropism [2, 3].

4.1.2 Anatomy of ANS

The ANS is anatomically and functionally divided into two complementary systems, the sympathetic nervous system (SNS) and the parasympathetic nervous system (PNS). The main center that processes ANS functions is the hypothalamus in the

C. G. Videla (✉)
Neurology Division, Hospital Italiano de Buenos Aires, Buenos Aires, Argentina
e-mail: guillermo.videla@hospitalitaliano.org.ar

C. G. Musso, A. Covic (eds.), *Organ Crosstalk in Acute Kidney Injury*,
https://doi.org/10.1007/978-3-031-36789-2_4

midbrain. Temperature regulation, fluid regulation, neurohumoral control, and response to stress are some of its functions.

The anterior hypothalamus controls temperature and the posterior hypothalamus is involved in water regulation [4].

The neural circuit of the ANS is composed of two neurons. The cell body of the first neuron, preganglionic, is in the central nervous system (CNS) and the second one, postganglionic, is peripheral. Both systems have efferent pathways through peripheral ganglia. One anatomic difference is that in the SNS the ganglia are located close to the CNS, next to the thoracolumbar spine, and in the PNS the ganglia are situated near or inside the innervated organs [5].

The SNS contains the first neuron body within the lateral gray column of the spinal cord from level T1 to level L2. The preganglionic neuron axon travels a short distance to the ganglion and synapses and activates nicotinic receptors on postganglionic neurons using acetylcholine as neurotransmitters. The postganglionic neuronal axon travels a large distance to the target site and uses norepinephrine to activate adrenergic receptors [2, 6, 7].

The PNS has a cranial and a pelvic portion. The cranial preganglionic neuron body is located in the brainstem and its axons travel through cranial nerves III, VII, IX, and X; the pelvic portion leaves the SNC through nerves from S2 to S4 spine level. The ganglia of the parasympathetic system are close to the target organ, and hence the postganglionic neurons have short axons. Both parasympathetic neurons are cholinergic. The renal innervation of the parasympathetic nervous system is almost nil and plays only a secondary role in contrast to the sympathetic nervous system [3].

4.2   Mechanism of Action

The synapse is the way in which the nervous system communicates with a second neuron (postganglionic) or an effector cell. There are several types of synapses: chemical, electrical, or mixed, the chemical type being the most common in humans [8].

4.2.1   Chemical Synapse

This type of synapse comprises an axon terminal and a target cell, usually a dendrite of a second neuron. The typical synapse consists of a presynaptic element, the synaptic cleft (20–50 nm), and the postsynaptic element. The typical presynaptic element is the axonal bouton and contains mitochondria which supply the energy for this process, as well as vesicles where neurotransmitters are stored. The arrival of an electric signal called "action potential" depolarizes the presynaptic terminal, opening an electric dependent calcium channel. The resulting influx of calcium into the cell initiates a sequence of events that cause synaptic vesicles to merge with the presynaptic membrane and to release their neurotransmitter into the cleft. These molecules diffuse through the cleft and bind to the receptors of the postsynaptic membrane, triggering a biochemical or electrochemical reaction in the target cell [9].

4.2.2   Neurotransmitters

The ANS controls the target organs through chemical messengers known as neurotransmitters [1, 10].

Acetylcholine (Ach), norepinephrine, and epinephrine are the main neurotransmitters involved in the ANS. Preganglionic neurons of both divisions of the ANS utilize Ach as neurotransmitters, as well as postganglionic neurons of the PNS. Postganglionic neurons of the sympathetic system utilize norepinephrine or epinephrine [1, 11].

4.2.3   Catecholamines

Norepinephrine and epinephrine are biogenic amines, also called catecholamines. They have small differences in their chemical structure; norepinephrine has a hydrogen atom attached to the nitrogen that is replaced in the epinephrine by a methyl group. The norepinephrine synthesis process occurs in postganglionic neurons of the sympathetic nervous system. Norepinephrine is the main neurotransmitter used by the SNS and it is synthesized from phenylalanine through a series of enzymatic steps. Most of them take place in the neuron cytoplasm and the final conversion from dopamine to norepinephrine occurs inside the neurotransmitter vesicle. Finally, norepinephrine can be converted into epinephrine by the action of the enzyme phenylethanolamine N-methyltransferase with S-adenosyl-L-methionine as cofactor [2, 12, 13].

$$\text{Phenylalanine} \rightarrow \text{Tyrosine} \rightarrow \text{L} - \text{DOPA} \rightarrow \text{Dopamine} \rightarrow \text{Norepinephrine} \rightarrow \text{Epinephrine}$$

Once in the synapse, norepinephrine binds and activates postsynaptic receptors. Subsequently, norepinephrine is unbound from the receptors and follows two pathways: it is absorbed back into the presynaptic cell, via reuptake through the norepinephrine transporter and repackaged into new vesicles for future release, or it is metabolized and degraded into various inactive metabolites and excreted in the urine, as vanillylmandelic acid or 3-Methoxy-4-hydroxyphenylglycol (MHPG) is the major metabolite of norepinephrine in the brain. Monoamine oxidase and catechol-o-methyltransferase are the enzymes involved in this process [14].

Norepinephrine exerts its effects by binding and activating specific receptors located on the surface of the cell. There are two main types: the alpha- and beta-adrenergic receptors with different subtypes. Alpha receptors are divided into α_1 and α_2 and beta receptors into β_1, β_2, and β_3. These receptors are G protein-coupled receptors using a second messenger system.

Alpha-1 and all beta receptors have an excitatory effect; in contrast, alpha-2 receptors located in the presynaptic membrane have an inhibitory effect during activation by decreasing the amount of norepinephrine released.

Epinephrine plays a secondary role as a neurotransmitter but has an important systemic effect because it is released directly into circulation by chromaffin cells of the adrenal gland. The adrenal medulla functions as a sympathetic ganglion in direct communication with the systemic circulation. The splanchnic nerves of the SNS synapse with the gland cells and stimulate them to release epinephrine. The direct release of epinephrine into the bloodstream allows the sympathetic nervous system to have systemic effects along all the organs which have adrenergic receptors. Adrenal gland stimulation acts as an amplifier of the stress response [15].

4.2.4   Acetylcholine (ACh)

Acetylcholine (ACh) is an organic molecule which functions as a neurotransmitter. Its chemical structure consists of an ester of acetic acid and choline. It is not considered a biogenic amine. All the neural pathways and organs that are affected by ACh are cholinergic [16].

There are two main locations where ACh acts as a neurotransmitter: in the neuromuscular junction, triggering muscle contraction, and in the ANS. ACh is released by all preganglionic neurons of the ANS and is the primary neurotransmitter of the PNS.

Synaptic transmission through ANS ganglia is similar in both the SNS and the PNS. Both preganglionic neurons of the SNS and PNS are cholinergic. Acetylcholine (ACh) is stored in synaptic vesicles and released by a calcium- (Ca^{2+}) dependent process upon nerve terminal depolarization. Once released, ACh interacts with postsynaptic receptors to depolarize the postsynaptic membrane. The principal ganglionic receptors are excitatory nicotinic ACh receptors. ACh binds and opens the ion channel, allowing sodium and calcium to generate a depolarization and induce an excitatory postsynaptic potential.

4.2.5   Nitric Oxide (NO)

NO is a gaseous diatomic molecule which exerts an action on brain blood flow. There is a hypothesis stating that it also acts as a neurotransmitter in the brain modulating the sympathetic nerve activity and thereby blood pressure and renal nerve activation. NO could act as a neurotransmitter and a neuromodulator with an inhibiting action in the central sympathetic activity. NO works as a retrograde neurotransmitter in synapses and has an important role in the regulation of metabolic status of neurons and dendritic spine growth. It is possible that a low level of NO could increase sympathetic nerve activity and vice versa [17].

4.3 Sympathetic Nervous System and Kidneys

The CNS communicates with the kidneys through a densely innervated net of efferent and afferent nerves. The main innervated kidney structures are blood vessels, tubules, the renal pelvis, and the glomeruli.

The adrenal gland and the kidneys receive more nerve supply than any other abdominal organ. The renal plexus' nerve axons come from the celiac ganglion, inferior and posterior renal ganglia, superior mesenteric ganglion, and thoracic splanchnic nerves. From the plexus the nerves run over the superior and inferior parts of the renal artery, following the anatomical vascular subdivision [18].

The SNS is the most important nervous innervation of the kidneys. Renal sympathetic nerves play a crucial role in blood pressure regulation; in fact during hypertension elevated renal sympathetic nerve activity is commonly found. The increased activity of the renal sympathetic nerves elevates the blood pressure by three mechanisms: (1) increasing tubular reabsorption of water and urinary sodium; (2) reducing renal blood flow and glomerular filtration rate; and (3) through renin releasing from the juxtaglomerular apparatus, activating the renin-angiotensin-aldosterone (RAAS) cascade [2].

The neural efferent nerves are distributed along the renal artery and the vein, following the different vascular segments, with more evident action in the renal cortex and outer medulla and a secondary role in the inner medulla. A weak stimulation (low frequency) of the efferent nerves releases renin and reduces the blood flow of the outer cortex; a higher stimulation increases the renin release and reduced urinary sodium; finally a maximum level of stimulus releases higher quantities of renin and reduces sodium excretion, renal blood flow, and glomerular filtration rate [19].

The efferent nerves are sympathetic postganglionic axons and have norepinephrine as their neurotransmitter. There are different types of receptors: α1-adrenoreceptors are located on the renal vasculature, nephrons, and proximal tubules. Their activation produces vasoconstriction, sodium reabsorption, glycogenesis, and prostaglandins.

α2-receptors play a similar role to α1 but they also mediate diuresis at the collecting duct. β1-adrenoreceptors are located on the juxtaglomerular cells, nephrons, distal tubules, and collecting ducts where they stimulate renin secretion and suppress potassium secretion. In contrast, β2-adrenoreceptors are located only at the proximal and distal tubules and collecting ducts. β-adrenoreceptors activation mediates reabsorption of Ca + and magnesium in the cortex, and of sodium chloride (NaCl) in the cortex and medulla.

4.4 Central Nervous System Control of Renal Function

The sympathetic premotor nuclei located at the brainstem and hypothalamus, including the rostral ventrolateral (RVLM) and ventromedial medulla, rule the neuronal activity of renal SNS. The rostral ventrolateral medulla is the pressor site of the brain. Seventy percent of the RVLM descending projections are sympathetic excitatory pathways and direct to C1 preganglionic neurons in the intermediolateral cell column of the spinal cord. From there, via postganglionic neurons, they innervate the kidneys and modulate SNS renal activity [1, 2].

Afferent sensory renal nerves are unmyelinated. Chemo- and mechanoreceptors stimulate afferent nerves from the kidney and modulate the activity of the RVLM and paraventricular nucleus (PVN), completing a circuit. The mechano-receptors are activated by changes of size of the renal pelvic wall. A gradual increase in renal pelvic pressure directly increases renal sensory fibers activity. The chemoreceptors react to the presence of ischemic metabolites and uremic toxins.

Most renal afferent nerves originate in the proximal ureter, around large vessels, and the smooth muscle layer of the renal pelvis [20].

Afferent sensory nerve fibers contain substance P and calcitonin gene-related peptide as primary neurotransmitters.

In contrast, parasympathetic system activation, similar to massage of the carotid sinus, stimulates the *nucleus tractus solitarius* (NTS), which projects to the caudal ventrolateral medulla nucleus and produces an inhibitory effect on the RVLM, decreasing sympathetic renal activity.

Finally, there is a local mechanism called the renorenal reflex, which consists of an inhibitory reflex where stretch stimulus of afferent nerves decreases efferent renal activity, producing compensation. It acts as an inhibitory response in normal conditions; unfortunately, when renal function is impaired, this reflex is attenuated and loses preponderancy.

4.5 Acute Kidney Injury and Special Conditions

Acute kidney injury is defined as a rapid loss of kidney function. Neurohumoral activation with increased (SNS) activity plays a crucial role during this event [21].

4.6 Septic Acute Renal Injury

Septic shock is characterized by inflammation, systemic vasodilation, hypotension, and increased SNS activity. There is overproduction of pro-inflammatory cytokines such as tumor necrosis factor-alpha (TNF-α), interleukins, and activation of RAAS. This is also known as the "cytokine storm" [22]. Pro-inflammatory cytokines and angiotensin II can reach the brain by crossing the brain–blood-barrier. Once in the brain they produce a stimulation of sympathetic nuclei as PVN, RVLM, and NTS causing an increase of sympathetic activity in the body. The synergy combination of decreased systemic blood and renal arterial vasoconstriction due to elevated sympathetic activity induces renal ischemia and abrupt loss of renal function [23, 24].

Some implications of this physiopathology synergism are important in the treatment of sepsis and prevention of renal damage.

For example, norepinephrine, an α-adrenergic agonist, is the standard treatment for septic hypotension but in excess can lead to an increase in sympathetic renal activity and can produce a decrease of renal blood flow and local renal damage.

During events of ischemia-reperfusion, as in cardiac surgery, increased renal sympathetic activity triggers fibrogenesis, tubular atrophy, and inflammatory cascade. Treatments directed at the inhibition of norepinephrine such as clonidine or moxonidine (central sympatholytic effect) could prevent or limit renal damage [25].

In addition, by increasing parasympathetic activity through stimulation of vagal or splenic nerves, both cholinergic pathways produce an anti-inflammatory effect and ameliorate renal damage during this type of procedure.

4.7 Conclusions

Sympathetic renal activity plays a crucial role in maintaining a correct renal homeostasis. Afferent renal nerves send information from the renal parenchyma to the nervous system. Central autonomic nuclei influence the level of sympathetic activity of the kidneys through renal afferent nerves. Different levels of renal sympathetic nerve activity could play a protective role or lead to damage of the renal parenchyma. A group of molecules called neurotransmitters are the final keys for all this activity. Norepinephrine is the most important adrenergic neurotransmitter and plays a crucial part in renal vasoconstriction and in water and sodium reabsorption.

An adequate knowledge of the location and type of action of the different neurotransmitters will allow the development of better therapeutic strategies [26]. Treatments aimed at regulation of the neurotransmitters and, through these, sympathetic renal activity will lead to prevention of renal damage or improved recovery after an injury [23].

References

1. Kumagai H, Oshima N, Matsuura T, Iigaya K, Imai M, Onimaru H, et al. Importance of rostral ventrolateral medulla neurons in determining efferent sympathetic nerve activity and blood pressure. Hypertens Res. 2012;35:132–41. https://doi.org/10.1038/hr.2011.208.

2. DiBona GF. Neural control of the kidney: functionally specific renal sympathetic nerve fibers. Am J Physiol Regul Integr Comp Physiol. 2000;279:R1517–24. https://doi.org/10.1152/ajpregu.2000.279.5.R1517.

3. McCorry LK. Physiology of the autonomic nervous system. Am J Pharm Educ. 2007;71(4):78. https://doi.org/10.5688/aj710478.

4. Glick DB. The autonomic nervous system. In: Miller RD, Eriksson LI, Fleisher LA, et al., editors. Miller's anesthesia. 7th ed. Philadelphia: Elsevier; 2011. p. 261–304.

5. Nurse CA. Neurotransmitter and neuromodulatory mechanisms at peripheral arterial chemoreceptors. Exp Physiol. 2010;95:657–67.

6. Gibbins I. Functional organization of autonomic neural pathways. Organogenesis. 2013;9(3):169–75.

7. Nathan PW, Smith MC. The location of descending fibers to sympathetic preganglionic vasomotor and sudomotor neurons in man. J Neurol Neurosurg Psychiatry. 1987;50:1253–62.

8. Jessell TM, Kandel ER. Synaptic transmission: a bidirectional and self-modifiable form of cell-cell communication. Cell. 1993:721–30. https://doi.org/10.1016/S0092-8674(05)80025-X.

9. Pereda AE. Electrical synapses and their functional interactions with chemical synapses. Nat Rev Neurosci. 2014;15(4):250–63. https://doi.org/10.1038/nrn3708.

10. Kelly RB. Storage and release of neurotransmitters. Cell. 1993:7243–53. https://doi.org/10.1016/S0092-8674(05)80027-3.

11. Burnstock G. The changing face of autonomic neurotransmission. Acta Physiol Scand. 1986;126(1):67–91. https://doi.org/10.1111/j.1748-1716.1986.tb07790.x.

12. Rang HP, Ritter JM, Flower R, Henderson G. Chapter 14: Noradrenergic transmission. In: Rang & Dale's pharmacology. Elsevier Health Sciences; 2014. 177–96. ISBN 978-0-7020-5497-6.

13. Musacchio JM. Chapter 1: Enzymes involved in the biosynthesis and degradation of catecholamines. In: Iverson L, editor. Biochemistry of biogenic amines. Springer; 2013. 1–35. ISBN 978-1-4684-3171-1.

14. Eisenhofer G, Kopin IJ, Goldstein DS. Catecholamine metabolism: a contemporary view with implications for physiology and medicine. Pharmacol Rev. 2004;56(3):331–49. https://doi.org/10.1124/pr.56.3.1.

15. Joseph Feher (2012) The adrenal medulla and integration of metabolic control. In: Quantitative human physiology. Elsevier 916-923

16. Tiwari P, Dwivedi S, Singh MP, Mishra R, Chandy A. Basic and modern concepts on cholinergic receptor: a review. Asian Pac J Trop Dis. 2013;3(5):413–20. https://doi.org/10.1016/S2222-1808(13)60094-8.

17. Garthwaite J, Boulton CL. Nitric oxide signaling in the central nervous system. Annu Rev Physiol. 1995;57(1):683–706. https://doi.org/10.1146/annurev.ph.57.030195.003343.

18. Barajas L, Liu L, Powers K. Anatomy of the renal innervation: intrarenal aspects and ganglia of origin. Can J Physiol Pharmacol. 1992;70:735–49. https://doi.org/10.1139/y92-098.

19. Johns EJ, Kopp UC, DiBona GF, Terjung R. Neural control of renal function. Compr Physiol. 2011;1(2):731–67.

20. Mulder J, Hokfelt T, Knuepfer MM, Kopp UC. Renal sensory and sympathetic nerves reinnervate the kidney in a similar time dependent fashion following renal denervation in rats. Am J Physiol Regul Integr Comp Physiol. 2013;304:R675–82. https://doi.org/10.1152/ajpregu.00599.2012.

21. Hering D, Winklewski PJ. R1 autonomic nervous system in acute kidney injury. Clin Exp Pharmacol Physiol. 2017;44(2):162–71. https://doi.org/10.1111/1440-1681.12694.

22. Johnston GR, Webster NR. Cytokines and the immunomodulatory function of the vagus nerve. Br J Anaesth. 2009;102:453–62.

23. Barrett CJ, Navakatikyan MA, Malpas SC. Long-term control of renal blood flow: what is the role of the renal nerves? Am J Physiol Regul Integr Comp Physiol. 2001;280:R1534–45. https://doi.org/10.1152/ajpregu.2001.280.5.R1534.

24. Fujii T, Kurata H, Takaoka M, et al. The role of renal sympathetic nervous system in the pathogenesis of ischemic acute renal failure. Eur J Pharmacol. 2003;481:241–8.

25. Bonventre JV, Zuk A. Ischemic acute renal failure: an inflammatory disease? Kidney Int. 2004;66:480–5.
26. Hering D, Marusic P, Walton AS, Lambert EA, Krum H, Narkiewicz K, et al. Sustained sympathetic and blood pressure reduction 1 year after renal denervation in patients with resistant hypertension. Hypertension. 2014;64(1):118–24. https://doi.org/10.1161/HYPERTENSIONAHA.113.03098.

Chapter 5
Cytokines, Chemokines, Inflammasomes, Myokines and Complement-Related Factors in Acute Kidney Injury

Eloina Del Carmen Zarate-Peñata, Ornella Fiorillo-Moreno, Catherine Meza-Torres, and Elkin Navarro-Quiroz

5.1 Cytokines in Acute Kidney Injury (AKI)

Cytokines are soluble mediators composed of glycoproteins or low-molecular weight proteins produced during the initiation or effector phase of the immune response. Their role is to mediate and regulate the amplitude and duration of immune/inflammatory responses. Therefore, cytokines contribute to the immuno-pathogenesis of acute kidney injury (AKI) [1, 2]. In AKI, injured endothelial cells and tubular cells go through morphological and/or functional changes that result in their activation and consequential cytokines production. Leukocytes, including neutrophils and macrophages, natural killer cells, and lymphocytes, infiltrate the kidneys and contribute to the production of AKI. Consequently, the quantity and type of cytokine production from all of the above mentioned cells contribute to the generation of different patterns of expression and activation of proinflammatory and anti-inflammatory cytokines, key components of both the onset and extension of inflammation in AKI [3].

During the early initiation phase of AKI, epithelial and endothelial cells upregulate their proinflammatory cytokine production, which includes TNF-α, IFNγ,

E. D. C. Zarate-Peñata · O. Fiorillo-Moreno
Basic and Biomedical Sciences, Universidad Simón Bolívar, Barranquilla, Colombia

C. Meza-Torres
College of Health Sciences, Medicine Program, Corporation University Rafael Nuñez, Cartagena, Colombia

E. Navarro-Quiroz (✉)
Basic and Biomedical Sciences, Universidad Simón Bolívar, Barranquilla, Colombia

Life Sciences Research Center, Universidad Simón Bolívar, Barranquilla, Colombia

Fundación Universidad San Martin, School of Medicine, Puerto Colombia, Colombia
e-mail: elkin.navarro@unisimon.edu.co

TGF-β, IL-2, and IL-6. Other pro-inflammatory cytokines such as IL-1β and IL-18 are produced through activation of the caspase 1 signaling pathway [4, 5]. Another important cytokine that contributes to the pathogenesis of AKI is IL-20 [6].

Experimental and clinical evidence has demonstrated the role of these cytokines in worsening renal function and mortality in patients with AKI [7]. The mentioned molecules and their effect on renal function in AKI patients are described below.

5.1.1 *Tumor Necrosis Factor-Alpha (TNF-α)*

TNF-α is a potent pleiotropic mediator of the inflammatory response in the kidney. It is produced by various cells, including macrophages, podocytes, mesangial cells, and tubular epithelial cells [8]. The major TNF-α-activated pathways center on caspase, nuclear factor-κB (NF-κB), and mitogen-activated protein kinase (MAPK). The NF-κB and MAPK signaling pathways induce secondary responses by increasing the expression levels of several proinflammatory cytokines that further activate TNF-α [9]. It has been proposed that renal function and blood pressure regulation could be partially influenced by different TNF-α concentrations within the kidney, while high circulating TNF-α levels have been reported to be associated with adverse clinical outcomes in patients with AKI [7, 10].

TNF-α alters renal hemodynamics and nephron transport, affecting both the activity and expression of transporters. It is also involved in organ damage by stimulating immune cell infiltration and apoptosis in epithelial cells, tubular cells, and mesangial cells. This phenomenon could be diminished by blocking TNF-α [11–14]. TNF-α stimulates the expression of MCP-1 and IL-8, as well as the expression of molecular adhesion molecules such as ICAM- in mesangial cells, tubular epithelial cells, and podocytes to promote the infiltration of neutrophils and monocytes. Moreover, it increases reactive oxygen species (ROS) production in mesangial cells. TNF-α correlates positively with albuminuria, and inflammatory biomarkers levels [10]. TNF-α induces loss of glomerular endothelial cell fenestration, leading to decreased GFR and albumin leakage. TNF-α-mediated damage to the glomerular endothelium is an important determinant of acute kidney injury in sepsis [15].

On the other hand, functionally relevant polymorphisms within the promoter region of the *TNF* gene that affect transcriptional activity have previously been associated with the severity and mortality of patients, including those with AKI requiring dialysis [16, 17], such as the *TNFA* gene polymorphism rs1800629. This polymorphism was found to be associated with markers of renal disease severity and distant organ dysfunction among patients with AKI. Carriers of the minor A allele rs1800629 of *TNFA* have higher levels of filtration markers, including higher serum creatinine and cystatin C, and higher markers of urinary tubular injury, including KIM-1 and π-GST [17].

5.1.2 Interferon Gamma (IFNγ)

IFNγ is the only member of the type II interferons. This cytokine is pleiotropically produced by activated immune cells, including natural killer (NK) cells. Its proinflammatory functions in renal disease include the following: (a) activation of M1 macrophages [18, 19], (b) modulation of effector T-cell responses [20], (c) induction of major histocompatibility complex class I and II molecules for antigen presentation [21], and (d) positive regulation of chemokines that increase immune cell infiltration [22]. In addition, interferon-γ production by human tubule-interstitial NK [bright] CD56 cells has been reported to contribute to renal fibrosis and progression of chronic kidney disease (CKD) [23].

5.1.3 Transforming Growth Factor-Beta (TGF-β)

TGF-β, a key profibrotic growth factor, is activated in AKI and is associated with cellular responses leading to the development of CKD. The persistently injured dedifferentiated tubular epithelial cell is an important mediator of the transition from AKI to CKD. TGF-β signaling can perpetuate proximal tubule injury through dedifferentiation, cell cycle arrest, and increased susceptibility to apoptosis. In addition, TGF-β signaling promotes macrophage chemotaxis, endothelial injury, and myofibroblast differentiation after AKI. Future studies blocking TGF-β signaling after cessation of AKI are needed to better define its role in the progression from acute to chronic kidney damage [24, 25].

5.1.4 Interleukin 1-Beta (IL-1β)

IL-1β is a member of the interleukin 1 family of cytokines. This cytokine is produced by activated macrophages as a proprotein, which is proteolytically processed to its active form by caspase 1 (CASP1). The inflammasome-driven release of interleukin IL-1β is a central element of many forms of sterile inflammation, and has been shown to promote the initiation and progression of kidney disease by activating tubule-interstitial fibrosis of the kidney by inducing a metabolic change in platelet-derived growth factor receptor (PDGFRβ) + renal stromal cells [26]. IL-1β has been shown to have a direct effect on the production of neutrophil gelatinase-associated lipocalin (NGAL), a biomarker of AKI by tubular epithelial cells [27, 28].

5.1.5   *Interleukin 2 (IL-2)*

IL-2 is a pleiotropic cytokine, first described as a T-cell growth factor, a potent mitogen that controls the differentiation and homeostasis of proinflammatory and anti-inflammatory T cells central to determining the molecular details of immune regulation. This cytokine has been described as a mediator of inflammation in AKI [2], as well as the role of T lymphocytes in affecting the pathogenesis and magnitude of AKI. In particular, helper T lymphocytes 17 enhance tissue injury by recruiting neutrophils and other inflammatory cells, whereas regulatory T cells, in contrast, reduce renal injury and facilitate repair. Interestingly, evidence supports parenchymal-local T-cell interactions as essential in producing T-cell phenotypic changes that affect long-term renal and patient survival [29]. It has also demonstrated an association of T-cell-derived inflammatory cytokines with AKI and mortality after cardiac surgery [30]. On the other hand, it has been described that acute respiratory failure associated with COVID-19 leads to a strong imbalance of circulating immune mediators including IL-2 [31].

5.1.6   *Interleukin 6 (IL-6)*

IL-6 is a cytokine that can be produced by renal resident cells, including tubular epithelial cells, podocytes, and mesangial cells under some stimuli such as TNF-α and IL-1β. This cytokine mediates a proinflammatory response that partially contributes to the generation of renal damage. It increases early in the serum of patients with AKI and has been described to predict short-term renal function and mortality in patients with AKI [32, 33]. Animal studies demonstrate that IL-6 induces collagen I expression in the proximal tubular epithelial cells of mice through STAT3 phosphorylation. It plays a role in mesangial cell proliferation, which is associated with glomerular hypertrophy and stimulation of MCP-1 expression [34, 35]. In addition, it participates in high glucose-induced podocyte apoptosis by regulating the activation of caspase-3 and caspase-9, enhances the production of cell cycle inhibitors (p21 and p27) in podocytes [36], and improves the fibrotic response through TGF-β, collagen I, and collagen IV in the IRI-IRA model. IL-6 deficiency improves renal function and decreases neutrophil infiltration in IRI- and HgCl2-induced AKI models [37]. In addition, hepatocyte-mediated IL-6 production has been associated with NGAL production in plasma and urine during AKI [38]. On the other hand, patient studies demonstrate that IL-6 increased within 6 h in pediatric patients with AKI after cardiopulmonary bypass. This determines that the role of the kidney in IL-6 filtration and metabolism is consistent with the known role of the proximal tubule in protein metabolism, as failure to metabolize this cytokine in the proximal tubule causes an increase in both serum and urine, contributing to harmful systemic effects and increased mortality [39].

5.1.7 Interleukin 18 (IL-18)

IL-18 is a proinflammatory cytokine structurally similar to IL-1β, and is produced by proximal tubules, lymphocytes, neutrophils, and macrophages in ischemic AKI. IL-18 promotes IFN-γ production, and strongly induces a Th1 response in inflammatory kidney disease. Like IL-1β, this cytokine drives the same myeloid differentiation factor 88 (MyD88)/nuclear factor kappa B (NF-κB) [5]. AKI is usually diagnosed by increases in serum creatinine or blood urea nitrogen. In clinical studies of patients with AKI, some of these biomarkers (e.g., IL-18, kidney injury molecule 1 (KIM-1, and NGAL) have been shown to increase in urine before serum creatinine. IL-18 is both a mediator and a biomarker of ischemic AKI for three reasons: (a) its expression is increased in the kidney, (b) its inhibition is protective against AKI in mice, and (c) it is increased in urine in both mice and humans with AKI [40]. In response to stress, renal tubular cells acutely release IL-18 which recruits and activates neutrophils. Activation of IL-18 by caspase-1 results in the production of various cytokines and chemokines, activation of helper T cells, and lymphocyte proliferation. Activated renal endothelial cells express E selectin that binds to the β integrins of neutrophils and initiates the process of diapedesis. Neutrophils damage renal tissue by degranulation, release of IFN-γ, and recruitment of NK T cells [40]. Caspase-1-deficient mice were shown to be protected against ischemic AKI [41], which exerts proinflammatory effects associated with increased IL-1β, IL-18, IL-6, and neutrophil infiltration in the kidney [42].

5.1.8 Interleukin 20 (IL-20)

IL-20 is a cytokine which belongs to the IL-10 family and shares structural homology with other members (IL-10, IL-19, IL-24, and IL-26). It is secreted by immune cells and activated epithelial cells such as keratinocytes, and binds to two types of receptor complexes, IL-20R1/IL-20R2 and IL-22R1/IL-20R2. Both heterodimer receptor complexes signal in part through JAK-STAT pathways [43]. Studies have indicated that this cytokine is involved as a pathogenic factor in renal epithelial cell injury in AKI [6, 44], mainly in CKD and diabetic nephropathy [45]. IL-20 acts on interstitial fibroblasts, renal epithelial cells, mesangial cells, and podocytes, and contributes to the progression of renal disease. It enhances inflammatory response, renal fibrosis, and cell apoptosis, through receptors IL-20R1 and IL-20R2 [6] that activate initiator and effector caspases such as caspase-9 in human proximal tubular epithelial HK-2 cells and caspase-3 in tubular epithelial cells (TKPTS and M-1) by upregulating the proapoptotic protein BAD, respectively. Thus, IL-20 induces programmed cell death of human renal epithelial cells by creating an imbalance in proapoptotic and prosurvival molecules that ultimately activates the mitochondria-dependent apoptosis pathway, and increases the expression of cytokines such as IL-1β and TGF-β1, a key inducer for renal fibrogenesis [45].

5.2 Immunoregulation by Cytokines in AKI

The inflammatory molecules described in the previous section are finely regulated by multiple inhibitors and antagonists such as IL-10, CSF1, IL-4, IL-13, and GM-CSF. These molecules have been shown to participate in tissue recovery and immune regulation by M2 macrophages [18, 19, 46–48]. Specifically, the anti-inflammatory cytokine IL-10 limits the severity of the pathobiological effects of proinflammatory cytokines (TNF-α, IL-1, IL-6, IL-8, and IFN-γ). Dysregulation of this mechanism and the accumulation of an excessive number of cytokines are responsible for the immunopathogenesis of AKI [1]. The production of these data is complemented by experiments in murine models where neutralization or blockade of IL-10 leads to elevated levels of TNF-α and IL-6 and supplying IL-10 exogenously improves survival and reduces inflammatory cytokines. It also shows a protective effect against ischemic and cisplatin-induced renal injury and leukocyte infiltration and through the induction of NGAL [49]. In addition, higher plasma IL-10 concentration has been associated with a lower risk of all-cause mortality following cardiac surgery after adjustment for clinical and demographic factors as well as renal function [32].

Colony-stimulating factor 1 (CSF1) is a secreted cytokine that induces hematopoietic stem cells to differentiate into macrophages or other related cell types. The epithelia of renal tubules represent the primary site of damage in AKI, a process initiated and propagated by macrophage infiltration. The role of resident renal macrophages and dendritic cells in the recovery of AKI after diphtheria toxin (DT)-induced ischemia/reperfusion injury has been investigated via CSF-1 signaling [47, 48]. CSF1 mediates the polarization of renal macrophages and dendritic cells during the recovery phase of AKI. The kidney, and specifically the proximal tubule, is a major source of intrarenal CSF-1 production in response to AKI [47]. In addition, IL-4/IL-13 induces polarization of kidney-resident macrophages/dendritic cells to a tissue-repairing phenotype ("M2a") that heals wounds, while IL-10 promotes polarization to a regulatory, anti-inflammatory phenotype ("M2c") [50]. Macrophage and granulocyte colony-stimulating factor (GM-CSF) play a crucial role in the phenotype of mononuclear phagocytes in the kidney after injury because it promotes the acquisition of characteristics in Mϕ M2 more commonly associated with dendritic cells (DCs). The abovementioned factors likely promote the resolution of inflammation and effective renal repair, probably due to the elimination of apoptotic cells and the phenotypic shift from M1 to M2 [51].

5.2.1 Chemokines in AKI

Chemokines, also known as chemotactic cytokines, are small, low-molecular weight (8–17 kDa) proteins belonging to the cytokine family. They are frequently mentioned due to the fact that they were initially identified because of their ability to activate, attract, and guide inflammatory cells in their migration to sites of inflammation [52]. In ischemia-reperfusion kidney injury, an essential feature of the innate immune response is the rapid accumulation of neutrophils and monocytes/ macrophages that regulate the pathological changes from AKI to chemokine/ chemokine receptor-mediated CKD [53]. Several chemokine families show a strong association with AKI, including the CXCL-IL-8/CXCL8 subfamily, Gro-α/CXCL1 and MIP-2/Gro-β/CXCL2, which act primarily on neutrophils, CXCL10 on Th1 cells and CXCL16 on macrophages. The CCL subfamily (MCP-1/CCL2), the CX3CL subfamily (fractalkine/CX3CL1) that have specific effects on monocytes and monocyte-derived lineages, and RANTES/CCL5 that operate more broadly to attract cells, monocytes and lymphocytes [52, 54, 55].

Chemokine production is induced by cytokines, complement activation, reactive oxygen species, and NF-κB and Toll-like receptors (TLR)-related signaling pathways [56, 57]. The effects of chemokines and their receptors have been reported to contribute to tissue injury in animal models of inflammatory kidney disease. The chemokine CXCL8/IL-8 can bind to G protein-coupled receptors (CXCR1 and CXCR2) expressed on neutrophils. CXCL8/IL-8 is vital in triggering local infiltration during renal inflammation and can be upregulated by IL-1β and TNF-α [58, 59]. CXCL8 expression in renal tissues and serum was reduced by G31P antagonist action, in this manner maintaining renal function and alleviating sepsis-induced AKI by its anti-inflammatory and anti-apoptotic effects through the NF-κB and JAK2/STAT3 pathways [58]. Similarly, CXCL1/CXCR2 regulates cisplatin-induced inflammatory responses through the P38 and NF-κB signaling pathways in vitro and in vivo. Cisplatin-induced AKI mice lacking the CXCL1 or CXCR2 gene show attenuation of renal injury and decreased proinflammatory effects. Meanwhile, inhibition of CXCR2 signaling with the CXCR2 receptor antagonist (repertaxin) could partly attenuate cisplatin-induced AKI [60]. Another study demonstrated that CXCL16 plays a crucial role in the pathogenesis of cisplatin-induced AKI through the regulation of renal tubular epithelial cell apoptosis and decreased caspase-3 activation. CXCL16 deficiency inhibited macrophage and T-cell infiltration in kidneys after cisplatin treatment, which was associated with reduced expression of proinflammatory cytokines in kidneys [61]. CXCL16 also contributes to chronic kidney injury and fibrosis by recruiting bone marrow-derived fibroblast precursors and fibrocytes, macrophages, and T cells in the kidney [61–63].

Another receptor mediating leukocyte trafficking is CXCR3, to which CXCL10, also known as interferon-γ inducible protein 10 (IP-10), binds to exert its biological function as chemoattraction, cell growth facilitation, and angiostatic effects. Studies have shown that renal resident mesangial cells, renal tubular epithelial cells, podocytes, endothelial cells, and infiltrating inflammatory cells express CXCL10 and CXCR3 under inflammatory conditions. In addition, CXCL10 has been shown to be an important biomarker of disease severity and can be used as a prognostic indicator for a variety of renal diseases. Urine determination of CXCR3-activating chemokines, such as CXCL9 and CXCL10, is promising for the early diagnosis of acute, humoral, cellular, or mixed rejection. One study showed that AKI is significantly associated with elevated urinary CXCL10 and CXCL9 levels in children after hematopoietic cell transplantation [64, 65]. In addition, these mediators may improve the diagnosis of humoral rejection in conjunction with the determination of donor-specific studies [66].

Chemokine (C-X3-C motif) receptor 1 (CX3CR1) is ubiquitously expressed in most tissues on circulating mononuclear leukocytes and lymphocytes. Fractalkine, also known as CX3CL1, is the only CX3CR1 ligand that combines the properties of chemoattractant (T cell and monocyte) and adhesion molecules. Therefore, the CX3CL1/CX3CR1 axis is a new type of leukocyte migration controller. The chemokine (C-X3-C motif) receptor 1 (CX3CR1) is ubiquitously expressed in most tissues on circulating mononuclear leukocytes and lymphocytes. Fractalkine, also known as CX3CL1, is the sole CX3CR1 ligand that blends the properties of chemotactic (T cell and monocyte) and adhesion molecules. Thus, the CX3CL1/CX3CR1 axis represents a new kind of leukocyte migration controller. A variety of recently published studies exploring the connection between the CX3CL1/CX3CR1 axis and kidney diseases and disorders, including diabetic nephropathy, renal allograft rejection, infectious kidney diseases, IgA nephropathy, fibrotic kidney disease, lupus nephritis and glomerulonephritis, acute kidney injury (AKI), and renal carcinoma, have showcased its role in both promoting renal pathopoiesis and in other cases reducing renal pathopoiesis. Thus, the CX3CL1/CX3CR1 axis is now considered a double-edged sword that could provide new insights into the pathogenesis and treatment of renal diseases and disorders [67]. The role of CX3CL1 and its ligand CX3CR1 in ischemic acute renal failure in mice has been investigated. CX3CR1 inhibition may reduce macrophage infiltration in the kidney and protect against AKI [68]. Fractalkine receptor (CX3CR1) expression is increased in patients with renal tubule-interstitial inflammation, and the strongest expression is localized at vascular sites close to macrophage inflammation. Fractalkine is a strong candidate for targeting mononuclear cell infiltration induced by vascular injury [69]. Expression of this receptor is increased in the endothelium of large blood vessels, capillaries, and glomeruli in ischemic AKI, and inhibition of the fractalkine receptor protects against ischemic AKI [68]. Fractalkine receptor expression is also increased in blood vessels of cisplatin-exposed mouse kidneys. However, fractalkine inhibition did not protect against functional and histological abnormalities in cisplatin-induced AKI in mice [70].

The presence of increased neutrophils in the kidney has been described both in animal models and in biopsies from patients with AKI. These cells are the target of CXCL2 chemokines, also known as macrophage inflammatory protein (MIP)-2α [53]. Neutralization of this chemokine suppresses neutrophil infiltration in the kidney after ischemia-reperfusion injury and in lipopolysaccharide (LPS), and Shiga toxin type 2-induced inflammatory models [71, 72]. Importantly, these cells accumulate in the peritubular capillary network of the outer medulla as soon as 30 min after ischemia-reperfusion [73], and adhere to endothelial cells with the help of specific adhesion molecules (intercellular adhesion molecule-1 and P-selectin). In addition, together with platelets and red blood cells, they also cause capillary plugging, leading to vascular congestion. Neutrophils release proteases, myeloperoxidase, and cytokines, which together with the generation of reactive species can aggravate the injury and damage endothelial and epithelial cells in the outer medulla [74–77]. CXCL1/CXCL2 regulates the early phase of neutrophil recruitment in LPS-induced inflammation [72].

Because there is a reciprocal relationship between cytokines and chemokines in renal inflammation, the IL-6/sIL-6R complex has been shown to have a strong synergistic effect on the synthesis and release of MCP-1 (CCL2) in human mesangial cells [35]. MCP-1 binds to the CCR2 receptor and is encoded by the CCL2 gene. Activation of this gene acts in AKI [78]. Higher plasma CCL2 level is associated with increased AKI and risk of death after a cardiac operation. Therefore, MCP-1 could be used as a biomarker to identify high-risk patients for potential AKI prevention strategies in the setting of cardiac operations [79]. Because an inflammatory effect of CCL2 is related to renal inflammatory injury, down-regulation of CCL2 may have beneficial therapeutic potential for renal injury [80]. A recent study found that another chemokine with CC motif as CCL14 contributes to the development of persistent renal damage, maladaptive repair, and risk of non-recovery of renal function [81]. In AKI, CCL14 can be released from injured tubular epithelial cells by activation of inflammatory mediators (e.g., by stimulation of TNF-α receptor activity) [82].

Another member of the CC chemokine family, RANTES (Regulated on Activation Normal T cell Expressed and Secreted, also known as CCL5), is secreted by various tissues and has been shown to simultaneously orchestrate the recruitment of various immune cells, such as neutrophils, monocytes, and lymphocytes [83]. RANTES is one of the inflammatory mediators implicated in IRI-related diseases because of its potent chemoattractant effect, and its strong ability to recruit immune cells resulting in significant inflammatory damage. This mediator has been observed to increase in renal tubular cells, further aggravating renal injury by recruiting inflammatory cells and leading to loss of renal function after IRI [84]. Studies show that RANTES expression in renal tubular cells undergoing hypoxia is controlled at the transcriptional level by NF-κB [84].

5.2.2 Inflammasome

Inflammasomes are multiprotein complexes that serve as a platform for caspase activation to regulate cytokine maturation, inflammation, and cell death. Inflammasome activation is one of the earliest innate immune events that occur in the host response against infection, and may also promote the development of adaptive immune responses. Activation of the inflammasome can occur by tissue injury or damage by non-microbial particles; thus, the inflammasome is involved in the response to various microbial and non-microbial diseases, including various organs (lung, heart, liver, and kidneys) [85]. Activation of the canonical inflammasome involves pattern recognition receptors (PRRs) that detect PAMP or DAMP. PRRs are expressed on the cell membrane or in the cytosol of a wide variety of cells, but predominantly on leukocytes. Five families of PRRs have been described: Toll-like receptors (TLRs), nucleotide-binding oligomerization domain (NOD)-like receptors (NLRs), Rig-I-like receptors, C-type lectin receptors, and absent in melanoma-like receptors 2 (AIM2) (ALRs). Proteins of the NLR and ALR families form inflammasome. Pathogen recognition receptors play a central role in the innate immune response and inflammatory processes in the kidney, thus increasing the interest in the functions of the inflammasome in renal diseases. In experimental models of AKI, the inflammasome and the expression of its genes have been linked to the pathogenesis of this disease and also to diabetic kidney disease, through canonical and non-canonical inflammasome activation. Polymorphisms associated with the NLRP1 gene have been shown to decrease the risk of developing diabetic kidney disease in type 1 diabetics [86, 87]. In addition, the inflammasome-dependent innate immunity pathway has been identified as being associated with the pathogenesis of severe pediatric renal parenchymal infections [88].

5.2.3   Canonical Inflammasome

The canonical inflammasome consists of a group of multiprotein complexes of NLR or ALR, PRR, ASC, and caspase 1 proteins. These, in turn, regulate the activation of caspase 1, resulting in the maturation and production of the cytokine IL-1β and IL-18 described above. Activation of the canonical inflammasome depends on PRR types, which may play a physiological role after sensing microbial agents and molecular patterns associated with damage [89]. Pathogen recognition patterns do not have transmembrane domains; they are distributed in the cytosol and rely primarily on interacting proteins through a pyrin domain (PYD) and/or caspase recruitment domain (CARD) to enable their proteolytic function. NLRP1 [90], NLRP3, NLRP2, NLRC4, NLRP6, NLRP9b, pyrin13, AIM2, and IFI16 trigger the formation of caspasa-1 activators in vitro and in vivo [91–93].

5.2.4   NLRP3

NLPR3 was first described in 2002 [94], as a protein oligomer complex with a molecular weight of 700 kD. This tripartite protein consists of an amino-terminal pyrin domain (PYD), a central oligomerization and nucleotide-binding domain (NOD), known as the NACHT domain, and a C-terminal leucine-rich repeat domain [93]. The PYD domain of NLRP3 interacts with the PYD domain of ASC to initiate assembly of the inflammasome. The NOD domain has ATPase activity that is required for NLRP3 oligomerization after activation [94].

In some cells of the immune system and even in macrophages, activation of the canonical NLRP3 inflammasome pathway generally requires two steps: priming and activation [95]. The priming step is stimulated by the binding of PAMP and/or

DAMP to TLR and/or cytokine receptors, which may involve the activation of nuclear factor-κB (NF-κB). Following these events, downstream gene regulation has been observed by increasing the expression of genes and substrates associated with the inflammasome, such as proIL-1β. After priming, the activation step occurs inducing assembly of the inflammasome and activation of caspases. NLRP3 inflammasome activation can occur by interaction with bacterial and viral nucleic acids, LPS, and damage-associated molecular patterns such as ATP, uric acid and β-amyloid peptides, changes in ion flux, mitochondrial dysfunction, and production of reactive oxygen species and lysosomal damage [91, 96, 97].

Unlike typical pathogen recognition receptors that recognize defined ligands, NLRP3 and other inflammasome-forming genes may function primarily by sensing changes in cell and/or tissue homeostasis [98].

5.2.5 Non-Canonical Inflammasomes

Non-canonical inflammasome activation has been associated primarily with caspase-11, caspase-4, caspase-5, and caspase-8. Murine caspase-11, also called caspase-4, has been shown to be a critical regulatory factor in caspase-1 activation in bacterial infections. In an LPS-stimulated monocyte model, it was observed that human caspase-4/caspase-5 can regulate the release of inflammatory cytokines by binding LPS directly through CARD domains [99]. This binding induces production of IL-1β [100]. In the non-canonical pathway, inflammasomes assemble first due to the detection of PAMP or DAMP by pathogen recognition receptors, resulting in the activation of caspase-11, which in turn has two types of effects. The activation of caspase-11 directly leads to macrophage death, and also functions as a binding partner in caspase-1 activation, leading to the release of pro-IL-1β and pro-IL-18 and subsequent pyroptosis, which may indicate that caspase-11 can regulate caspase-1 activation [101, 102]. A further study also found that LPS-induced caspase-11 in mice or caspase-4 in humans can trigger gasdermin D cleavage (GSDMD) and subsequent insertion into the cell membrane, leading to pyroptosis. In addition, caspase-11-mediated response to cytoplasmic LPS activates GSDMD, which is essential for pyroptosis and IL-1β secretion [103]. Although the mechanism of GSDMD and its relationship with IL-1β remains only partially investigated, these studies have provided new insights for both canonical and non-canonical signaling pathways in inflammasome activation.

5.2.6 Inflammasomes in AKI

As described above, AKI is characterized by a rapid decline in renal function and involves an increase in metabolites such as creatinine [104]. Some of the factors that can trigger AKI are sepsis, ischemia reperfusion, chemotherapy, and contrast agents

[105–107]. AKI can also occur with exposure of the body to harmful factors such as LPS and cisplatin, which have the ability to activate innate immunity and inflammasomes [108].

A study published in 2014 showed that activation of NLRP3 inflammasomes mediated by mitochondrial reactive oxygen species (mROS) aggravates kidney injury [108]. Wen et al. demonstrated that the inflammasome (NLRP3) is activated by mitochondrial reactive oxygen species (mROS) during ischemia/reperfusion (I/R) injury through direct interactions between the inflammasome and thioredoxin-interacting protein (TXNIP). It was evidenced that activation of the inflammasome NOD-like receptor protein 3 was induced by I/R injury, peaking at day 3 after reperfusion. Consistent with this observation, deletion of NLRP3 significantly attenuated I/R-induced renal injury and markers of inflammasome activation [109].

SIRT family proteins also play a certain role in the inflammatory response. SIRT1 reduces ROS production and exerts its anti-inflammatory effect, although whether it can directly regulate inflammation remains controversial [110]. In an AKI model of sepsis, SIRT3 was shown to have a protective effect on renal mitochondrial injury by reducing ROS production and decreasing IL-1β and IL-18 release [111]. In order to look at the mechanisms underlying the effect of SIRT3 on sepsis-induced AKI, the possible involvement and modulation of autophagy by AMPK and mTOR was emphasized. AKI was induced by CLP in SIRT3 KO mice. Examination of serum and kidney tissues after treatment with selective inhibitors indicated the involvement of autophagy and modulation by AMPK and mTOR activation as seen by the protective effects of SIRT3 on kidney function and structure [112]. The use of cisplatin is often limited by the presence of AKI during chemotherapy [113]. Research shows that cisplatin can inhibit autophagy and activate NLRP3, leading to kidney injury [114]. However, SIRT3 can protect against renal injury caused by cisplatin by inducing autophagy [113]. In a rhabdomyolysis-induced AKI (RIAKI) model, activation and assembly of NLRP3 inflammasomes preceded the infiltration of renal immune cells, such as macrophages [115]. Anisodamine shows a protective role in RIAKI by inhibiting endoplasmic reticulum stress related to thioredoxin interacting protein (TXNIP)/inflammasome NLRP3 [116]. The NLRP3 inflammasome could also mediate contrast agent-induced AKI by regulating cell apoptosis; indeed, NLRP3 inhibition could reduce the rate of apoptosis and ROS production in contrast agent-induced AKI [117, 118].

The ALR family is named after its best characterized member, AIM2 (absent in melanoma 2). The release of endogenous DNA from necrotic cells is thought to be a common phenomenon in organ injury. The DNA-sensing AIM2 inflammasome has been implicated in the pathogenesis of sterile brain injury in mice [119], human autoimmune thyroiditis, glomerulonephritis related to human hepatitis B virus [120], and human and mouse systemic lupus erythematosus [121]. However, a comprehensive evaluation of AIM2 in kidney disease has not been performed. In 2018, we reported that AIM2 contributes to kidney injury in human CKD and in the UUO mouse model, finding that AIM2 is constitutively expressed in glomerular podocytes and, to a lesser extent, in TECs in healthy human kidneys. AIM2 expression was increased in tubular epithelium and infiltrating leukocytes in renal biopsy samples from patients with DKD or hypertensive nephrosclerosis compared to healthy kidney samples. In UUO mice, renal inflammasome activation was restricted to leukocytes, especially monocyte-derived macrophages. Bone marrow chimera studies revealed that myeloid cells were the predominant reservoir for IL-1β processing in the UUO model. Activation of the AIM2 inflammasome contributed to the recruitment of proinflammatory macrophages leading to kidney injury and fibrosis. In addition, multiphoton intravital microscopy showed monocyte-derived macrophages phagocytizing cellular debris, including necrotic DNA, in UUO kidneys. In this model, necrotic DNA is likely a strong DAMP for AIM2 inflammasome activation. Ongoing studies are investigating the biology of AIM2 in the glomerular compartment. To date, no non-canonical functions of AIM2 in the kidney have been described [122].

The NLRC4 inflammasome has been implicated in humans and DKD1 mice. NLRC4-deficient mice with diabetes and a high-fat diet exhibit enhanced hyperglycemia and diabetic glomerular changes compared with diabetic wild-type controls. Although the mechanisms that result in reduced blood glucose levels in NLRC4 knockout mice are unknown, it has been suggested that the canonical inflammasome and IL-1β pathways play a role [123]. Importantly, SIRT3 specifically regulates NLRC4, but not NLRP3 or AIM2 inflammasomes. SIRT3-mediated NLRC4 deacetylation increases the assembly of NLRC4 inflammasome, thereby promoting the activation of NLRC4 inflammasome and production of IL-1β [124]. NLRC4 expression is enhanced after IR injury, which is related to T-cell immunoglobulin domain and mucin domain-containing molecule-3 (Tim-3) signaling. The administration of RMT3–23, a Tim-3 neutralizing antibody, can reduce NLRC4 expression and macrophage infiltration. This suggests that Tim-3-mediated NLRC4 inflammasome activation participates in I/R-induced AKI [125]. Although studies concerning the role of NLRC4 in AKI are scarce, this finding presents a novel perspective on the potential action of NLRC4 in I/R-induced AKI.

NLRC5 is a newly identified member of the NLR family that acts as a transcriptional activator of major histocompatibility complex (MHC) class I genes [126]. In mice with I/R injury or cisplatin-induced nephrotoxicity, NLRC5 was shown to negatively regulate the expression of carcinoembryonic antigen-related cell adhesion molecule 1 (CEACAM1), which activates the ERK1/2 and AKT anti-apoptotic signaling pathways, and exacerbates kidney injury. NLRC5-induced downregulation of CEACAM1 in AKI also resulted in CD4+ T-cell activation, which was likely mediated by T-cell receptor-CD3 complex signaling [127, 128]. Findings from bone marrow chimera studies also suggest that NLRC5 expressed in renal resident cells plays an important role in tubular injury and renal dysfunction in AKI. In addition, NLRC5 is expressed in the glomeruli of DKD patients and was shown to contribute to DKD progression in mice by promoting inflammation and fibrosis in part through effects on NF-κB and TGFβ-SMAD signaling pathways in mesangial cells and macrophages [129].

5.3   Complement-Related Factors in AKI

The complement system is one of the essential components of the immune system. It consists of more than 40 intracellular proteins, which can be either associated with the membrane or circulating in the blood. While activated, the complement system can exert its function in serum, tissues, locally, or intracellularly. It performs three very important physiological functions: defending the host against infection, being an essential factor in innate and adaptive immunity, and being involved in the elimination of apoptotic/necrotic, ischemic, or damaged cells [130]. Complement activation can occur through three different pathways: the classical pathway (CP), the lectin pathway (LP), and the alternative pathway (AP). Each pathway generates protein complexes that can cleave the C3 protein, which is generally considered to be the central protein of the complement cascade. Many studies, such as clinical and pre-clinical models, demonstrate that complement activation contributes to the pathogenesis of AKI by generating multiple proinflammatory fragments [131, 132]. Furthermore, complement activation within the injured kidney is a proximal trigger of many downstream inflammatory events within the renal parenchyma that exacerbate injury to the kidney. Complement activation may also account for the systemic inflammatory events that contribute to remote organ injury and patient mortality [131]. Complement activation in AKI occurs mainly through the CP, which plays an important role in the pathophysiology of the disease, as well as through the LP and AP [131–133]. Complement C1q is the initiator of CP and induces leukocyte infiltration by secretion of cytokines and chemokines, leading to inflammation of the vascular wall. C1q can induce the production of reactive oxygen species (ROS) and activation of the complement system, and can cause renal vascular endothelial cell dysfunction and renal medullary ischemia and hypoxia, thus demonstrating its role in the incidence of renal injury [134].

In addition, there is increased generation of C3 and its fragments in renal cells by activation of the CP and AP. Single nucleotide RNA sequencing studies in renal tissue from mice with unilateral ureteral obstruction show that increased synthesis of complement C3 and C5 occurs mainly in renal tubular epithelial cells (proximal and distal). In contrast, increased expression of complement receptors C3ar1 and C5ar1 occurs in interstitial cells, including immune cells, such as monocytes/macrophages, suggesting compartmentalization of complement components during renal injury [133]. Biopsies of human kidneys with histologic evidence of acute tubular necrosis (ATN) also demonstrated C3 deposits along the tubular basement membrane [135]. Similar to what is seen in rodents, patchy tubule-interstitial C3 was seen in histologically normal kidneys, but the extent of deposition was increased in kidneys with ATN.

In the human and mouse kidney, complement activity is regulated by soluble and cell surface complement regulatory proteins (CRPs). Some examples of CRPs are decay accelerating factor (CD55), membrane cofactor protein (CD47), complement receptor type 1 (CR1), CD59, clusterin, and factor H. These are expressed in various renal microanatomical compartments such as glomerular capillaries, peritubular capillaries, proximal tubules, collecting ducts, medullary interstitium, and glomerular cells (endothelial, epithelial, and mesangial) [136]. For example, a study with CD47-deficient mice showed normalization of d-7 creatinine scores, reduced weight loss, and increased survival, consistent with protection from initial renal parenchymal injury [137]. CD55-deficient but not CD59-deficient mice exhibited increased renal I/R injury as indicated by significantly elevated blood urea nitrogen levels, histological scores, and neutrophil infiltration. Surprisingly, although CD59 deficiency alone was inconsequential, CD55/CD59 double deficiency greatly exacerbated I/R injury. Severe I/R injury in double-deficient mice was accompanied by endothelial deposition of C3 and membrane attack complex (MAC) and medullary capillary thrombosis. Thus, CD55 and CD59 act synergistically to inhibit complement-mediated renal I/R injury, and abrogation of their function leads to MAC-induced microvascular injury and dysfunction that may exacerbate the initial ischemic insult [138]. In mice, C3aR and C5aR deficiency reduces renal production of inflammatory mediators after I/R injury, and both C3a and C5a contribute to renal I/R injury, C5a being the molecule with the more pathological role [139]. In a mouse model with glycerol-induced AKI, C5a and C5a receptor (C5aR) expressions were significantly increased, as was the expression of inflammatory cytokines, such as IL-1β, IL-6, and TNF-α. Treatment with C5aR antagonists prevented renal injury [140]. Other complement-related factors that activate complement are factor B (cfB) and and factor H, which is essential for inhibiting AP. Factor B is significantly upregulated in the kidney and may contribute to acute tubular injury in an animal model of sepsis, mediated by TLR3/4 through the NF-κB pathway [141, 142]. FH-deficient mice have diffused glomerular capillary wall C3 staining; yet, they completely lack "normal" tubular C3 staining. Within minutes after being transplanted into a wild-type host (following cold ischemia of 45–60 min), kidneys from FH-deficient mice begin to generate C3 around tubules [143].

Importantly, complement inhibitor drugs have been used successfully in small and large animal models of ischemia-reperfusion injury and may represent new notable therapeutic approaches [144, 145] for patients with or at high risk of developing AKI. New advances have been shown with the use of eculizumab, a C5 fragment inhibitor, and C1INH, a recombinant C1 fraction inhibitor. They exert a protective effect in kidney disease and ischemia reperfusion injury and have been shown by the use of eculizumab. The action mechanism of eculizumab relies on the prevention of cleavage and formation of C5a and C1INH on the prevention of activation of the classical and lectin pathway complement activation [146, 147]. In addition, treatment with an inhibitory monoclonal antibody against mouse factor B, a necessary element of the alternative pathway, inhibits complement activation in the kidney after ischemia-reperfusion and protects mice from necrotic and apoptotic tubular injury [148]. Monoclonal anti-factor B and anti-properdin antibodies selectively block the alternative pathway, thereby preventing the pathological effects of this complement pathway in AKI while leaving the other complement pathways intact [149]. Crry inhibitor, a complement regulatory protein, is expressed in proximal renal tubules on the basolateral membrane, and a loss of Crry polarity in the tubular epithelium results in activation of the alternative pathway on the basolateral side of tubular cells. Mice with low levels of this protein are more susceptible to ischemia, which explains the protective function of Crry expression [150]. Importantly, the effects of these inhibitors in patients during acute episodes of the disease and during the peri-transplant period will be useful in identifying their effects on the course of AKI.

In conclusion, cytokines, chemokines, inflammasomes, myokines, and complement-related factors are essential elements in organic crosstalk.

References

1. Radi ZA. Immunopathogenesis of acute kidney injury. Toxicol Pathol. 2018;46(8):930–43.
2. Akcay A, Nguyen Q, Edelstein CL. Mediators of inflammation in acute kidney injury. Mediat Inflamm. 2009;2009:1–12.
3. Ortega L. Role of cytokines in the pathogenesis of acute and chronic kidney disease, glomerulonephritis, and end-stage kidney disease. Int J Interferon Cytokine Mediat Res. 2010;2:49–62.
4. Scheer JM. Chapter 505 - Caspase-1. In: Rawlings ND, Salvesen G, editors. Handbook of proteolytic enzymes. 3rd ed. San Diego, CA: Academic Press; 2013. p. 2237–43. https://www.sciencedirect.com/science/article/pii/B9780123822192005032.
5. Hirooka Y, Nozaki Y. Interleukin-18 in inflammatory kidney disease. Front Med. 2021;8:639103.
6. Lin TY, Hsu YH. IL-20 in acute kidney injury: role in pathogenesis and potential as a therapeutic target. Int J Mol Sci. 2020;21(3):1009. https://doi.org/10.3390/ijms21031009.
7. Kadiroglu AK, Sit D, Atay AE, Kayabasi H, Altintas A, Yilmaz ME. The evaluation of effects of demographic features, biochemical parameters, and cytokines on clinical outcomes in patients with acute renal failure. Ren Fail. 2007;29(4):503–8.
8. Al-Lamki RS, Mayadas TN. TNF receptors: signaling pathways and contribution to renal dysfunction. Kidney Int. 2015;87(2):281–96.
9. Sabio G, Davis RJ. TNF and MAP kinase signalling pathways. Semin Immunol. 2014;26(3):237–45.
10. Gupta J, Mitra N, Kanetsky PA, Devaney J, Wing MR, Reilly M, et al. Association between albuminuria, kidney function, and inflammatory biomarker profile in CKD in CRIC. Clin J Am Soc Nephrol. 2012;7(12):1938–46.
11. Peralta Soler A, Mullin JM, Knudsen KA, Marano CW. Tissue remodeling during tumor necrosis factor-induced apoptosis in LLC-PK1 renal epithelial cells. Am J Phys. 1996;270(5 Pt 2):F869–79.
12. Guo YL, Baysal K, Kang B, Yang LJ, Williamson JR. Correlation between sustained c-Jun N-terminal protein kinase activation and apoptosis induced by tumor necrosis factor-alpha in rat mesangial cells. J Biol Chem. 1998;273(7):4027–34.
13. Meldrum KK, Meldrum DR, Hile KL, Yerkes EB, Ayala A, Cain MP, et al. p38 MAPK mediates renal tubular cell TNF-alpha production and TNF-alpha-dependent apoptosis during simulated ischemia. Am J Physiol Cell Physiol. 2001;281(2):C563–70.
14. Ramseyer VD. Tumor necrosis factor-α: regulation of renal function and blood pressure. Am J Physiol Ren Physiol. 2013;304(10):F1231–42.
15. Xu C, Chang A, Hack BK, Eadon MT, Alper SL, Cunningham PN. TNF-mediated damage to glomerular endothelium is an important determinant of acute kidney injury in sepsis. Kidney Int. 2014;85(1):72–81.
16. Jaber B. Cytokine gene promoter polymorphisms and mortality in acute renal failure. Cytokine. 2004;25(5):212–9.

17. Susantitaphong P, Perianayagam MC, Tighiouart H, Liangos O, Bonventre JV, Jaber BL. Tumor necrosis factor alpha promoter polymorphism and severity of acute kidney injury. Nephron Clin Pract. 2013;123(1–2):67–73.
18. Cantero-Navarro E, Rayego-Mateos S, Orejudo M, Tejedor-Santamaria L, Tejera-Muñoz A, Sanz AB, et al. Role of macrophages and related cytokines in kidney disease. Front Med. 2021;8:688060.
19. Han HI, Skvarca LB, Espiritu EB, Davidson AJ, Hukriede NA. The role of macrophages during acute kidney injury: destruction and repair. Pediatr Nephrol. 2019;34(4):561–9.
20. Kitching AR, Holdsworth SR, Tipping PG. IFN-gamma mediates crescent formation and cell-mediated immune injury in murine glomerulonephritis. J Am Soc Nephrol. 1999;10(4):752–9.
21. Takei Y, Sims TN, Urmson J, Halloran PF. Central role for interferon-gamma receptor in the regulation of renal MHC expression. J Am Soc Nephrol. 2000;11(2):250–61.
22. Kassianos AJ, Wang X, Sampangi S, Afrin S, Wilkinson R, Healy H. Fractalkine-CX3CR1-dependent recruitment and retention of human CD1c+ myeloid dendritic cells by in vitro-activated proximal tubular epithelial cells. Kidney Int. 2015;87(6):1153–63.
23. Law BMP, Wilkinson R, Wang X, Kildey K, Lindner M, Rist MJ, et al. Interferon-γ production by tubulointerstitial human CD56bright natural killer cells contributes to renal fibrosis and chronic kidney disease progression. Kidney Int. 2017;92(1):79–88.
24. Gewin LS. Transforming growth factor-β in the acute kidney injury to chronic kidney disease transition. Nephron. 2019;143(3):154–7.
25. Chung S, Overstreet JM, Li Y, Wang Y, Niu A, Wang S, et al. TGF-β promotes fibrosis after severe acute kidney injury by enhancing renal macrophage infiltration. JCI Insight. 2018;3(21):e123563.
26. Otto G. IL-1β switches on kidney fibrosis. Nat Rev Nephrol. 2018;14(8):475.
27. Bonnemaison ML, Marks ES, Boesen EI. Interleukin-1β as a driver of renal NGAL production. Cytokine. 2017;91:38–43.
28. Konno T, Nakano R, Mamiya R, Tsuchiya H, Kitanaka T, Namba S, et al. Expression and function of interleukin-1β-induced neutrophil gelatinase-associated Lipocalin in renal tubular cells. PLoS One. 2016;11(11):e0166707.
29. Dellepiane S, Leventhal JS, Cravedi P. T cells and acute kidney injury: a two-way relationship. Front Immunol. 2020;11:1546. https://doi.org/10.3389/fimmu.2020.01546.
30. Moledina DG, Mansour SG, Jia Y, Obeid W, Thiessen-Philbrook H, Koyner JL, et al. Association of T cell–derived inflammatory cytokines with acute kidney injury and mortality after cardiac surgery. Kidney Int Rep. 2019;4(12):1689–97.
31. Medeiros T, Guimarães GMC, Carvalho FR, Alves LS, Faustino R, Campi-Azevedo AC, et al. Acute kidney injury associated to COVID-19 leads to a strong unbalance of circulant immune mediators. Cytokine. 2022;157:155974.
32. Zhang WR, Garg AX, Coca SG, Devereaux PJ, Eikelboom J, Kavsak P, et al. Plasma IL-6 and IL-10 concentrations predict AKI and long-term mortality in adults after cardiac surgery. J Am Soc Nephrol. 2015;26(12):3123–32.
33. Shimazui T, Nakada T, Tateishi Y, Oshima T, Aizimu T, Oda S. Association between serum levels of interleukin-6 on ICU admission and subsequent outcomes in critically ill patients with acute kidney injury. BMC Nephrol. 2019;20(1):74. https://doi.org/10.1186/s12882-019-1265-6.
34. Ruef C, Budde K, Lacy J, Northemann W, Baumann M, Sterzel RB, et al. Interleukin 6 is an autocrine growth factor for mesangial cells. Kidney Int. 1990;38(2):249–57.
35. Coletta I, Soldo L, Polentarutti N, Mancini F, Guglielmotti A, Pinza M, et al. Selective induction of MCP-1 in human mesangial cells by the IL-6/sIL-6R complex. Exp Nephrol. 2000;8(1):37–43.
36. Kim DI, Park SH. Sequential signaling cascade of IL-6 and PGC-1α is involved in high glucose-induced podocyte loss and growth arrest. Biochem Biophys Res Commun. 2013;435(4):702–7.

37. Nechemia-Arbely Y, Barkan D, Pizov G, Shriki A, Rose-John S, Galun E, et al. IL-6/IL-6R axis plays a critical role in acute kidney injury. J Am Soc Nephrol. 2008;19(6):1106–15.

38. Skrypnyk NI, Gist KM, Okamura K, Montford JR, You Z, Yang H, et al. IL-6-mediated hepatocyte production is the primary source of plasma and urine neutrophil gelatinase–associated lipocalin during acute kidney injury. Kidney Int. 2020;97(5):966–79.

39. Dennen P, Altmann C, Kaufman J, Klein CL, Andres-Hernando A, Ahuja NH, et al. Urine interleukin-6 is an early biomarker of acute kidney injury in children undergoing cardiac surgery. Crit Care. 2010;14(5):R181.

40. Edelstein CL. Biomarkers of acute kidney injury. Adv Chronic Kidney Dis. 2008;15(3):222–34.

41. Melnikov VY, Ecder T, Fantuzzi G, Siegmund B, Lucia MS, Dinarello CA, et al. Impaired IL-18 processing protects caspase-1-deficient mice from ischemic acute renal failure. J Clin Invest. 2001;107(9):1145–52.

42. Faubel S, Lewis EC, Reznikov L, Ljubanovic D, Hoke TS, Somerset H, et al. Cisplatin-induced acute renal failure is associated with an increase in the cytokines interleukin (IL)-1beta, IL-18, IL-6, and neutrophil infiltration in the kidney. J Pharmacol Exp Ther. 2007;322(1):8–15.

43. Wegenka UM. IL-20: biological functions mediated through two types of receptor complexes. Cytokine Growth Factor Rev. 2010;21(5):353–63.

44. Li HH, Hsu YH, Wei CC, Lee PT, Chen WC, Chang MS. Interleukin-20 induced cell death in renal epithelial cells and was associated with acute renal failure. Genes Immun. 2008;9(5):395–404.

45. Chang MS, Hsu YH. The role of IL-20 in chronic kidney disease and diabetic nephropathy: pathogenic and therapeutic implications. J Leukoc Biol. 2018;104(5):919–23.

46. Lee SA, Noel S, Sadasivam M, Hamad ARA, Rabb H. Role of immune cells in acute kidney injury and repair. Nephron. 2017;137(4):282–6.

47. Wang Y, Chang J, Yao B, Niu A, Kelly E, Breeggemann MC, et al. Proximal tubule-derived colony stimulating factor-1 mediates polarization of renal macrophages and dendritic cells, and recovery in acute kidney injury. Kidney Int. 2015;88(6):1274–82.

48. Zhang MZ, Yao B, Yang S, Jiang L, Wang S, Fan X, et al. CSF-1 signaling mediates recovery from acute kidney injury. J Clin Invest. 2012;122(12):4519–32.

49. Jung M, Sola A, Hughes J, Kluth DC, Vinuesa E, Viñas JL, et al. Infusion of IL-10-expressing cells protects against renal ischemia through induction of lipocalin-2. Kidney Int. 2012;81(10):969–82.

50. Zhang MZ, Wang X, Wang Y, Niu A, Wang S, Zou C, et al. IL-4/IL-13-mediated polarization of renal macrophages/dendritic cells to an M2a phenotype is essential for recovery from acute kidney injury. Kidney Int. 2017;91(2):375–86.

51. Mylonas KJ, Anderson J, Sheldrake TA, Hesketh EE, Richards JA, Ferenbach DA, et al. Granulocyte macrophage-colony stimulating factor: a key modulator of renal mononuclear phagocyte plasticity. Immunobiology. 2019;224(1):60–74.

52. Chung ACK, Lan HY. Chemokines in renal injury. J Am Soc Nephrol. 2011;22(5):802–9.

53. Furuichi K, Kaneko S, Wada T. Chemokine/chemokine receptor-mediated inflammation regulates pathologic changes from acute kidney injury to chronic kidney disease. Clin Exp Nephrol. 2009;13(1):9–14.

54. Holdsworth SR, Tipping PG. Leukocytes in glomerular injury. Semin Immunopathol. 2007;29(4):355–74.

55. Gao J, Wu L, Wang S, Chen X. Role of chemokine (C–X–C motif) ligand 10 (CXCL10) in renal diseases. Mediat Inflamm. 2020;2020:e6194864.

56. Segerer S, Nelson PJ, Schlöndorff D. Chemokines, chemokine receptors, and renal disease: from basic science to pathophysiologic and therapeutic studies. J Am Soc Nephrol. 2000;11(1):152–76.

57. Thurman JM, Lenderink AM, Royer PA, Coleman KE, Zhou J, Lambris JD, et al. C3a is required for the production of CXC chemokines by tubular epithelial cells after renal Ishemia/reperfusion. J Immunol. 2007;178(3):1819–28.

58. Zhou Y, Xu W, Zhu H. CXCL8(3–72) K11R/G31P protects against sepsis-induced acute kidney injury via NF-κB and JAK2/STAT3 pathway. Biol Res. 2019;52:29. https://doi.org/10.1186/s40659-019-0236-5.
59. Yu C, Qi D, Sun JF, Li P, Fan HY. Rhein prevents endotoxin-induced acute kidney injury by inhibiting NF-κB activities. Sci Rep. 2015;5:11822.
60. Liu P, Li X, Lv W, Xu Z. Inhibition of CXCL1-CXCR2 axis ameliorates cisplatin-induced acute kidney injury by mediating inflammatory response. Biomed Pharmacother. 2020;122:109693.
61. Liang H, Zhang Z, He L, Wang Y. CXCL16 regulates cisplatin-induced acute kidney injury. Oncotarget. 2016;7(22):31652–62.
62. Chen G, Lin SC, Chen J, He L, Dong F, Xu J, et al. CXCL16 recruits bone marrow-derived fibroblast precursors in renal fibrosis. J Am Soc Nephrol. 2011;22(10):1876–86.
63. Xia Y, Entman ML, Wang Y. Critical role of CXCL16 in hypertensive kidney injury and fibrosis. Hypertens Dallas Tex 1979. 2013;62(6):1129–37.
64. Erez DL, Denburg MR, Afolayan S, Jodele S, Wallace G, Davies SM, et al. Acute kidney injury in children after hematopoietic cell transplantation is associated with elevated urine CXCL10 and CXCL9. Biol Blood Marrow Transplant J Am Soc Blood Marrow Transplant. 2020;26(7):1266–72.
65. Erez DL, Sullivan KE, Denburg M, Bunin NJ, Jodele S, Afolayan S, et al. Urinary CXCL10 and CXCL9 are associated with acute kidney injury in children after hematopoietic stem cell transplantation: results of a discovery and validation cohort. Biol Blood Marrow Transplant. 2019;25(3, Supplement):S185–6.
66. Aouad Y, Pizarro MS, Fernández-Fernández B, Ramos AM, Ortiz A. Inflamación renal en el trasplante: ¿existen biomarcadores? Nefrol Engl Ed. 2016;7:14–21.
67. Zhuang Q, Cheng K, Ming Y. CX3CL1/CX3CR1 Axis, as the therapeutic potential in renal diseases: friend or foe? Curr Gene Ther. 2017;17(6):442–52.
68. Oh DJ, Dursun B, He Z, Lu L, Hoke TS, Ljubanovic D, et al. Fractalkine receptor (CX3CR1) inhibition is protective against ischemic acute renal failure in mice. Am J Physiol-Ren Physiol. 2008;294(1):F264–71.
69. Cockwell P, Chakravorty SJ, Girdlestone J, Savage COS. Fractalkine expression in human renal inflammation. J Pathol. 2002;196(1):85–90.
70. Lu LH, Oh DJ, Dursun B, He Z, Hoke TS, Faubel S, et al. Increased macrophage infiltration and fractalkine expression in cisplatin-induced acute renal failure in mice. J Pharmacol Exp Ther. 2008;324(1):111–7.
71. Roche JK, Keepers TR, Gross LK, Seaner RM, Obrig TG. CXCL1/KC and CXCL2/MIP-2 are critical effectors and potential targets for therapy of Escherichia coli O157:H7-associated renal inflammation. Am J Pathol. 2007;170(2):526–37.
72. De Filippo K, Dudeck A, Hasenberg M, Nye E, van Rooijen N, Hartmann K, et al. Mast cell and macrophage chemokines CXCL1/CXCL2 control the early stage of neutrophil recruitment during tissue inflammation. Blood. 2013;121(24):4930–7.
73. Li L, Huang L, Sung SSJ, Vergis AL, Rosin DL, Rose CE, et al. The chemokine receptors CCR2 and CX3CR1 mediate monocyte/macrophage trafficking in kidney ischemia–reperfusion injury. Kidney Int. 2008;74(12):1526–37.
74. Okusa MD, Linden J, Huang L, Rieger JM, Macdonald TL, Huynh LP. A2A adenosine receptor-mediated inhibition of renal injury and neutrophil adhesion. Am J Physiol-Ren Physiol. 2000;279(5):F809–18.
75. Li L, Okusa MD. Blocking the immune response in ischemic acute kidney injury: the role of adenosine 2A agonists. Nat Clin Pract Nephrol. 2006;2(8):432–44.
76. Jang HR, Rabb H. The innate immune response in ischemic acute kidney injury. Clin Immunol. 2009;130(1):41–50.
77. Bolisetty S, Agarwal A. Neutrophils in acute kidney injury: not neutral any more. Kidney Int. 2009;75(7):674–6.

78. Munshi R, Johnson A, Siew ED, Ikizler TA, Ware LB, Wurfel MM, et al. MCP-1 gene activation marks acute kidney injury. J Am Soc Nephrol. 2011;22(1):165–75.
79. Moledina DG, Isguven S, McArthur E, Thiessen-Philbrook H, Garg AX, Shlipak M, et al. Plasma monocyte chemotactic protein-1 is associated with acute kidney injury and death after cardiac operations. Ann Thorac Surg. 2017;104(2):613–20.
80. Jung YJ, Lee AS, Nguyen-Thanh T, Kim D, Kang KP, Lee S, et al. SIRT2 regulates LPS-induced renal tubular CXCL2 and CCL2 expression. J Am Soc Nephrol. 2015;26(7):1549–60.
81. Hoste E, Bihorac A, Al-Khafaji A, Ortega LM, Ostermann M, Haase M, et al. Identification and validation of biomarkers of persistent acute kidney injury: the RUBY study. Intensive Care Med. 2020;46(5):943–53.
82. Bagshaw SM, Al-Khafaji A, Artigas A, Davison D, Haase M, Lissauer M, et al. External validation of urinary C-C motif chemokine ligand 14 (CCL14) for prediction of persistent acute kidney injury. Crit Care. 2021;25(1):185. https://doi.org/10.1186/s13054-021-03618-1.
83. Charo IF, Ransohoff RM. The many roles of chemokines and chemokine receptors in inflammation. N Engl J Med. 2006;354(6):610–21.
84. Yu TM, Palanisamy K, Sun KT, Day YJ, Shu KH, Wang IK, et al. RANTES mediates kidney ischemia reperfusion injury through a possible role of HIF-1α and LncRNA PRINS. Sci Rep. 2016;6:18424.
85. Lamkanfi M, Dixit VM. Mechanisms and functions of inflammasomes. Cell. 2014;157(5):1013–22.
86. Shahzad K, Bock F, Dong W, Wang H, Kopf S, Kohli S, et al. Nlrp3-inflammasome activation in non-myeloid-derived cells aggravates diabetic nephropathy. Kidney Int. 2015;87(1):74–84.
87. Soares JLS, Fernandes FP, Patente TA, Monteiro MB, Parisi MC, Giannella-Neto D, et al. Gain-of-function variants in NLRP1 protect against the development of diabetic kidney disease: NLRP1 inflammasome role in metabolic stress sensing? Clin Immunol. 2018;187:46–9.
88. Cheng CH, Lee YS, Chang CJ, Lin JC, Lin TY. Genetic polymorphisms in inflammasome-dependent innate immunity among pediatric patients with severe renal parenchymal infections. PLoS One. 2015;10(10):e0140128.
89. Rathinam VAK, Chan FKM. Inflammasome, inflammation, and tissue homeostasis. Trends Mol Med. 2018;24(3):304–18.
90. Martinon F, Burns K. The inflammasome: a molecular platform triggering activation of inflammatory caspases and processing of proIL-β. Mol Cell. 2002;10(2):417–26. https://doi.org/10.1016/s1097-2765(02)00599-3.
91. Sharma D, Kanneganti TD. The cell biology of inflammasomes: mechanisms of inflammasome activation and regulation. J Cell Biol. 2016;213(6):617–29.
92. Mulay SR. Multifactorial functions of the inflammasome component NLRP3 in pathogenesis of chronic kidney diseases. Kidney Int. 2019;96(1):58–66.
93. Franchi L, Warner N, Viani K, Nuñez G. Function of nod-like receptors in microbial recognition and host defense. Immunol Rev. 2009;227(1):106–28.
94. Vajjhala PR, Mirams RE, Hill JM. Multiple binding sites on the pyrin domain of ASC protein allow self-association and interaction with NLRP3 protein. J Biol Chem. 2012;287(50):41732–43.
95. Rathinam VAK, Vanaja SK, Fitzgerald KA. Regulation of inflammasome signaling. Nat Immunol. 2012;13(4):333–2.
96. He Y, Hara H, Núñez G. Mechanism and regulation of NLRP3 inflammasome activation. Trends Biochem Sci. 2016;41(12):1012–21.
97. Hoseini Z, Sepahvand F, Rashidi B, Sahebkar A, Masoudifar A, Mirzaei H. NLRP3 inflammasome: its regulation and involvement in atherosclerosis. J Cell Physiol. 2018;233(3):2116–32.
98. Vilaysane A, Chun J, Seamone ME, Wang W, Chin R, Hirota S, et al. The NLRP3 inflammasome promotes renal inflammation and contributes to CKD. J Am Soc Nephrol. 2010;21(10):1732–44.

99. Viganò E, Diamond CE, Spreafico R, Balachander A, Sobota RM, Mortellaro A. Human caspase-4 and caspase-5 regulate the one-step non-canonical inflammasome activation in monocytes. Nat Commun. 2015;6:8761.
100. Non-canonical activation of inflammatory caspases by cytosolic LPS in innate immunity | Elsevier Enhanced Reader [Internet]. 3 August 2022. https://reader.elsevier.com/reader/sd/pii/S0952791515000084?token=035A6ADC7E38FCB083AFC98725556A361E0AFB01FB4D10FDE704B75679FE63D84C9533A3A8E5E63579008BF679651D39&originRegion=us-east-1&originCreation=20220803121837
101. Kayagaki N, Warming S, Lamkanfi M, Walle LV, Louie S, Dong J, et al. Non-canonical inflammasome activation targets caspase-11. Nature. 2011;479(7371):117–21.
102. Broz P, Ruby T, Belhocine K, Bouley DM, Kayagaki N, Dixit VM, et al. Caspase-11 increases susceptibility to salmonella infection in the absence of caspase-1. Nature. 2012;490(7419):288–91.
103. Shi J, Zhao Y, Wang K, Shi X, Wang Y, Huang H, et al. Cleavage of GSDMD by inflammatory caspases determines pyroptotic cell death. Nature. 2015;526(7575):660–5.
104. Levey AS, James MT. Acute kidney injury. Ann Intern Med. 2017;167(9):ITC66–80.
105. Gómez H, Kellum JA. Sepsis-induced acute kidney injury. Curr Opin Crit Care. 2016;22(6):546–53.
106. Yang K, Li WF, Yu JF, Yi C, Huang WF. Diosmetin protects against ischemia/reperfusion-induced acute kidney injury in mice. J Surg Res. 2017;214:69–78.
107. Fähling M, Seeliger E, Patzak A, Persson PB. Understanding and preventing contrast-induced acute kidney injury. Nat Rev Nephrol. 2017;13(3):169–80.
108. Leemans JC, Kors L, Anders HJ, Florquin S. Pattern recognition receptors and the inflammasome in kidney disease. Nat Rev Nephrol. 2014;10(7):398–414.
109. Liu D, Xu M, Ding LH, Lv LL, Liu H, Ma KL, et al. Activation of the Nlrp3 inflammasome by mitochondrial reactive oxygen species: a novel mechanism of albumin-induced tubulointerstitial inflammation. Int J Biochem Cell Biol. 2014;57:7–19.
110. Wen Y, Liu YR, Tang TT, Pan MM, Xu SC, Ma KL, et al. mROS-TXNIP axis activates NLRP3 inflammasome to mediate renal injury during ischemic AKI. Int J Biochem Cell Biol. 2018;98:43–53.
111. Yeung F, Hoberg JE, Ramsey CS, Keller MD, Jones DR, Frye RA, et al. Modulation of NF-kappaB-dependent transcription and cell survival by the SIRT1 deacetylase. EMBO J. 2004;23(12):2369–80.
112. Zhao W, Zhang L, Sui M, Zhu Y, Zeng L. Protective effects of sirtuin 3 in a murine model of sepsis-induced acute kidney injury. Sci Rep. 2016;6(1):33201. https://www.scinapse.io
113. Zhao W, Zhang L, Chen R, Lu H, Sui M, Zhu Y, et al. SIRT3 protects against acute kidney injury via AMPK/mTOR-regulated autophagy. Front Physiol. 2018;9:1526.
114. Huang TH, Wu TH, Guo YH, Li TL, Chan YL, Wu CJ. The concurrent treatment of Scutellaria baicalensis Georgi enhances the therapeutic efficacy of cisplatin but also attenuates chemotherapy-induced cachexia and acute kidney injury. J Ethnopharmacol. 2019;243:112075.
115. Qu X, Gao H, Tao L, Zhang Y, Zhai J, Song Y, et al. Autophagy inhibition-enhanced assembly of the NLRP3 inflammasome is associated with cisplatin-induced acute injury to the liver and kidneys in rats. J Biochem Mol Toxicol. 2018;33:e22208.
116. Komada T, Usui F, Kawashima A, Kimura H, Karasawa T, Inoue Y, et al. Role of NLRP3 inflammasomes for rhabdomyolysis-induced acute kidney injury. Sci Rep. 2015;5(1):10901.
117. Shen J, Wang L, Jiang N, Mou S, Zhang M, Gu L, et al. NLRP3 inflammasome mediates contrast media-induced acute kidney injury by regulating cell apoptosis. Sci Rep. 2016;6(1):34682.
118. Tan X, Zheng X, Huang Z, Lin J, Xie C, Lin Y. Involvement of S100A8/A9-TLR4-NLRP3 inflammasome pathway in contrast-induced acute kidney injury. Cell Physiol Biochem Int J Exp Cell Physiol Biochem Pharmacol. 2017;43(1):209–22.

119. Denes A, Coutts G, Lénárt N, Cruickshank SM, Pelegrin P, Skinner J, et al. AIM2 and NLRC4 inflammasomes contribute with ASC to acute brain injury independently of NLRP3. Proc Natl Acad Sci U S A. 2015;112(13):4050–5.

120. Zhen J, Zhang L, Pan J, Ma S, Yu X, Li X, et al. AIM2 mediates inflammation-associated renal damage in hepatitis B virus-associated glomerulonephritis by regulating caspase-1, IL-1β, and IL-18. Mediat Inflamm. 2014;2014:190860. https://doi.org/10.1155/2014/190860.

121. Zhang W, Cai Y, Xu W, Yin Z, Gao X, Xiong S. AIM2 facilitates the apoptotic DNA-induced systemic lupus erythematosus via arbitrating macrophage functional maturation. J Clin Immunol. 2013;33(5):925–37.

122. Komada T, Chung H, Lau A, Platnich JM, Beck PL, Benediktsson H, et al. Macrophage uptake of necrotic cell DNA activates the AIM2 inflammasome to regulate a proinflammatory phenotype in CKD. J Am Soc Nephrol. 2018;29(4):1165–81.

123. Yuan F, Kolb R, Pandey G, Li W, Sun L, Liu F, et al. Involvement of the NLRC4-Inflammasome in diabetic nephropathy. PLoS One. 2016;11(10):e0164135.

124. Guan C, Huang X, Yue J, Xiang H, Shaheen S, Jiang Z, et al. SIRT3-mediated deacetylation of NLRC4 promotes inflammasome activation. Theranostics. 2021;11(8):3981–95.

125. Guo Y, Zhang J, Lai X, Chen M, Guo Y. Tim-3 exacerbates kidney ischaemia/reperfusion injury through the TLR-4/NF-κB signalling pathway and an NLR-C4 inflammasome activation. Clin Exp Immunol. 2018;193(1):113–29.

126. Meissner TB, Li A, Biswas A, Lee KH, Liu YJ, Bayir E, et al. NLR family member NLRC5 is a transcriptional regulator of MHC class I genes. Proc Natl Acad Sci. 2010;107(31):13794–9.

127. Li Q, Wang Z, Zhang Y, Zhu J, Li L, Wang X, et al. NLRC5 deficiency protects against acute kidney injury in mice by mediating carcinoembryonic antigen–related cell adhesion molecule 1 signaling. Kidney Int. 2018;94(3):551–66.

128. Nagaishi T, Pao L, Lin SH, Iijima H, Kaser A, Qiao SW, et al. SHP1 phosphatase-dependent T cell inhibition by CEACAM1 adhesion molecule isoforms. Immunity. 2006;25(5):769–81.

129. Luan P, Zhuang J, Zou J, Li H, Shuai P, Xu X, et al. NLRC5 deficiency ameliorates diabetic nephropathy through alleviating inflammation. FASEB J. 2018;32(2):1070–84.

130. Martin M, Blom AM. Complement in removal of the dead - balancing inflammation. Immunol Rev. 2016;274(1):218–32.

131. McCullough JW, Renner B, Thurman JM. The role of the complement system in acute kidney injury. Semin Nephrol. 2013;33(6):543–56. https://doi.org/10.1016/j.semnephrol.2013.08.005.

132. Franzin R, Stasi A, Fiorentino M, Stallone G, Cantaluppi V, Gesualdo L, et al. Inflammaging and complement system: a link between acute kidney injury and chronic graft damage. Front Immunol. 2020;11:734.

133. Portilla D, Xavier S. Role of intracellular complement activation in kidney fibrosis. Br J Pharmacol. 2021;178(14):2880–91.

134. Skoglund C, Wetterö J, Bengtsson T. C1q regulates collagen-dependent production of reactive oxygen species, aggregation and levels of soluble P-selectin in whole blood. Immunol Lett. 2012;142(1):28–33.

135. Thurman JM, Lucia MS, Ljubanovic D, Holers VM. Acute tubular necrosis is characterized by activation of the alternative pathway of complement. Kidney Int. 2005;67(2):524–30.

136. Brar JE, Quigg RJ. Complement activation in the tubulointerstitium: AKI, CKD, and in between. Kidney Int. 2014;86(4):663–6.

137. El-Rashid M, Ghimire K, Sanganeria B, Lu B, Rogers NM. CD47 limits autophagy to promote acute kidney injury. FASEB J. 2019;33(11):12735–49. https://doi.org/10.1096/fj.201900120RR.

138. Yamada K, Miwa T, Liu J, Nangaku M, Song WC. Critical protection from renal ischemia reperfusion injury by CD55 and CD59. J Immunol. 2004;172(6):3869–75.

139. Peng Q, Li K, Smyth LA, Xing G, Wang N, Meader L, et al. C3a and C5a promote renal ischemia-reperfusion injury. J Am Soc Nephrol. 2012;23(9):1474–85.

140. Zhang Z. Association of C5a/C5aR pathway to activate ERK1/2 and p38 MAPK in acute kidney injury – a mouse model. Rev Romana Med Lab. 2022;30:31–40.
141. Li D, Zou L, Feng Y, Xu G, Gong Y, Zhao G, et al. Complement factor B production in renal tubular cells and its role in sodium transporter expression during polymicrobial sepsis. Crit Care Med. 2016;44(5):e289–99.
142. Zou L, Feng Y, Li Y, Zhang M, Chen C, Cai J, et al. Complement factor B is the downstream effector of TLRs and plays an important role in a mouse model of severe sepsis. J Immunol. 2013;191(11):5625–35.
143. Alexander JJ, Wang Y, Chang A, Jacob A, Minto AWM, Karmegam M, et al. Mouse podocyte complement factor H: the functional analog to human complement receptor 1. J Am Soc Nephrol. 2007;18(4):1157–66.
144. Castellano G, Melchiorre R, Loverre A, Ditonno P, Montinaro V, Rossini M, et al. Therapeutic targeting of classical and lectin pathways of complement protects from ischemia-reperfusion-induced renal damage. Am J Pathol. 2010;176(4):1648–59.
145. Lu F, Chauhan AK, Fernandes SM, Walsh MT, Wagner DD, Davis AE. The effect of C1 inhibitor on intestinal ischemia and reperfusion injury. Am J Physiol Gastrointest Liver Physiol. 2008;295(5):G1042–9.
146. Danobeitia JS, Ziemelis M, Ma X, Zitur LJ, Zens T, Chlebeck PJ, et al. Complement inhibition attenuates acute kidney injury after ischemia-reperfusion and limits progression to renal fibrosis in mice. PLoS One. 2017;12(8):e0183701.
147. Barnett ANR, Asgari E, Chowdhury P, Sacks SH, Dorling A, Mamode N. The use of eculizumab in renal transplantation. Clin Transpl. 2013;27(3):E216–29.
148. Thurman JM, Royer PA, Ljubanovic D, Dursun B, Lenderink AM, Edelstein CL, et al. Treatment with an inhibitory monoclonal antibody to mouse factor B protects mice from induction of apoptosis and renal ischemia/reperfusion injury. J Am Soc Nephrol. 2006;17(3):707–15.
149. Miwa T, Sato S, Gullipalli D, Nangaku M, Song WC. Blocking properdin, the alternative pathway, and anaphylatoxin receptors ameliorates renal ischemia-reperfusion injury in decay-accelerating factor and CD59 double-knockout mice. J Immunol. 2013;190(7):3552–9.
150. Thurman JM, Ljubanović D, Royer PA, Kraus DM, Molina H, Barry NP, et al. Altered renal tubular expression of the complement inhibitor Crry permits complement activation after ischemia/reperfusion. J Clin Invest. 2006;116(2):357–68.

Chapter 6
Genetic, Epigenetics, and Cell Adhesion in Acute Kidney Injury

Eloina Del Carmen Zarate-Peñata, Lorena Gómez-Escorcia,
Estefania Zapata, Roberto Navarro-Quiroz, Ornella Fiorillo-Moreno,
Katherine Zarate, Yezit Bello, Jaime Luna-Carrascal, Milton Quintana-Sosa,
Marlon Múnera, and Elkin Navarro-Quiroz

E. D. C. Zarate-Peñata · J. Luna-Carrascal
Life Sciences Research Centre, Universidad Simon Bolivar, Barranquilla, Colombia

Faculty of Basic and Biomedical Sciences, Universidad Simon Bolivar, Barranquilla,
Colombia
e-mail: eloina.zarate@unisimon.edu.co; jaime.luna@unisimon.edu.co

E. Zapata · O. Fiorillo-Moreno · Y. Bello · M. Quintana-Sosa
Life Sciences Research Centre, Universidad Simon Bolivar, Barranquilla, Colombia
e-mail: estafania.zapata@unisimon.edu.co; ornella.fiorillo@unisimon.edu.co;
yezit.bello@unisimon.edu.co; milto.quintana@unisimon.edu.co

L. Gómez-Escorcia
Centro de Investigaciones clinicas, Clinica de la costa, Barranquilla, Colombia
e-mail: lgomez@clinicadelacosta.co

R. Navarro-Quiroz · E. Navarro-Quiroz (✉)
Life Sciences Research Centre, Universidad Simon Bolivar, Barranquilla, Colombia

Faculty of Basic and Biomedical Sciences, Universidad Simon Bolivar, Barranquilla,
Colombia

Fundación Universidad San Martin, School of medicine, Puerto Colombia, Colombia
e-mail: rnqcri@ibmb.csic.es; elkin.navarro@unisimon.edu.co

K. Zarate
School of Medicine, Universidad Simon Bolivar, Barranquilla, Colombia
e-mail: katherine.zarate@unisimon.edu.co

M. Múnera
School of Medicine, Universidad Rafael Nuñez, Cartagena, Colombia
e-mail: marlon.munera@curnvirtual.edu.co

C. G. Musso, A. Covic (eds.), *Organ Crosstalk in Acute Kidney Injury*,
https://doi.org/10.1007/978-3-031-36789-2_6

6.1 Introduction

Acute kidney injury (AKI) is a syndrome that can be caused by multiple factors associated with various etiologies and pathophysiological processes leading to a decrease in kidney function, which has a potential systemic effect [1]. The cellular response in both physiological and AKI contexts is mediated by a combination of genetic and epigenetic factors that modulate the transcriptional programs of different cell types in the kidney.

Epigenetic mechanisms can regulate gene expression and pretranscriptionally, transcriptionally, posttranscriptionally, and postralationally. Pretranscriptional epigenetic mechanisms include DNA methylation and histone modifications that modulate different states of chromatin compaction through chromatin remodelers such as the SWI/SNF complex, which allows the assembly of the transcriptional machinery. Once transcription is initiated, epigenetic mechanisms control the production of different types of RNAs such as splicing, circRNAs, and modifications at the 5′ and 3′ ends. Furthermore, post-transcriptionally microRNAs can regulate the translation and degradation of mRNAs. The second section of this chapter will articulate the experimental and clinical evidence for some of these mechanisms in renal cells in the context of AKI.

6.2 Epigenetics of Cell Adhesion and Migration in AKI

The kidneys interact systemically through the circulatory system in a dynamic and bidirectionally with all other organ systems, receiving, processing, filtering, and excreting potentially dangerous water-soluble substances. Furthermore, they secrete some hormones with which vital processes are regulated, such as arterial pressure, blood pH, and water homeostasis. Lastly, the kidney metabolizes amino acids and lipids into glucose, in this manner providing 10% of the body's bioenergetics in fasting states. The coexistence of various types of kidney function alterations generates disruptions in bidirectional dynamics, which leads to the onset of AKI and AKI progression.

Renal vascular endothelial cells are a selective barrier that regulates the trafficking of inflammatory molecules and cells to nephrons through a series of molecular connections that expand from the cell surface to the nucleus. This promotes cell migration, a process highly regulated by several molecules, such as integrins and selectins [2]. These molecules modulate migration of neutrophils to a specific anatomical site such as the kidney [3]. As an inflammatory response, endothelium stimulates an increase in infiltration of immune cells [3]. This is an immune response where molecules, such as cadherins, can act as inducers of cell adhesion and stimulate effect mechanisms of activated T cells promoting cytotoxic responses [4]. Cellular traffic in the kidney is modulated by cadherin, integrin, and selectins. In this case, there are several examples of cadherins (L-CAM, A-CAM, E-CAM,

M-CAM, and P-cadherins), and the expression of each one is related to a tissue. For example, L-CAM is expressed in epithelial cells, whereas P-cadherins are expressed in placenta [5]. The loss in cadherin expression leads to impairment of actin filaments and an altered microfilament arrangement. In the human adult kidney, A-CAM is the major adhesion molecule present in this organ, affecting its morphogenesis [6]. Cadherins are not expressed in similar ways in the entire kidney; in some structures like podocytes, their expression is lower, or null, compared to other anatomical sites. Moreover, during a disease the scenario can be altered, meaning that cadherins can be expressed again [6]. Additionally, cadherins are implicated in regeneration and injury reparation mechanisms by inducing cellular migration to a damaged site. In this scenario, neutrophils play a pivotal role during nephrotoxic processes induced by metals, drugs, and venom components. In this aspect, intracellular adhesion molecule-1 (ICAM-1), integrins, and selectins modulate recruitment of leukocytes and inflammatory responses that are associated with nephrotoxic injury [7]. Moreover, molecules such as E-selectin ligand basigin/CD147 are responsible for neutrophil recruitment in renal ischemia/reperfusion [7]. For this reason, some molecules implicated in cell adhesion are considered targets for therapies in renal diseases.

Other cadherins, such as vascular cell adhesion molecule-1 (VCAM-1) and ICAM-1, have been proposed as biomarkers for monitoring clinical conditions of patients suffering from lupus nephritis (LN) [8]. Considering that in some AKI diseases vascular endothelium is affected by inflammation, molecular adhesion can vary in this process. Cell adhesion molecules are expressed by the vascular endothelium and are essential for attracting inflammatory cells to areas of injury. ICAM-1 and VCAM-1 are two examples of the immunoglobulin superfamily proteins; their expression on endothelial cells increases in response to systemic or local inflammation, which is typically accompanied by higher levels of TNF-α and IL-1β. The ensuing robust adherence, spreading, and transmigration of leukocytes across endothelial cells are all encouraged by these substances [9, 10].

AKI is an inflammatory condition where molecules such as transcription factors, pro-inflammatory cytokines, chemokines, adhesion molecules, Toll-like receptors, adipokines, and nuclear receptors are overexpressed. In this immunological context, other adhesion molecules also mediate cellular trafficking, in this case cell adhesion molecule-1 (CADM1) protein, an isoform SP4 present in renal distal tubes [11]. CADM1 is modulated by post-proteolytic cleavage (α- and β-shedding), an important mechanism involved in the regulation of renal disease. The reduction in CADM1 expression specifically induces apoptosis in renal tubular epithelial cells (TEC). These cells, which line the renal tubules, perform the essential function of reabsorbing water and other substances from urine. The phenomenon of apoptosis in TEC is often observed in situations of AKI [11].

It is important to mention that when sepsis leads to AKI, there is already advanced cell migration and infiltration, such as neutrophils. This migration occurring with sepsis has been seen to be modulated by two β2-integrins: LFA-1 and Mac-1. In addition, other molecules have been identified as part of neutrophil migration: E-selectin and P-selectin. Both of these are involved in neutrophil recruitment into the kidney after induction of sepsis [12]. The role of E-selectin and P-selectin in neutrophil migration has been tested in animal models, where their blockade leads to a considerable decrease in neutrophil migration [12].

Renal autoregulation integrates intrarenal mechanisms that stabilize renal blood flow and glomerular filtration rate during changes in renal perfusion pressure through the joint action of myogenic response and macula densa tubuloglomerular feedback, both of which are altered in AKI. Extracellular stimuli such as angiotensin II, hypoxia, aldosterone, and mechanical stretch trigger a variety of cell type-specific signaling cascades, such as the cAMP response elements and TET2 [13]. These proteins can modulate methylation states in regulatory and promoter sequences in DNA such as the IFNγ-responsive element in C3 promoter [14], IL-1–IL-6 response element and NF-κB binding site 2 in C3 promoter [15], and gene promoters such as Slc22a12 [16], CALCA [17], and KLK1 [18]. This leads to the demethylation of regulated/promoter regions in DNA by recruiting other molecules such as histone deacetylases (HDAC) that add methyl groups to histones, inducing a permissive chromatin structure [19]. The mentioned permissive structure allows for the binding of specific transcription factors such as HIF1α, NF-kB, and p53, which transcribe a variety of genes, among them miR-127 [20], miR-489 [21], miR-146a [22, 23], miR-375 [24], and miR-34a [25, 26], which post-transcriptionally modulate KIF3B, IRAK1, PARP1, SIRT1, and HNF1β, mainly in their 3′-untranslated region (3′-UTR). It is also possible that the interaction between miRNAs and mRNA occurs within the coding region or in the 5′-UTR of the mRNA [27]. It has also been shown that miR–mRNA interaction, mainly in the 5′-UTR, can enhance mRNA translation and can increase mRNA translation [28]. This is the reason for the urgency to improve molecular characterization in each patient, given the heterogeneous possibilities of different combinations of the described epigenetic mechanisms associated with AKI. This picture in AKI becomes even more complex while adding the possibilities of combinations of patient genetic factors. The abovementioned will be described in the next sections.

6.2.1 *Why Polymorphic Variants Might Better Explain the Interplay Between Acute Kidney Disease and Its Effect on Patients*

Individual single nucleotide polymorphisms (SNPs) constitute the most common genetic variant found in the modern human genome [29]. SNPs that have functional implications for gene expression levels are called regulatory SNPs (rSNPs) [30], while those that affect alternative translation, splicing, efficiency to enhance or inhibit expression, mRNA stability, and protein function (without altering its structure) [31] are called structural RNA SNPs (srSNPs). Several studies have identified these polymorphisms associated with different common diseases, for example, hypertension, obesity, rheumatoid arthritis, and acute kidney disease [32].

6.2.2 Some Genes and Polymorphic Variants That Could Exacerbate Acute Kidney Injury

Genetic variability and susceptibility determine the severity of AKI and may be strongly related to multiple environmental factors of the exposome involved in various pathophysiological mechanisms for the resolution of AKI disease.

6.2.3 Polymorphism Associated with Inflammatory Responses

6.2.3.1 Tumor Necrosis Factor-α (TNF-α)

Tumor necrosis factor (TNF-α) could initiate cascade processes within kidney cells and induce the production of proinflammatory mediators with cytokine alternation [33, 34]; furthermore, polymorphisms such as *rs1800629* and r*s1799964* [35] could be associated with TNF-α gene expression in patients with increased occurrence of AKI disease [36]. The presence or absence of these polymorphisms would influence the regulation of hemodynamic and excretory function in the kidney by inducing renal vasoconstriction and hyperfiltration [37]. Increased serum creatinine level has been associated with renal damage, as well as with the urinary renal damage molecule (KIM-1) [38]. The intensity of the manifestation of proinflammatory reactions may determine the severity of AKI, and therefore an evaluative genetic scheme to assess the presence of such TNF-α-associated polymorphisms should be considered.

6.2.3.2 Interleukin 6 (IL6) and Interleukin 10 (IL10)

IL6 has been demonstrated to induce a cell-mediated immune reaction that causes renal damage [39]. Interleukin-6 serves as a biomarker for predicting AKI [40]. Accordingly, three promoter polymorphisms have been identified within the *IL6* genes, namely the *rs1800795*, *rs1800796*, and *rs1800797* polymorphisms, which influence cytokine expression and secretion [41]. Consequently, the low-penetrance AA genotype of the IL 10 rs1800896 polymorphism has been linked to AKI [42], along with the combined genotype of *rs1800629* GG + *rs1800896* AA [43]. IL-10 has a key role in restraining excessive inflammatory responses [44], which could enhance innate immunity and promote tissue repair mechanisms to maintain tissue homeostasis during inflammation and infection [45].

6.2.3.3   Human Leukocyte Antigen–Major Histocompatibility Complex (HLA-DR)

The immune system is characterized by the presence of monocytes that initiate phagocytic processes, the presentation of antigens, and the production of cytokines that are mediated by certain cell surface molecules [46]. The major histocompatibility complex cell surface receptor has a key receptor, the human leukocyte antigen (HLA-DR) [47], which allows antigen presentation to T cells and is crucial for the initiation of an immune response [48]. Locating polymorphisms within the histocompatibility system has been an arduous task. However, a comparison with other HLA genes has found that the SNP (rs7192) [49] may be associated with the HLA-DR ~ HLA-DQ haplotypes and may indicate a conformational extension of the proteins involved in the histocompatibility system [50]. We have identified 20 novel SNP positions in the intronic sequences within the 7711 bp region represented in IPD-IMGT/HLA. This polymorphism gives rise to at least 22 new alleles within HLA-DRA, together with intronic 3′UTR patterns corresponding to the HLA-DRA ~ HLA-DRB345 ~ HLA-DRB1 ~ HLA-DQB1 haplotypes, which could be candidates for AKI compression in the near future.

6.2.4   Polymorphisms Associated with Vascular Hemodynamic Response and Cellular Metabolic Homeostasis

Vascular endothelial growth factor (VEGF) is a protein that promotes angiogenesis, blood flow between stacked vessels, and cell differentiation [51]. In terms of genetics, AKI and VEGF are associated with the genotypic rs3025039 polymorphism [52], which according to some studies could be related to severe sepsis in patients with acute kidney injury [53].

Critical cytochrome b245, which belongs to the CYBA gene, plays an important role in the hemodynamic processes of renal system metabolism [54]. The rs885 polymorphism is found within the CYBA complex. It is an allele in the cytochrome b245 α (CYBA) gene that could be correlated with AKI and mortality in hospitalized patients compared to GG genotype, A-A-G-G haplotype of rs4782390, rs4673, rs3794624, and rs8854 polymorphisms, which were associated with increased vulnerability to this outcome. On the other hand, other polymorphic variants have been explored as possible determinants of AKI disease severity, with processes compatible with oxidative stress and the activation of NADPH oxidase, an enzyme complex that produces mainly superoxide.

6.3   Conclusion

Given the current knowledge on AKI, defining a set of combinations of genetic variations, of epigenetic mechanisms in the modulation of, e.g., cell adhesion molecules, thus manifesting the urgency of integrated exploration at different levels and scales, will improve the understanding of this syndrome. Consequently, this will allow better patient stratification that will contribute to personalized approaches that maximize their response to treatment and will ultimately lead to a patient-specific preventive medicine.

References

1. Hoste EAJ, Kellum JA, Selby NM, Zarbock A, Palevsky PM, Bagshaw SM, et al. Global epidemiology and outcomes of acute kidney injury. Nat Rev Nephrol. 2018;14(10):607–25. https://www.nature.com/articles/s41581-018-0052-0.
2. Cell adhesion by integrins | Physiological reviews [Internet]. [cited August 15, 2022]. https://journals.physiology.org/doi/full/10.1152/physrev.00036.2018.
3. Elangbam CS, Qualls CW, Dahlgren RR. Cell adhesion molecules—update. Vet Pathol. 1997;34(1):61–73. https://doi.org/10.1177/030098589703400113.
4. Maître JL, Heisenberg CP. Three functions of cadherins in cell adhesion. Curr Biol. 2013;23(14):R626–33. https://www.ncbi.nlm.nih.gov/pmc/articles/PMC3722483/.
5. Brady HR. Leukocyte adhesion molecules: potential targets for therapeutic intervention in kidney diseases. Curr Opin Nephrol Hypertens. 1993;2(2):171–82.
6. Müller GA, Müller CA, Markovic-Lipkovski J. Adhesion molecules in renal diseases. Ren Fail. 1996;18(5):711–24.
7. Kato N, Yuzawa Y, Kosugi T, Hobo A, Sato W, Miwa Y, et al. The E-selectin ligand basigin/CD147 is responsible for neutrophil recruitment in renal ischemia/reperfusion. J Am Soc Nephrol. 2009;20(7):1565–76.
8. Yu KY, Yung S, Chau MK, Tang CS, Yap DY, Tang AH, et al. Clinico-pathological associations of serum VCAM-1 and ICAM-1 levels in patients with lupus nephritis. Lupus. 2021;30(7):1039–50.
9. Remuzzi G, Bertani T. Pathophysiology of progressive nephropathies. N Engl J Med. 1998;339(20):1448–56.
10. Wada J, Makino H. Inflammation and the pathogenesis of diabetic nephropathy. Clin Sci (Lond). 2013;124(3):139–52.
11. Kato T, Hagiyama M, Takashima Y, Yoneshige A, Ito A. Cell adhesion molecule-1 shedding induces apoptosis of renal epithelial cells and exacerbates human nephropathies. Am J Physiol Renal Physiol. 2018;314(3):F388–98.
12. Herter JM, Rossaint J, Spieker T, Zarbock A. Adhesion molecules involved in neutrophil recruitment during sepsis-induced acute kidney injury. J Innate Immun. 2014;6(5):597–606.
13. Yang Q, Li X, Li R, Peng J, Wang Z, Jiang Z, et al. Low shear stress inhibited endothelial cell autophagy through TET2 downregulation. Ann Biomed Eng. 2016;44(7):2218–27.
14. Pratt JR, Parker MD, Affleck LJ, Corps C, Hostert L, Michalak E, et al. Ischemic epigenetics and the transplanted kidney. Transplant Proc. 2006;38(10):3344–6.
15. Parker MD, Chambers PA, Lodge JPA, Pratt JR. Ischemia-reperfusion injury and its influence on the epigenetic modification of the donor kidney genome. Transplantation. 2008;86(12):1818–23.

16. Endo K, Kito N, Fukushima Y, Weng H, Iwai N. A novel biomarker for acute kidney injury using TaqMan-based unmethylated DNA-specific polymerase chain reaction. Biomed Res. 2014;35(3):207–13.

17. Mehta TK, Hoque MO, Ugarte R, Rahman MH, Kraus E, Montgomery R, et al. Quantitative detection of promoter hypermethylation as a biomarker of acute kidney injury during transplantation. Transplant Proc. 2022;38(10):3420–6. https://www.sciencedirect.com/science/article/pii/S0041134506013947.

18. Kang SW, Shih P-AB, Mathew RO, Mahata M, Biswas N, Rao F, et al. Renal kallikrein excretion and epigenetics in human acute kidney injury: expression, mechanisms and consequences. BMC Nephrol. 2022;12(1):27. https://doi.org/10.1186/1471-2369-12-27.

19. O'Connor DT. Response of the renal kallikrein-kinin system, intravascular volume, and renal hemodynamics to sodium restriction and diuretic treatment in essential hypertension. Hypertension. 1982;4(5 Pt 2):III72–8.

20. Aguado-Fraile E, Ramos E, Sáenz-Morales D, Conde E, Blanco-Sánchez I, Stamatakis K, et al. miR-127 protects proximal tubule cells against ischemia/reperfusion: identification of kinesin family member 3B as miR-127 target. PLoS One. 2012;7(9):e44305. https://journals.plos.org/plosone/article?id=10.1371/journal.pone.0044305.

21. Wei Q, Liu Y, Liu P, Hao J, Liang M, Mi Q-S, et al. MicroRNA-489 induction by hypoxia–inducible factor–1 protects against ischemic kidney injury. J Am Soc Nephrol. 2016;27(9):2784–96. https://www.ncbi.nlm.nih.gov/pmc/articles/PMC5004659/.

22. Dai Y, Jia P, Fang Y, Liu H, Jiao X, He JC, et al. miR-146a is essential for lipopolysaccharide (LPS)-induced cross-tolerance against kidney ischemia/reperfusion injury in mice. Sci Rep. 2016;6(1):27091. https://www.nature.com/articles/srep27091.

23. Amrouche L, Desbuissons G, Rabant M, Sauvaget V, Nguyen C, Benon A, et al. MicroRNA-146a in human and experimental ischemic AKI: CXCL8-dependent mechanism of action. J Am Soc Nephrol. 2022;28(2):479–93. https://jasn.asnjournals.org/content/28/2/479.

24. Hao J, Lou Q, Wei Q, Mei S, Li L, Wu G, et al. MicroRNA-375 is induced in cisplatin nephrotoxicity to repress hepatocyte nuclear factor 1-β. J Biol Chem. 2022;292(11):4571–82. https://www.ncbi.nlm.nih.gov/pmc/articles/PMC5377773/.

25. Lee CG, Kim JG, Kim HJ, Kwon HK, Cho IJ, Choi DW, et al. Discovery of an integrative network of microRNAs and transcriptomics changes for acute kidney injury. Kidney Int. 2022;86(5):943–53. https://www.sciencedirect.com/science/article/pii/S0085253815304051.

26. MicroRNA-34a is induced via p53 during cisplatin nephrotoxicity and contributes to cell survival. Molecular Medicine. Full Text [Internet]. [15 August 2022]. https://molmed.biomedcentral.com/articles/10.2119/molmed.2010.00002.

27. Fabbri M. MicroRNAs and miRceptors: a new mechanism of action for intercellular communication. Philos Trans R Soc Lond Ser B Biol Sci. 2022;373(1737):20160486. https://www.ncbi.nlm.nih.gov/pmc/articles/PMC5717440/.

28. Vasudevan S, Tong Y, Steitz JA. Switching from repression to activation: microRNAs can up-regulate translation. Science. 2007;318(5858):1931–4.

29. Sherman RM, Salzberg SL. Pan-genomics in the human genome era. Nat Rev Genet. 2020;21(4):243–54.

30. Degtyareva AO, Antontseva EV, Merkulova TI. Regulatory SNPs: altered transcription factor binding sites implicated in complex traits and diseases. Int J Mol Sci. 2021;22(12):6454.

31. Manning KS, Cooper TA. The roles of RNA processing in translating genotype to phenotype. Nat Rev Mol Cell Biol. 2017;18(2):102–14.

32. Zhao B, Lu Q, Cheng Y, Belcher JM, Siew ED, Leaf DE, et al. A genome-wide association study to identify single-nucleotide polymorphisms for acute kidney injury. Am J Respir Crit Care Med. 2017;195:482–90.

33. Shalkami AGS, Hassan MIA, Abd El-Ghany AA. Perindopril regulates the inflammatory mediators, NF-κB/TNF-α/IL-6, and apoptosis in cisplatin-induced renal dysfunction. Naunyn Schmiedeberg's Arch Pharmacol. 2018;391(11):1247–55.

34. Chen L, Deng H, Cui H, Fang J, Zuo Z, Deng J, et al. Inflammatory responses and inflammation-associated diseases in organs. Oncotarget. 2018;9(6):7204–18.
35. Wu S, Wang MG, Wang Y, He JQ. Polymorphisms of cytokine genes and tuberculosis in two independent studies. Sci Rep. 2019;9(1):1–11.
36. Hashad DI, Elsayed ET, Helmy TA, Elawady SM. Study of the role of tumor necrosis factor-α(-308G/A) and interleukin-10 (-1082 G/A) polymorphisms as potential risk factors to acute kidney injury in patients with severe sepsis using high-resolution melting curve analysis. Ren Fail. 2017;39(1):77–82.
37. Saad RA, Afsah I, Akl A. Drug handling by elderly kidney: a prospective review to senile kidney physiology. Open Urol Nephrol J. 2022;10(1):15. https://doi.org/10.15406/unoaj.2022.10.00317.
38. Wajda J, Dumnicka P, Kolber W, Sporek M, Maziarz B, Ceranowicz P, et al. The marker of tubular injury, kidney injury molecule-1 (KIM-1), in acute kidney injury complicating acute pancreatitis: a preliminary study. J Clin Med. 2020;9(5):1–12.
39. Jordan SC, Ammerman N, Choi J, Kumar S, Huang E, Toyoda M, et al. Interleukin-6: an important mediator of allograft injury. Transplantation. 2020;104(12):2497–506. https://doi.org/10.1097/TP.0000000000003249.
40. Albert C, Haase M, Albert A, Kropf S, Bellomo R, Westphal S, et al. Urinary biomarkers may complement the Cleveland score for prediction of adverse kidney events after cardiac surgery: a pilot study. Ann Lab Med. 2020;40(2):131–41.
41. Omoyinmi E, Forabosco P, Hamaoui R, Bryant A, Hinks A, Ursu S, et al. Association of the IL-10 gene family locus on chromosome 1 with juvenile idiopathic arthritis (JIA). PLoS One. 2012;7(10):e47673. https://doi.org/10.1371/journal.pone.0047673. PMID: 23094074, PMCID: PMC3475696.
42. Alves LV, Martins SR, Simões e Silva AC, Cardoso CN, Gomes KB, Mota APL. TNF, IL-6, and IL-10 cytokines levels and their polymorphisms in renal function and time after transplantation. Immunol Res. 2020;68(5):246–54.
43. Ivanova M, Manolova I, Stoilov R, Stanilova S. The synergistic role of TNFA – 308G/A and IL10–1082A/G polymorphisms in ankylosing spondylitis. Rheumatol Int. 2021;41(12):2215–24.
44. Rocha S, Valente MJ, Coimbra S, Catarino C, Rocha-Pereira P, Oliveira JG, et al. Interleukin 6 (rs1800795) and pentraxin 3 (rs2305619) polymorphisms-association with inflammation and all-cause mortality in end-stage-renal disease patients on dialysis. Sci Rep. 2021;11(1):14768.
45. Ortega-Loubon C, Martínez-Paz P, García-Morán E, Tamayo-Velasco Á, López-Hernández FJ, Jorge-Monjas P, et al. Genetic susceptibility to acute kidney injury. J Clin Med. 2021;10(14):1–33.
46. Kurts C, Ginhoux F, Panzer U. Kidney dendritic cells: fundamental biology and functional roles in health and disease. Nat Rev Nephrol. 2020;16(7):391–407.
47. Houseman M, Huang MYY, Huber M, Staiger M, Zhang L, Hoffmann A, et al. Flow cytometry-based high-throughput RNAi screening for miRNAs regulating MHC class II HLA-DR surface expression. Eur J Immunol. 2022;52:1452. https://doi.org/10.1002/eji.202149735.
48. Franzin R, Netti GS, Spadaccino F, Porta C, Gesualdo L. Oncology and the occurrence of AKI: where do we stand? Front Immunol. 2020;8(11):574271. https://doi.org/10.3389/fimmu.2020.574271.
49. Kanchan K, Clay S, Irizar H, Bunyavanich S, Mathias RA. Current insights into the genetics of food allergy. J Allergy Clin Immunol. 2021;147(1):15–28.
50. Wolin A, Lahtela EL, Anttila V, Petrek M, Grunewald J, van Moorsel CHM, et al. SNP variants in major histocompatibility complex are associated with sarcoidosis susceptibility-a joint analysis in four European populations. Front Immunol. 2017;8:422. https://doi.org/10.3389/fimmu.2017.00422.
51. Darden J, Payne LB, Zhao H, Chappell JC. Excess vascular endothelial growth factor-A disrupts pericyte recruitment during blood vessel formation. Angiogenesis. 2019;22(1):167–83.

52. Vilander LM, Vaara ST, Kaunisto MA, Pettilä V, Laru-Sompa R, Pulkkinen A, et al. Common inflammation-related candidate gene variants and acute kidney injury in 2647 critically ill Finnish patients. J Clin Med. 2019;8:342. https://doi.org/10.3390/jcm803034.
53. Song Y, Yang Y, Liu L, Liu X. Association between five polymorphisms in vascular endothelial growth factor gene and urinary bladder cancer risk: a systematic review and meta-analysis involving 6671 subjects. Gene. 2019;698:186–97.
54. Katakami N, Kaneto H, Matsuoka TA, Takahara M, Osonoi T, Saitou M, et al. Accumulation of oxidative stress-related gene polymorphisms and the risk of coronary heart disease events in patients with type 2 diabetes – an 8-year prospective study. Atherosclerosis. 2014;235(2):408–14.

Chapter 7
Organs Crosstalk Perspective

Carlos Guido Musso, Victoria Paula Musso-Enz, Olivia Maria Capalbo, and Guido Mateo Musso-Enz

7.1   Introduction

The great philosopher Immanuel Kant introduced the notion that the interpretation of a final reality (noumen) can never be fully attained, but rather is understood as a biased representation of it (phenomenon). The epistemological concept agrees that the interpretation of something is only a partial version of it, and in addition states that it is an inexact reconstruction of it. Each interpreter has its own conceptual schema, experiences, points of view, and even unique cognitive ability. Therefore, to acknowledge or understand something is fragmentary (an inaccurate copy), as the interpreter always has structural restrictions and cannot grasp the uniqueness of the universe, or at least cannot see it in exactly the same way as another individual. Whenever science finds a problem resolution while working on a renowned and classical point of view, it should shift its perspective in order to overcome any fragmentary or reduced mindset. This is why an awareness should arise that a scientific interpretative model is only a representation to aid in problem solving, and not an exact reproduction of reality [1, 2].

C. G. Musso (✉)
Physiology Department, Instituto Universitario del Hospital Italiano de Buenos Aires, Buenos Aires, Argentina

Facultad de Ciencias de la Salud, Universidad Simón Bolivar, Barranquilla, Colombia
e-mail: carlos.musso@hospitalitalino.org.ar

V. P. Musso-Enz · O. M. Capalbo
Physiology Department, Instituto Universitario del Hospital Italiano de Buenos Aires, Buenos Aires, Argentina
e-mail: victoria.musso@hospitalitaliano.org.ar; olivia.capalbo@hospitalitaliano.org.ar

G. M. Musso-Enz
Facultad de Medicina, Universidad Católica Argentina, Buenos Aires, Argentina

C. G. Musso, A. Covic (eds.), *Organ Crosstalk in Acute Kidney Injury*,
https://doi.org/10.1007/978-3-031-36789-2_7

In this way, the medical interpretation of health and sickness from a physiological and pathophysiological point of view is still outdated. The reductionist concept portrays organs as machines which work together with neighbor organs in order to orchestrate body functions and maintain homeostasis, or work discordantly in a sickness scenario. Henceforth, diseases are allowed to freely develop and establish, because under this disintegrative viewpoint there is no way to foresee them before actual organ damage [3]. Fortunately, there is an encouraging new perspective brought by a relatively new scientific discipline called *biosemiotics*.

7.2 Biosemiotics: Life as a Dialogue

Semiotics is the science involved in the study of signs and the meaning that any sign entails. Jesper Hoffmeyer, a leading figure in the field of biosemiotics, stated that semiosis is essential for the phenomenon of life because it is based not on molecules themselves but their function as signs which make life possible, because every single living being integrates a semiotic system itself [4, 5]. Establishing a parallelism between the chemical signs within an organism and the linguistic sign of the Saussureian model of human language, it can be said that a molecule (e.g., a hormonal chemical messenger) represents a linguistic sound, while its action (in this example, intracellular changes) equals the linguistic meaning or concept of that sound [6]; like words in anthroposemiotics (human intercommunication) [5]. Acknowledging the presence of language in all forms of nature and its complexity is, as philosopher Martin Heidegger once stated, the essence of the Being [7].

Biosemiotics studies the broad language of nature. The pathway from a sign to its meaning is packed by a set of codes and conventions in order to translate a received sensory signal into its corresponding response or reaction, as well as adaptors which aid in the step-process of this representation. This concept is present in many different fields. For example, cytosemiotics delves into cell intercommunication, with thermal, mechanical, electrical, or chemical signs. There is also an external semiosis (*exosemiosis*), where there is an exchange between an organism and the environment, and an *endosemiosis*, where the information exchange occurs within the organism at its different levels (cellular, tissues, organ systems, etc.) [4, 5].

7.3 Biosemiotics: Health and Disease as a Process

The perspective brought by biosemiotics is that the organism is formed by a biologic space (cells, organs, organ system) and a biosemiotic space (flow of cytokines, neurotransmitters, hormones, which act as *signals*) [3] (Fig. 7.1). There is a structural and functional difference between these two spaces. The biologic space

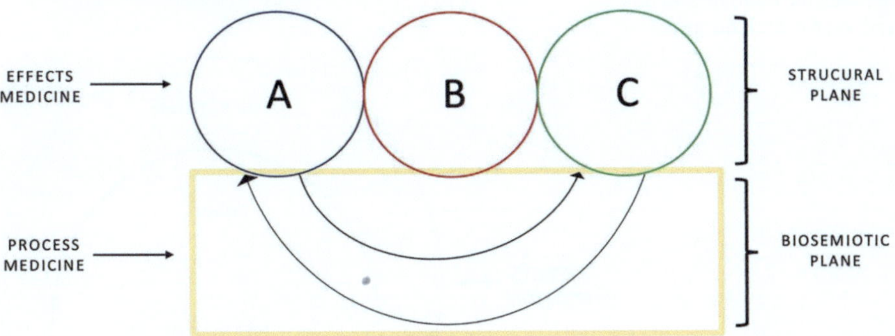

Fig. 7.1 Crosstalk in biologic and biosemiotic spaces. **A, B, C**: organ system, organs, tissues, or cells

has a slow velocity and a heavier density, while the biosemiotics space has a faster velocity and a lighter density. Therefore, the body organs (and the vital process itself) are the result of an interrelation between a dense and slow pulse and a light and fast one. Delving further, each biological layer (cell, tissues, organs) is also the result of the dialogues between the underlying and superficial layers. The way an organism works is hence the result of the information flow and dialogues established in the biosemiotics space and thereafter in the biologic space. This constitutes the constant bidirectional nature of the organs not only providing communication signals but as a result of the dialogues in the body as a whole. Visually, and referring to the works of the great artists (e.g., Dante Alighieri, William Butler Yeats), this concept can be portrayed as a lemniscate figure, which represents how the process flows both vertically (ascendant and descendent) and laterally (biologically and biosemiotically) [8–10] (Fig. 7.2).

This vast convoluted network arising from biosemiotics differs drastically from the pathophysiological structuralist and simplistic point of view which interprets organs simply as parts of a big machine, which can overall work in a healthy or diseased way [11]. On the other hand, biosemiotics provides a perspective where health or sickness is the effect of a physiological or pathological dialogue between every biological level of complexity respectively, and where the disruption of the biological space is preceded by the biosemiotic one. These dialogues are the essence of existence.

7.4 Organic Intercommunication: The Crosstalk Perspective

The aforementioned language and communication between biologic and biosemiotic spaces is broad and varies depending on the level of complexity involved. These layers can be depicted as a series of steps: on the lower and basic steps the cellular

Fig. 7.2 Interaction between the biologic space and the biosemiotic space

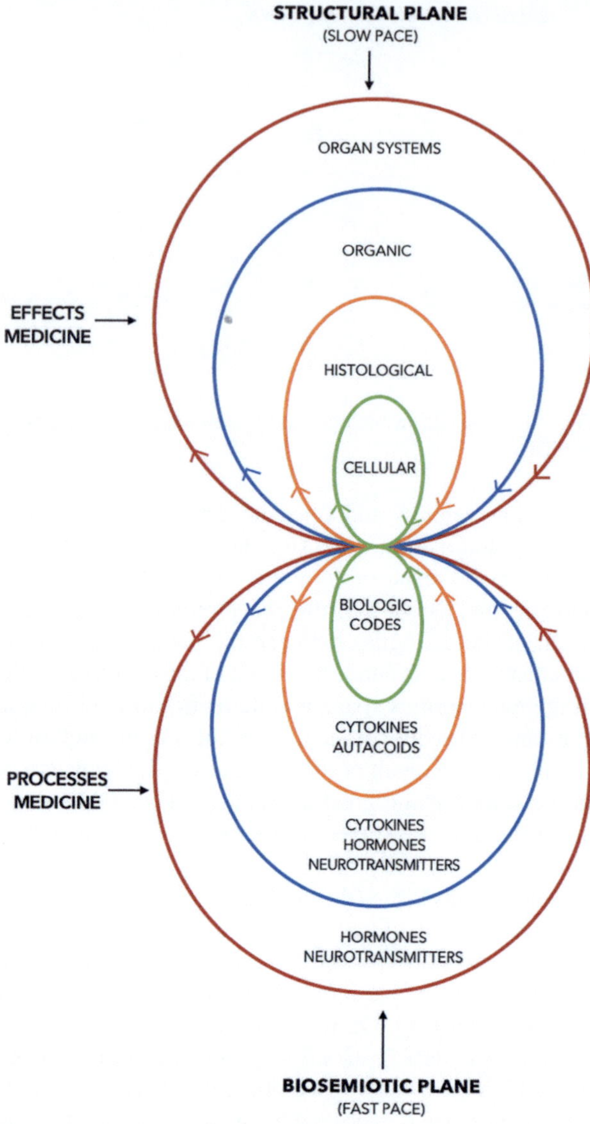

space can be found, followed by the tissue level, and then the organic level. Genetic code acts on the first step, while an immense number of mediators (e.g., cytokines, prostaglandins, and innumerable autacoids) communicate at the tissue level. Moreover, organs interrelate with neurotransmitters and hormones, which can travel long distances through nerves or the bloodstream in order to deliver their message. Inorganic substances such as oxygen and carbon dioxide are also messengers in this context [3–7, 12–14] (Fig. 7.2).

It should be pointed out that the different biological spaces (BS) are not closed structures, but are rather in continual communication by crosstalk established between two or more BS, and even at different complexity levels. The type of information flow in this crosstalk is what determines salutogenesis or pathogenesis, as they can act directly on the target organ, or indirectly as a second messenger on another organ. At the same time, it is considered that the organ which receives the communication can provide two types of responses: a fast response by any structure (organ) and a slow response that requires transcription and expression of genes [3–5].

Bearing the crosstalk concept in mind, modern medicine needs to shift its structuralist perspective (effect medicine) toward determining how crosstalk acts on the different biological layers, and hence how it is altered during sickness. In this biosemiotic medicine perspective, it is possible to detect organic pathologic crosstalk before structural damage occurs. This could lead to early diagnosis of diseases with the advantage of reaching an early treatment and better prognosis [3].

7.5 Conclusion

Acknowledging the existence of a continual communication and flow of information between biological and biosemiotics spaces of all levels of complexity, and hence the presence of organic crosstalk, will allow physicians to foresee organ damage in multiple sickness scenarios. The shift from effect medicine to process medicine will help to determine not only effective treatment strategies but also to plan preventive care.

References

1. Musso CG. The epistemology of introspection: the inner key to scientific research. Arch Argent Pediatr. 2019;117(6):356–9.
2. Musso CG, Musso-Enz VP, Musso-Enz GM, Olivia Capalbo MO, Porrini S. Organic crosstalk: a new perspective in medicine. Biosemiotics. 2021;14:829–37.
3. Musso CG. Biosemiotic medicine: from an effect-based medicine to a process-based medicine. Arch Argent Pediatr. 2020;118(5):e449–53.
4. Barbieri M. From biosemiotics to code biology. Biol Theory. 2014;9:239–49.
5. Barbieri M. The semantic theory of language. Biosystems. 2020;190:104100.
6. Musso CG. The organ language. Evidencia; 2005.
7. Porrini S. The others. Operational metaphysics in the 20th and 21st centuries. Madrid: Matrioska; 2020.
8. Lamúa A. The secrets of infinity. Barcelona: Ilusbooks; 2012.
9. Purce J. The mystic spiral. London: Thames & Hudson; 2017.
10. Yeats BW. A vision. London: MacMillan & Co; 1937.
11. McPhee S, Hammer G. Pathophysiology of disease. New York: McGraw Hill Medical; 2010.
12. Musso CG, Rosell C, Gonzalez-Torres H, Ordonez JD, Aroca-Martinez G. Primary prevention for acute kidney injury in ambulatory patients. Postgrad Med. 2020;132(8):746–8.

13. Domenech P, Perez T, Saldarini A, Uad P, et al. Kidney-lung pathophysiological crosstalk: its characteristics and importance. Int Urol Nephrol. 2017;49(7):1211–5.
14. Capalbo O, Giuliani S, Ferrero-Fernández A, Casciato P, et al. Kidney-liver pathophysiological crosstalk: its characteristics and importance. Int Urol Nephrol. 2019;51(12):2203–7.

Chapter 8
Kidney–Brain Crosstalk in Acute Kidney Injury

Micaela Patti, Florencia Grynszpan, Victoria Ristagno-Ruiz,
and Carlos Guillermo Videla

8.1 Introduction

The brain, the all-encompassing receptor, processor, and effector of our organism, receives countless signals from the body which are highly essential during injury: from initial pain interpretation, to involuntarily commanding adequate adaptations to attain homeostasis and recovery. Despite its crucial role, however, its physiological activity is challenged by apparent distant events that, due to organ crosstalk, have an impact on its functioning.

Patients with acute kidney injury (AKI) usually develop changes in the central and peripheral nervous systems, which lead to several neurologic signs and symptoms of fluctuating nature. Headache, visual abnormalities, tremor, asterixis, multifocal myoclonus, chorea, seizures, cognitive impairment, and coma are some of the most frequent manifestations. These neurological disorders can be caused by uremic toxin accumulation, electrolyte imbalance, drug toxicity, and the effects of renal replacement therapy. Kidney failure generates changes in the central and peripheral nervous systems. Furthermore, chronic hemodialysis can be associated with dialysis dementia, an indicator of global cerebral cortex dysfunction [1].

On the other hand, acute brain injury can generate neurohumoral changes that directly impact the kidney by increasing the activity of the renal sympathetic nervous system. This impairs vasopressin release and renin-angiotensin-aldosterone system (RAAS) activation, which generates changes in the sodium and water balance, leading to an inadequate renal blood flow and glomerular filtration. Severe

M. Patti · F. Grynszpan · V. Ristagno-Ruiz
Physiology Department, Instituto Universitario del Hospital Italiano de Buenos Aires,
Buenos Aires, Argentina

C. G. Videla (✉)
Neurology Division, Hospital Italiano de Buenos Aires, Buenos Aires, Argentina
e-mail: guillermo.videla@hospitalitaliano.org.ar

"""

brain injury resulting in cerebral death also entails renal consequences such as haemodynamic instability, hormonal imbalance, endothelial activation, and an exacerbation in the immune response which triggers an inflammatory cascade, not only in the kidneys, but also in several organs.

A thorough analysis of the various pathological scenarios and mechanisms of damage will help to understand the communication pathways between the kidneys and the brain during acute injury to elucidate the pathophysiology behind the patient's clinical deterioration, hence preparing physicians for possible complications.

8.2 Pathological Crosstalk

8.2.1 Inflammation

In recent years, the importance of the subsequent inflammatory response that arises from acute kidney injury (AKI) has been established. Damage elicits a pro-inflammatory cytokine generation, but also decreases cytokine clearance, therefore increasing the levels of soluble mediators capable of traveling through the bloodstream and initiating inflammatory responses in distant organs. Progress in biomolecular technologies allowed the identification of specific mediators that are primarily involved in the AKI inflammatory response. Granulocyte colony-stimulating (G-CSF) factor, interleukin-1B (IL-1B), interleukin-6 (IL-6), interleukin-8 (IL-8), tumor necrosis factor alpha (TNF-α), and keratinocyte-derived chemoattractant were specifically identified in AKI animal experimental models [2]. These small peptides cause leukocyte recruitment and activation, oxidative stress, activation of the complement cascade pathway, increased vascular permeability, and amplification of the humoral immune response.

Specialized brain cells, including neurons, astrocytes, microglia, and endothelial cells, have Toll-like receptors (TLRs) that command the innate immune response by recognizing pathogen associated molecular patterns (PAMPs) and damage-associated molecular patterns (DAMPs). PAMPs represent molecular patterns common in a series of microorganisms and help the innate immune system to detect organisms that do not belong to the human body. On the other hand, DAMPs are molecular fragments of human cells that are released during cell damage as a result of cellular death different from apoptosis. The importance of DAMPs recognition on behalf of the innate immune system relies upon the fact that these soluble inflammatory mediators not only reach the brain but are also produced in it as a part of the remote organ involvement during crosstalk. Meanwhile, cytokines such as TNF, interleukins, and interferon-alpha feed the ongoing inflammation and increase the expression of aquaporin 4 channels, allowing for the movement of water inside brain cells, which leads to swelling and brain edema [1]. Ischemic AKI leads to marked brain inflammatory changes evidenced by increased soluble inflammatory proteins: KC neutrophil chemoattractant, chemokine ligand 1 (CXCL-1), and G-CSF with increased expression of glial fibrillary acidic protein (GFAP). GFAP is a specific cellular marker of cerebral inflammation whose levels increase particularly after AKI, reflecting a pathological glial cell activation in this precise clinical situation. Increased KC and G-CSF in the brain likely represents increased neuronal production of these pro-inflammatory factors or an accumulation of these proteins through an altered blood–brain barrier arising from a systemic or renal source. Several studies evidenced changes in mRNA transcription proteins in the cerebral cortex, corpus callosum, hypothalamus, and hippocampus [3], showing how systemic inflammation initiating in the kidney evoked inflammation originating from brain cells.

This humoral route that distributes inflammatory mediators is also accompanied by a neuronal afferent route located at the site of injury that sends inflammatory signals to the brain. During AKI, there is an activation of the afferent renal sympathetic system, which has been evidenced to cause glial activation and pro-inflammatory gene expression [4]. Inflammation evoked in the brain not only plays a pathological role, but also represents an essential component of recuperation. The mentioned mediator release induces a *sickness behavior* which is responsible for the classic symptoms of fatigue, fever, loss of appetite, sleepiness, lethargy, and joint pain. This general malaise forces the organism to rest and recognize its priority for healing and recovery [5, 6].

Inflammation is not limited to kidney failure. In an opposite scenario, brain injury also elicits an inflammatory response. Pro-inflammatory cytokines are released during traumatic brain injury. For example, IL-6 and neutrophil gelatinase-associated lipocalin were specifically investigated in these cases, showing an increased level of serum and cerebrospinal fluid [7, 8]. Due to the ubiquitous spreading of these soluble mediators, they have the potential to alter renal tubular epithelial cells, and even cause apoptosis that can affect renal function and lead to AKI [9]. At the same time and in the context of brain injury, there is also an increased sympathetic response that causes renal vasoconstriction and blood flow restriction, further contributing to the loss of kidney function (see Chap. 4) (Fig. 8.1).

8.3 Blood–Brain Barrier

The brain, an immune-privileged tissue, is normally protected from toxins and potentially harmful substances that circulate in the bloodstream due to the blood–brain barrier (BBB). The BBB is a highly selective and semi-permeable barrier histologically formed of endothelial cells held together by tight junctions. Its core role is to prevent the indiscriminate entrance of certain solutes from the circulating blood to the central nervous system (CNS). Pericytes, microglia, astrocytes, and proteins from the extracellular cell matrix also contribute to the orchestrated function of allowing certain substances and solutes to enter the brain, while intelligently excluding microorganisms and other endogenous or exogenous

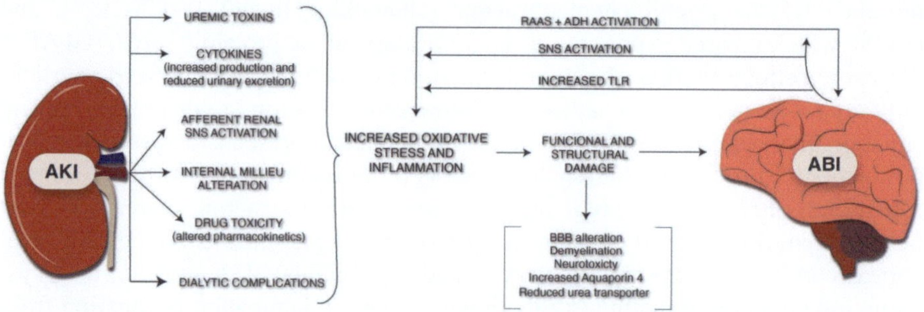

Fig. 8.1 Kidney–brain crosstalk. *AKI* acute kidney injury, *ABI* acute brain injury, *RAAS* renin-angiotensin-aldosterone system, *ADH* antidiuretic hormone, *BBB* blood brain barrier, *SNS* sympathetic nervous system, *TLR* Toll-like receptors

undesirable substances. The inflammatory response in AKI generates a disruption of the BBB. Also, a sudden reduction in renal function causes toxin accumulation and increased serum osmolality, which can directly stimulate vascular endothelial growth factor (VEGF) and increase oxygen reactive species, leading to endothelial damage. The released cytokines also contribute to endothelial injury by directly activating immune cells, therefore stimulating their responsive properties, and increasing endothelial permeability. The consequential entry of soluble mediators and harmful substances, such as retained urea and nitrogen, leads to an inflammatory response inside the brain, which modifies neuronal cell protein transcription and cellular activation, affecting brain function [1, 2].

The disruption of the BBB also implies that essential active transport proteins cannot exert their normal function. The sodium independent cationic amino acid transporter 1 (CAT1/SLC7A1) regulates L-arginine influx into the brain. Considering that L-arginine is the precursor for guanidine compounds, any interference with this transporter during AKI may potentially cause both the accumulation and the reduction of amino acids and neurotransmitters in the brain. Glutamate, aspartic acid, glycine, gamma aminobutyric acid (GABA), and taurine are actively exported out through excitatory amino acid transporters, and hence alterations in the BBB integrity in AKI can lead to amino acid accumulation within the CNS [1–3] (Fig. 8.1).

8.4 Oxidative Stress

Oxidative stress is a process which results from an imbalance between free radicals and antioxidant mechanisms available to neutralize them. Free radicals are produced in physiological processes such as cellular signaling or immune response and are key mediators in the inflammatory response against microorganisms and foreign pathogens. However, they can also damage healthy tissues and induce sterile inflammation. The organic compounds that are the most susceptible to being affected by oxidative stress are lipids. In this manner, cellular structures composed by a high proportion of lipidic products, such as cellular membranes, are greatly affected by these reactions. Likewise, neurons and nervous tissue, due to the lipidic myelin sheath, are especially prone to oxidative damage. Therefore, this makes lipid peroxidation the most sensitive marker of oxidative stress [10].

Oxidative stress plays a crucial role in AKI, causing remote organ damage as evidenced in several experimental studies. Out of all structures of the CNS, the frontal cortex and the hippocampus are particularly susceptible to this type of damage mechanism [10]. Heme-oxygenase-1 is an enzyme that suppresses oxidative stress, induces anti-inflammatory and antioxidant metabolites such as bilirubin, and upregulates cell cycle inhibitors. In a renal ischemia–reperfusion animal model with heme oxygenase-1 knock-out mice, it was evidenced that an augmented renal injury and inflammation increased local and systemic interleukin-6 levels, and augmented mortality in comparison with controls [11]. In the brain, all of this increases the susceptibility to ischemic damage by increasing the permeability of the BBB, which can cause brain edema, bleeding, inflammation, and ischemia–reperfusion injury. It is also known that uremia-induced oxidative stress generates an overactivation of N-methyl-D-aspartate (NMDA) receptors and increases nitric oxide synthesis, leading to formation of peroxynitrite and protein nitration. These alterations can promote cognitive decline through both biochemical and structural changes within the CNS [12] (Fig. 8.1).

8.5   Uremia

AKI is defined by an increase in serum creatinine, which reflects the decline in the glomerular filtration rate and thereby retention of waste products, including urea. Increased uremia is known to have diverse complications, in both acute and chronic kidney disease. Urea being an osmotically active solute, it causes water changes in intracellular and extracellular space, particularly when an abrupt increase in its concentrations occurs, and compensatory mechanisms have little time to act. Serositis, pericarditis, nausea, vomiting, coagulopathy, and, especially relevant here, uremic encephalopathy may develop. Finally, a global cerebral dysfunction occurs, and patients may present with altered mental status, delirium, hypervigilance or decreased alertness, hallucinations, disorganized speech, and disorientation. Coma is the end stage of this clinical syndrome.

Uremic encephalopathy is not only due to the elevated levels of urea, but is characterized by accumulation of other waste products which act as neurotoxins. Guanidine compounds, indoxyl sulfates, phenols, and indolic acid, among others, have been described. The pathophysiological mechanism involving this accumulation is organic anion transporters (OATs) responsible for the excretion of uremic toxins that can be found in the kidney and the brain. A reduction of the expression of various subtypes of these transporters during AKI has been observed, particularly a downregulation of cerebral OAT3. This results in a decreasing efflux of drugs and organic solutes from the brain [13, 14]. Other molecule transport channels that are altered during uremia are the aquaporins (AQP) and urea transporters (UTs). A decrease in UTs and a concomitant increase in AQP expression have been evidenced in the brain of uremic rats [15]. Although the exact mechanism is still unknown, it can be a cause of brain edema, and specifically can provide a pathophysiologic explanation basis for the dialysis disequilibrium syndrome. The dialysis disequilibrium syndrome is a complication that arises from an excessive decrease of blood urea in a CKD patient as a result of dialysis. The sudden modification in blood urea cannot be accompanied by the same extent of decrease in urea in brain cells. Therefore, the osmotic gradient between the brain cells and the blood will force water into the brain compartment due to osmosis, leading to brain swelling. This pathology presents with headache, muscle cramps, and restlessness in a patient with a history of a recent dialysis session [16, 17].

The precise pathophysiology of the symptoms caused by brain accumulation of uremic toxins is still partially unknown. However, several pathophysiological mechanisms have been hypothesized and experimentally studied. Impaired synaptic function can explain the clinical cerebral disorders. Guanidine compounds are found to be increased in the brain and cerebral spinal fluid in renal failure, and to act as sodium/potassium ATPase pump inhibitors, an essential pump for neuronal metabolism, as well as inhibiting the release of neurotransmitters such as GABA. This phenomenon leads to neurotransmitter imbalance, and consequently neuroexcitatory effects which were related to convulsions in rodent studies [18]. It can also stimulate leukocytes to produce lipopolysaccharides and TNF-α [19]. Indoxyl sulfate, another uremic solute, has been known to cause vascular inflammation and contribute to causing the mentioned neurological symptoms [20].

It is proposed that one of the damage mechanisms of these neurotoxins is oxidative stress, which is known to cause mitochondrial dysfunction. Acknowledging that urea is also a by-product of the purine metabolism that requires mitochondrial enzymes to work, an impaired function will hence increase the urea production. Moreover, it prevents cells from adequately utilizing ATP for physiological functions, leading to further oxidative stress, neuronal injury, and endothelial dysfunction. As previously mentioned, oxidative stress causes inflammation, disruption of the BBB, and neuronal lipid peroxidation and degeneration [10]. The maintenance of the myelin sheath is furthermore defective, as it was found that uremia inhibits the transketolase enzyme, essential for the lipidic axon covering formation [21]. This demyelination also occurs in the peripheral nervous system, leading to distal motor and sensory neuropathy characterized by burning sensations and weakness [16] (Fig. 8.1).

8.6 Metabolic Acidosis and Drug Toxicity

The kidney plays an imperative role in acid-base regulation, and a correct pH is crucial for an adequate internal milieu and homeostasis. Minimal but abrupt changes can have drastic effects on neuronal metabolism. Physiologically, the neurons depend upon movement of ions and electrical gradients in order to fire a response. When the kidney function diminishes and the remaining function is unable to eliminate acidic components, excess protons can activate ion channels, leading to an influx of sodium and calcium into the cell, and consequently causing a depolarization. This will not only lead to uncontrolled neuronal impulses, but can also cause cellular damage and cell death [22, 23]. Furthermore, acidosis also causes changes in free and bound concentrations of calcium and magnesium, which promote cellular ion fluxes and changes in electrical gradients as well. It is worth mentioning that these changes in protein binding involve not only ions, but also azotemic toxins and drugs with a high protein affinity. Apart from challenging its therapeutic effectiveness, this can also cause neurotoxicity. This happens with penicillin antibiotics, which compete for OAT transport channels. In an AKI scenario, a decreased clearance can lead to a penicillin-associated encephalopathy. This can also happen with tacrolimus and acyclovir, as well as with phenytoin, an anti-epileptic drug that acts on sodium channels recuperation on brain neurons, and hence altered pharmacokinetics can increase toxicity [24, 25].

Another deleterious effect of metabolic acidosis in the nervous system is the affectation of specific enzymes crucial for a correct functioning, such as glutamate dehydrogenase (GDH). This enzyme is involved in the metabolism of glutamate, the primary excitatory neurotransmitter in the brain. It catalyzes an oxidative deamination reaction and uses cofactors NAD(P)H and NAD(P)+, depending on the direction of the reaction. Acidosis has an impact on the affinity of GDH for these protons needed to act. A resultant increased affinity for ammonia [NH_4^+] causes oxidative deamination of glutamate and hence alters neurotransmitter balance, with an excess of ammonia cycling between neurons and astrocytes, affecting neuronal plasticity [26, 27] (Fig. 8.1).

8.7 Pathological Activation of Neurohormonal Systems

During AKI, neurohormonal systems, which under normal conditions function toward the maintenance of homeostasis, become activated and have pathological implications. For instance, the RAAS is one of the crucial roles the kidney plays to achieve a correct functioning of the organism by balancing sodium and potassium levels, regulating plasma volume and blood pressure. During AKI the RAAS is activated. Even if it is due to a hypovolemic AKI that needs a higher perfusion pressure, or as a response to inflammation and kidney cell damage, the subsequent circulating angiotensin II (Ang II) elicits responses that can perpetuate kidney and brain damage. Ang II has a vasoconstrictor effect on blood vessels, and oxygen reactive species increase the endothelial cell's sensitivity to this effect. Systemic inflammation is also responsible for increasing fibroblast growth factor 2 (FGF2) secretion, which furthermore increases vascular tone [28]. These hemodynamic changes can result in an impaired brain blood flow and increase the chances of brain ischemia and neuronal damage.

Ang II usually interacts with the parts of the brain which are free from the protection of the BBB, such as the circumventricular organs, which participate in the regulation of blood pressure. However, as previously discussed, AKI can lead to a disruption of the BBB, therefore permitting Ang II to reach the brain under this pathological condition. Angiotensin is known to modulate synaptic transmission in important areas such as the hypothalamus, hippocampus, and nucleus of the solitary tract. It was evidenced that it increases sympathetic transmissions as it promotes the release of norepinephrine, via the interaction with the Ang II receptor, the AT1 [29]. This receptor, together with the isoforms AT2 and AT4, is found in areas of the brain responsible for cognition and memory. By modulation of neurotransmitter balance (sympathetic, as well as glutamatergic and gamma-aminobutyric acid-ergic neurons), it is believed that it has detrimental effects on neuronal development and normal cognitive processes [30].

Another system that is altered during AKI is the calcium-phosphate metabolism and parathyroid hormone (PTH). Current hypotheses propose that the uremic state and acidosis characteristic of renal failure lead to an increase in the serum PTH and calcium levels [31]. Evidence of this effect in an acute setting varies and is far from being established. Hypocalcemia is a common condition during AKI. This may be due to phosphate sequestration in hyperphosphatemia, decreased 1,25 dihydroxy vitamin D kidney synthesis, cytokine upregulation of calcium sensing channels that interfere with the negative feedback mechanism, and skeletal resistance to PTH [32]. On the other hand, studies revealed that secondary hyperparathyroidism in AKI causes increased calcium levels in the cerebral cortex and synaptosomes. Acknowledging that calcium ions are important for electric gradient and neuronal action potential, an imbalance impairs nerve transmission and function [33]. The deleterious effects of an increased PTH are more pronounced in the chronic condition of kidney failure. In this setting, there are increases in GABA levels, as well as in fibroblast growth factor 23 (FGF23) and impaired dimethylarginine (ADMA) levels. The latter has been particularly associated with cognitive impairment and depression in patients with CKD [1, 34] (Fig. 8.1).

8.8 Protective Responses During Injury

Fortunately, the physiological kidney–brain communication pathways and crosstalk via the peripheral nervous system allow for adequate responses during injury that protects from extensive damage and remote organ failure. Afferent sensory nerves of the kidney send signals which are primarily integrated in the hypothalamus and the brainstem. On the other hand, efferent sympathetic fibers emerge from the medullary raphe nuclei, rostral ventrolateral and ventromedial medulla, and pontine cells of the hypothalamus [35]. The interaction between both pathways gives rise to the 'inhibitory renorenal reflex,' which controls the sodium equilibrium. It was evidenced that a high intake of sodium increases the afferent activity and consequently inhibits the efferent renal sympathetic impulses, leading to an increase in urinary sodium excretion. Conversely, a low sodium intake inhibits the afferent activity, resulting in an augmented efferent sympathetic activity which causes a decrease in sodium excretion in order to maintain an adequate blood volume [36, 37].

The cholinergic pathway has been identified as a potent immunomodulator, showing how the integration of sensory perceptive signals and efferent responses in the brain can offer protection during organ stress and damage. Although its implication in pathophysiological responses is not well established, it has been studied as an alternative treatment for various injury scenarios. It was proven that the cholinergic vagus nerve, the tenth cranial nerve, sends signals through the celiac plexus and spleen nerve. The consequent noradrenaline released in the neuron terminals, through the adrenergic receptors present in T lymphocytes and macrophages, inhibits the secretion of pro-inflammatory mediators, hence limiting the immune response [38, 39]. Rodent models of acute kidney ischemia and reperfusion injury were used to investigate the effect of neuroimmunomodulation and vagus nerve stimulation. Several studies evidenced that ultrasound prior to and during AKI significantly improved the renal injury and deleterious outcomes [40, 41].

Erythropoietin (EPO), a peptide hormone produced by renal tubular interstitial cells, has long been identified for its role in promoting hematopoiesis. It has also been studied as a potential nephroprotective agent in injury conditions [42, 43]. EPO acts as an anti-apoptotic agent, and some of its mechanisms that offer protection in cases of ischemic kidney injury are protecting the cytoskeleton, increasing nephrin expression in podocytes, and promoting proliferation of stromal cells [44]. As the EPO receptor (EPOR) is expressed in various other tissues apart from the kidney and the bone marrow, it can be inferred that these anti-inflammatory and anti-apoptotic effects can also be exerted in multiple other stressful conditions. The BBB and neurons have EPOR, and it has been demonstrated that during infarcts EPOR expression increases in vascular endothelium and microvessels of neuronal fibers [45]. It was proved that astrocytes also expressed the EPO genes during hypoxia [45–47]. All of this suggests that EPO has a protective role in the brain during hypoxic conditions. Another hypothesis sustaining this idea is that EPO can act as a vasodilator or vasoconstrictor, depending on the context in which it is being secreted. It has been found that it induces dilation in cases of cerebral ischemia and myocardial infarction. In vivo studies even evidenced that it can reverse the increased permeability that the VEGF has on the BBB [48]. In contrast, it has also been shown that it is involved in atherosclerosis and hypertension mechanisms. However, these opposite actions depend on the nitric oxide (NO) levels. EPO can promote NO synthesis during stressful conditions such as ischemia, while inhibiting its production in other situations [49]. The transcendence of this physiological crosstalk relies upon the fact that it has been studied as a potential neuroprotective agent in therapeutic strategies. In vitro studies demonstrated that EPO reduces neuron apoptosis in the presence of glycation end-products, suggesting a possible protection in diabetic patients [50]. However, other randomized trials that evaluated EPO treatment in brain trauma and neuroprotection were not as promising [51, 52].

8.9   Conclusion

The brain is the organ responsible for integrating all our organism's signals. Nervous impulses and hormonal mediators orchestrate the body's major purpose: survival. The complexity of the brain's anatomy and physiology with the presence of a particular circulation, neurotransmitters, neuroendocrine integration, the BBB, and afferent/efferent fibers makes it susceptible to damage, regardless of and beyond its anatomical proximity. Acute kidney injury and brain damage are commonly associated in critically ill patients. This is particularly the case because ischemia in either of them, given their function in controlling blood volume and pressure, can lead to reduced perfusion and hypoxic damage. However, numerous mechanisms are also involved in this pathological crosstalk. The combination of systemic inflammation and uremia present in kidney failure is responsible for eliciting brain inflammation, cytokine production, and endothelial damage, causing changes in neurotransmitter balance, altering synaptic function, and contributing to brain excitotoxicity. The subsequent disruption of the BBB is an essential mechanism of damage that leads to brain edema, drug toxicity, and impaired molecule trafficking due to the loss of normal transport channels. This is the basis of the neurological clinical picture present in patients with kidney failure. It should be noted that the communication in this pathological scenario further allows for a correct counteractive response aimed at limiting damage and favoring recovery. The extent of damage is therefore determined by the amount of damage that cannot be compensated by an adequate brain response.

References

1. Afsar B, Sag AA, Yalcin CE, Kaya E, Siriopol D, Goldsmith D, Covic A, Kanbay M. Brain-kidney cross-talk: definition and emerging evidence. Eur J Intern Med. 2016;36:7–12.
2. Nongnuch A, Panorchan K, Davenport A. Brain–kidney crosstalk. Crit Care. 2014;18:1–11. Accessed 15 Jul 2021.
3. Liu M, Liang Y, Chigurupati S, Lathia JD, Pletnikov M, Sun Z, Crow M, Ross CA, Mattson MP, Hamid R. Acute kidney injury leads to inflammation and functional changes in the brain. J Am Soc Nephrol. 2008;19:1360–70.
4. Grisk O. The sympathetic nervous system in acute kidney injury. Acta Physiol. 2020;228:e13404.

5. Hart BL. Biological basis of the behavior of sick animals. Neurosci Biobehav Rev. 1988;12:123–37.
6. Dantzer R, Kelley KW. Twenty years of research on cytokine-induced sickness behavior. Brain Behav Immun. 2007;2:153–60.
7. Civiletti F, Assenzio B, Mazzeo AT, Medica D, Giaretta F, Deambrosis I, Fanelli V, Ranieri VM, Cantaluppi V, Mascia L. Acute tubular injury is associated with severe traumatic brain injury: in vitro study on human tubular epithelial cells. Sci Rep. 2019;9:6090.
8. Morganti-Kossmann MC, Kossmann T, Wahl SM. Cytokines and neuropathology. Trends Pharmacol Sci. 1992;13:286–91.
9. Davenport A. Management of acute kidney injury in neurotrauma. Hemodial Int. 2010;14:27–31.
10. Kovalčíková A, Gyurászová M, Vavrincová-Yaghi D, Vavrinec P, Tóthová L, Boor P, Šebeková K, Celec P. Oxidative stress in the brain caused by acute kidney injury. Metab Brain Dis. 2018;33:961–7.
11. Li X, Hassoun HT, Santora R, Rabb H. Organ crosstalk: the role of the kidney. Curr Opin Crit Care. 2009;15:481–7.
12. Lu R, Kiernan MC, Murray A, Rosner MH, Ronco C. Kidney-brain crosstalk in the acute and chronic setting. Nat Rev Nephrol. 2015;11:707–19.
13. Schneider R, Sauvant C, Betz B, Otremba M, Fischer D, Holzinger H, Wanner C, Galle J, Gekle M. Downregulation of organic anion transporters OAT1 and OAT3 correlates with impaired secretion of para-aminohippurate after ischemic acute renal failure in rats. Am J Physiol Renal Physiol. 2007;292:1599–605.
14. Risso MA, Sallustio S, Sueiro V, Bertoni V, Gonzalez-Torres H, Musso CG. The importance of tubular function in chronic kidney disease. Int J Nephrol Renov Dis. 2019;12:257–62.
15. Trinh-Trang-Tan MM, Cartron JP, Bankir L. Molecular basis for the dialysis disequilibrium syndrome: altered aquaporin and urea transporter expression in the brain. Nephrol Dial Transplant. 2005;20:1984–8.
16. Burn DJ, Bates D. Neurology and the kidney. J Neurol Neurosurg Psychiatry. 1998;65:810–21.
17. Davenport A. Renal replacement therapy for the patient with acute traumatic brain injury and severe acute kidney injury. Contrib Nephrol. 2007;156:333–9.
18. Hooge RD, Peib YQ, Marescau B, De Deyn PP. Convulsive action and toxicity of uremic guanidino compounds: behavioral assessment and relation to brain concentration in adult mice. J Neurol Sci. 1992;112:96–105.
19. Glorieux GL, Dhondt AW, Jacobs P, Van Langeraert B, Lameire NH, De Deyn PP, Vanholder RC. In vitro study of the potential role of guanidines in leukocyte functions related to atherogenesis and infection. Kidney Int. 2004;65:2184–92.
20. Leong SC, Sirich TL. Indoxyl sulfate-review of toxicity and therapeutic strategies. Toxins. 2016;8:1–13.
21. Van Dijck A, Van Daele W, De Deyn PP. Uremic encephalopathy. Miscellanea on encephalopathies—a second look. InTech; 2021. p. 23–38.
22. Zha XM. Acid-sensing ion channels: trafficking and synaptic function. Mol Brain. 2013;6:13.
23. Samways DSK, Harkins AB, Egan TM. Native and recombinant ASIC1a receptors conduct negligible Ca^{2+} entry. Cell Calcium. 2009;45:319–25.
24. Vanholder R, Van Landschoot N, De Smet R, Schoots A, Ringoir S. Drug protein binding in chronic renal failure: evaluation of nine drugs. Kidney Int. 1988;33:996–1004.
25. Vilay AM, Churchwell MD, Mueller BA. Clinical review: drug metabolism and nonrenal clearance in acute kidney injury. Crit Care. 2008;12:235.
26. McKenna MC. Glutamate dehydrogenase in brain mitochondria: do lipid modifications and transient metabolon formation influence enzyme activity? Neurochem Int. 2011;59:525–33.
27. Pajęcka K, Wendel Nielsen C, Schousboe A, Waagepetersen HS, Plaitakis A. The effect of pH and ADP on ammonia affinity for human glutamate dehydrogenases. Metab Brain Dis. 2013;28:127–31.

28. Zhao L, Cao X, Li L, Wang X, Wang Q, Jiang S, Tang C, Zhou S, Xu N, Cui Y, Hu W, Fei L, Zheng Z, Chen L, Schmidt MO, Wei Q, Zhao J, Labes R, Patzak A, Wilcox CS, Fu X, Wellstein A, Yin La E. Acute kidney injury sensitizes the brain vasculature to Ang II (Angiotensin II) constriction via FGFBP1 (Fibroblast Growth Factor Binding Protein 1). Hypertension. 2020;76:1924–34.
29. Pan HL. Brain angiotensin II and synaptic transmission. Neuroscientist. 2004;10:422–31.
30. Malek M. Brain consequences of acute kidney injury: focusing on the hippocampus. Kidney Res Clin Pract. 2018;37:315–22.
31. Arieff AI, Massry SG. Calcium metabolism of brain in acute renal failure. Effects of uremia, hemodialysis, and parathyroid hormone. J Clin Invest. 1974;53:387–92.
32. Leaf DE, Christov M. Dysregulated mineral metabolism in AKI. Semin Nephrol. 2019;39:41–56.
33. Akman C, Ülker Çakır D, Bakırdöğen S, Balcı S. The effect of serum calcium levels on uremic encephalopathy in patients with acute kidney injury in the emergency department. Medicina. 2019;55:1–5.
34. Kielstein H, Suntharalingam M, Perthel R, Song R, Schneider SM, Martens-Lobenhoffer J, Jäger K, Bode-Böger SM, Kielstein JT. Role of the endogenous nitric oxide inhibitor asymmetric dimethylarginine (ADMA) and brain-derived neurotrophic factor (BDNF) in depression and behavioural changes: clinical and preclinical data in chronic kidney disease. Nephrol Dial Transplant. 2015;30:1699–705.
35. Solano-Flores LP, Rosas-Arellano MP, Ciriello J. Fos induction in central structures after afferent renal nerve stimulation. Brain Res. 1997;753:102–19.
36. Tanaka S, Okusa MD. Crosstalk between the nervous system and the kidney. Kidney Int. 2020;97:466–76.
37. Kopp UC, Cicha MZ, Smith LA. Endogenous angiotensin modulates PGE2-mediated release of substance P from renal mechanosensory nerve fibers. Am J Phys Regul Integr Comp Phys. 2002;282:19–30.
38. Bratton O, Martelli D, McKinley MJ, Trevaks D, Anderson CR, McAllen RM. Neural regulation of inflammation: no neural connection from the vagus to splenic sympathetic neurons. Exp Physiol. 2012;97:1180–5.
39. Martelli D, McKinley MJ, McAllen RM. The cholinergic anti-inflammatory pathway: a critical review. Auton Neurosci. 2014;182:65–9.
40. Gigliotti JC, Huang L, Bajwa A, Ye H, Mace EH, Hossack JA, Okusa MD. Ultrasound modulates the splenic neuroimmune axis in attenuating AKI. J Am Soc Nephrol. 2015;26:2470–81.
41. Wasilczuk KM, Bayer KC, Somann JP, Albors GO, Sturgis J, Lyle LT, Irazoqui PP. Modulating the inflammatory reflex in rats using low-intensity focused ultrasound stimulation of the vagus nerve. Ultrasound Med Biol. 2019;45:481–9.
42. Peng B, Kong G, Yang C, Ming Y. Erythropoietin and its derivatives: from tissue protection to immune regulation. Cell Death Dis. 2020;11(2):79. https://doi.org/10.1038/s41419-020-2276-8.
43. Suresh S, Rajvanshi PK, Noguchi CT. The many facets of erythropoietin physiologic and metabolic response. Front Physiol. 2020;10:1534. https://doi.org/10.3389/fphys.2019.01534.
44. Bi B, Guo J, Marlier A, Lin SR, Cantley LG. Erythropoietin expands a stromal cell population that can mediate renoprotection. Am J Physiol Renal Physiol. 2008;295(4):F1017–22. https://doi.org/10.1152/ajprenal.90218.2008.
45. Bernaudin M, Bellail A, Marti HH, Yvon A, Vivien D, Duchatelle I, Mackenzie ET, Petit E. Neurons and astrocytes express EPO mRNA: oxygen-sensing mechanisms that involve the redox-state of the brain. Glia. 2000;30:271–8.
46. Sirén AL, Knerlich F, Poser W, Gleiter CH, Brück W, Ehrenreich H. Erythropoietin and erythropoietin receptor in human ischemic/hypoxic brain. Acta Neuropathol. 2001;101:271–6.
47. Silachev DN, Isaev NK, Pevzner IB, Zorova LD, Stelmashook EV, Novikova SV, Zorov DB. The mitochondria-targeted antioxidants and remote kidney preconditioning ameliorate brain damage through kidney-to-brain cross-talk. PLoS One. 2012;7(12):e51553.

48. Martinez-Estrada OM, Rodriguez-Millan E, Vicente EG, Reina M, Vilaro S, Fabre M. Erythropoietin protects the in vitro blood-brain barrier against VEGF-induced permeability. Eur J Neurosci. 2003;18:2538–44.
49. Onal EM, Sag AA, Sal O, Yerlikaya B, Afsar B, Kanbay M. Erythropoietin mediates brain-vascular-kidney crosstalk and may be a treatment target for pulmonary and resistant essential hypertension. Clin Exp Hypertens. 2017;39:197–209.
50. Shen J, Wu Y, Xu JY, Zhang J, Sinclair SH, Yanoff M, Xu GT. ERK- and Akt-dependent neuroprotection by erythropoietin (EPO) against glyoxal-AGEs via modulation of Bcl-xL, Bax, and BAD. Invest Opthalmol Vis Sci. 2010;51:35–46.
51. Juul SE, Comstock BA, Wadhawan R, Mayock DE, Courtney SE, Robinson T, Heagerty PJ. A randomized trial of erythropoietin for neuroprotection in preterm infants. N Engl J Med. 2020;382:233–43.
52. Nichol A, French C, Little L, Haddad S, Presneill J, Arabi Y, Bellomo R. Erythropoietin in traumatic brain injury (EPO-TBI): a double-blind randomised controlled trial. Lancet. 2015;386:2499–506.

Chapter 9
Kidney–Lung Crosstalk in Acute Kidney Injury

Olivia Maria Capalbo and Ventura Simonovich

9.1 Introduction

The body's anatomical and physiological characteristics offer the perfect organ communication pathway for coordination and homeostasis in order to provide a suitable environment. Broadly speaking, the circulatory and nervous system are the two main routes for hormones, chemical messengers, neurotransmitters, and countless mediators to reach distant organs in this "crosstalk" scenario and cause remote changes in either physiological conditions or pathological organ-specific diseases.

The kidney and lung have several characteristics and similarities that outline how both are bound to reach one another. They have an extensive capillary network since they receive all of the cardiac output with the purpose of filtrating or oxygenating the blood, respectively. They also have similar cell polarization and salt-water channels. This allows orchestration of crucial functions such as acid-base management, erythropoietin production, renin-angiotensin-aldosterone system (RAAS) activation for an adequate vascular tone, and fluid balance [1, 2]. The importance of acknowledging this relies upon the fact that when either of these two organs is injured, the other might suffer too, and hence needs special consideration when planning clinical care.

Understanding the underlying pathological mechanisms of damage in each clinical situation that can lead to renal and/or respiratory failure can provide a solid foundation for recognizing the severity of any individual patient and what to expect from the clinical picture's evolution. Not only will it provide a greater awareness

O. M. Capalbo · V. Simonovich (✉)
Physiology Department, Instituto Universitario del Hospital Italiano de Buenos Aires, Buenos Aires, Argentina
e-mail: ventura.simonovich@hospitalitaliano.org.ar

© The Author(s), under exclusive license to Springer Nature Switzerland AG 2023
C. G. Musso, A. Covic (eds.), *Organ Crosstalk in Acute Kidney Injury*,
https://doi.org/10.1007/978-3-031-36789-2_9

and anticipation for any possible mortal complication, but it will also enlighten the way for new ways of prevention.

9.2 Pathophysiology

A broad spectrum of diseases and pathological conditions can account for the cause of acute kidney injury (AKI) or acute lung injury (ALI) in any severely ill patient. Reinforcing the concept that there is a continuous crosstalk between organs, any specific situation that injures one can in turn affect the other. For example, pneumonia being a risk factor for developing AKI, or in an AKI scenario developing lung dysfunction is the most adverse outcome [3, 4]. There are some conditions not necessarily arousing from either organ that affects both, such as sepsis with multiorgan dysfunction (MOD) [5, 6]. In any case, patients who have acute respiratory distress syndrome (ARDS) have a greater chance of developing AKI (and vice versa), and also patients with both conditions can duplicate their mortality rates [2, 7]. The need for mechanical ventilation (MV) is higher in patients with AKI, and in this clinical scenario, the in-hospital mortality rate dramatically increases, as MV is an independent predictor of mortality [8].

Firstly, ALI is characterized by rapid alveolar damage and inflammation at neutrophils expenses. When the latest are activated, they trigger the formation of oxygen reactive species, cytokines, and proteases. This leads to epithelial damage and an increase in the alveolar-capillary barrier's permeability [9]. ARDS includes bilateral radiographic opacities and reduced lung compliance with an increase in the physiological dead space that contributes to the characteristic hypoxemia of this setting. The Berlin definition also includes that the edema cannot be explained by cardiac failure or fluid overload. It also categorizes in mild, moderate, and severe, depending on the PaO_2/FiO_2 ratio of each patient [2, 10] (Table 9.1).

On the other hand, AKI develops due to an abrupt decline in kidney function that reflects the decrease of glomerular filtration rate (GFR) and retention of waste products such as creatinine and urea [11, 12]. It is diagnosed by a significant increase in serum creatinine and the reduction of urinary volume (Table 9.2).

There are little sensitive and quick biological markers that can be looked out for in these patients. The most commonly used markers to measure kidney function are serum creatinine and blood urea nitrogen (BUN). For ARDS, the diagnosis is based upon arterial blood gases. Recent experiments show that urine IL-6 and lung myeloperoxidase (MPO) activity are sensitive and rapid markers of kidney function and lung neutrophil activation, respectively. However they are still confined to studies in mice, enhancing the need for special attention and anticipation to the clinical deterioration symptoms or late markers [5].

Table 9.1 Definitions of acute respiratory distress syndrome

Acute respiratory distress syndrome
Berlin definition:
• Timing: respiratory symptoms within 1 week of known insult.
• Chest imaging (X-ray or CT scan): nodules or bilateral opacities not fully explained by effusion, lobar collapse, nor lung collapse.
• Cause of edema: not fully explained by cardiac cause or fluid overload with evidence form objective diagnostic tools.
Severity assessment:
• Mild: PaO_2/FiO_2 >200 mmHg but ≤300 mmHg with PEEP or CPAP ≥ 5 cm H_2O.
• Moderate: PaO_2/FiO_2 > 100 mmHg but ≤200 mmHg with PEEP or CPAP ≥ 5 cm H_2O.
• Severe: PaO_2/FiO_2 ≤ 100 mmHg with PEEP or CPAP ≥ 5 cm H_2O.
Causes:
• Sepsis.
• Major trauma and/or burn injuries.
• Near drowning.
• Viral pneumonitis.
• Pneumonia (bacterial infection or aspiration pneumonia).
• Inhalation injury (chemical fumes or smokes).
• Drug overdose (cocaine or opioids).
• Massive blood transfusions.

9.3 Renal-Induced Lung Damage

It is well known that AKI leads to accumulation of toxic substances such as urea, to fluid overload, electrolyte imbalance, and metabolic acidosis. In the lungs, this overall leads to altered lung mechanics and gas exchange, edema, and compensatory hyperventilation. Additionally, it is known that the kidney upregulates and secretes cytokines, hence kidney injury involves a systemic inflammation where chemokines produced act upon distant organs causing neutrophil infiltration, capillary leak, endothelial dysfunction, oxidative stress, among others. This proinflammatory state is being studied only recently and is opening many doors in understanding how and why the magnitude of the multi-organ damage in different scenarios [13, 14] (Fig. 9.1).

9.3.1 Cytokine Induced Damage

Cytokines are small peptides secreted by numerous cells that have autocrine, paracrine, and endocrine actions in order to modulate the immune system. Subfamilies include chemokines, lymphokines, interferon, interleukins, and all through cell signaling are responsible for events such as [15, 16]:

• Neutrophil and lymphocyte migration and adhesion

Table 9.2 Definitions of acute kidney injury

Acute kidney injury
Definition (KDIGO guidelines):
• Increase in serum creatinine by $\geq$0.3 mg/dL ($\geq$26.5 µmol/L) within 48 h, or
• Increase in serum creatinine to $\geq$1.5 times baseline within the prior 7 days, or
• Urine volume <0.5 mL/kg/h for 6 h.
Staging criteria:
• Stage 1: Increase in serum creatinine to 1.5–1.9 times baseline, **or** increase in serum creatinine by $\geq$0.3 mg/dL, **or** reduction in urine output to <0.5 mL/kg/h for 6–12 h.
• Stage 2: Increase in serum creatinine to 2.0–2.9 times baseline, **or** reduction in urine output to <0.5 mL/kg/h for $\geq$12 h.
• Stage 3: Increase in serum creatinine to 3.0 times baseline, **or** increase in serum creatinine to $\geq$4.0 mg/dl, **or** reduction in urine output to <0.3 mL/kg/h for $\geq$24 h, **or** anuria for $\geq$12 h, **or** the initiation of kidney replacement therapy, **or**, in patients <18 years, decrease in estimated glomerular filtration rate (eGFR) to <35 mL/min/1.73 m^2.
Causes:
• Hypovolemia (acute hemorrhage, diarrhea).
• Low arterial pressure (sepsis, anaphylaxis).
• Effective hypovolemia (systolic heart failure with reduced ejection fraction, decompensated liver disease with portal hypertension, hepatorenal syndrome).
• Nonsteroidal anti-inflammatory drugs.
• Iodinated radiocontrast media.
• Renal vascular disease (microangiopathy hemolytic anemia, thrombotic thrombocytopenic purpura-hemolytic uremic syndrome, malignant hypertension, scleroderma.
• Glomerular disease (nephritic or nephrotic pattern).
• Tubular or interstitial disease (ischemic or after nephrotoxic drug exposure).
• Obstructive nephropathy.

- Caspase activation and subsequent cell apoptosis
- Oxidative stress
- Changes in actin assembly and cytoskeleton (this leads to greater cellular gap and alteration of pulmonary endothelial-epithelial barrier)
- Increased vascular permeability
- Anti-inflammatory effects, which are usually unbalanced

Altogether are accountable for lung inflammation and ALI in the context of AKI. Blood testing and laboratory experiments help elucidate the specific effects of each cytokine. Taking into account the advancement of biological molecules and technology, counteracting or mimicking certain effects may eventually play a part in treatment and prevention [17].

IL-6 is a well-known and studied proinflammatory cytokine that rises in multiple acute and chronic conditions and serves as a reliable serum marker of inflammation. It stimulates the production of CXCL-1 and MIP-2, chemokines that through the CXCR2 receptor causes the infiltration of neutrophils which perpetuates cytokine production and the inflammatory response. It also causes lung endothelial cells to produce IL-8 which furthermore increases neutrophils in the alveolar space [1, 18].

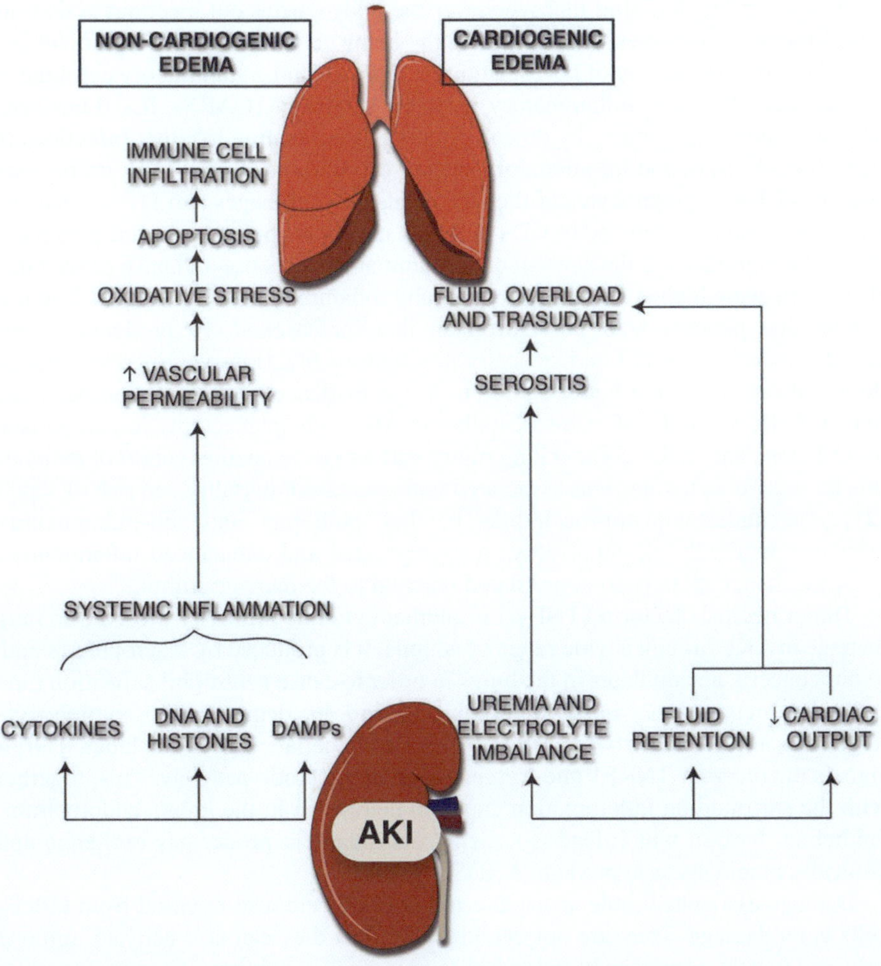

Fig. 9.1 Kidney–lung crosstalk during acute kidney injury (AKI). *DAMPs* damage-associated molecular pattern

It is proposed IL-8 plays a central role in the development of ALI in the context of AKI, as it was found to be increased in serum and bronchoalveolar fluid, and correlated with prolonged MV and mortality [19]. These two adverse outcomes were also shown in several studies in mice that measured and evidenced an increase in serum IL-6 after nephrectomy, ischemic AKI, or a sham operation [20]. Methodology in these studies also involved IL-6 deficient mice or neutralizing antibodies to block its action. In these cases, less lung inflammation, capillary leak, and reduced IL-8 levels were revealed, which were further restored when IL-6 was artificially injected, suggesting its crucial effect in inflammation and lung damage.

It is worth emphasizing that whenever the body carries out a certain action, its counteraction unleashes. IL-6, although being a proinflammatory cytokine, stimulates the production of IL-10, a quintessentially anti-inflammatory cytokine of the compensatory anti-inflammatory response syndrome (CARS). IL-10 has been shown to limit organ injury by downregulating inflammation in either infectious or noninfectious systemic inflammatory response syndrome (SIRS) [14]. Its primary source is CD4 T-lymphocytes of the spleen, also macrophages and B cells. Several studies with splenectomized or CD4 deficient mice have been conducted in order to mimic human AKI and the subsequent inflammatory response and have proven that IL-6 levels were higher, IL-10 lower, and lung inflammation was worse. In fact, it is known that patients with polymorphism that increases IL-10 production have reduced mortality in ALI and critically ill scenarios [4]. However, increased levels do not always foresee a better outcome. It was evidenced in splenectomized mice that IL-6, IL-8, and IL-10 were all higher in AKI with splenectomy in comparison to AKI alone and in this context lung injury was worse. In another cohort of patients, this increase in cytokines was associated with increased mortality and risk of sepsis [21]. The underlying approach may be that, both pro- and anti-inflammatory cytokines markedly elevated reflect a dysregulated and unbalanced inflammatory response, hence there is no coordinated reaction to the damage stimuli.

Tumor necrosis factor α (TNF-α) is another cytokine primarily involved in lung damage in AKI through a wide range of actions. It is produced by macrophages and, in our concern, accumulates in the lungs in order to cause neutrophil activation (and the subsequent release of more cytokines) and its degranulation, lymphocyte migration, and particularly activation of lung endothelial cells. In the latter, TNF-α signals the receptor TNRF1 and triggers the cell apoptotic pathway. This, together with the surrounding inflammation causes a disruption in the lung's endothelium-epithelium barrier, which leads to edema that unable a proper gas exchange and clinically manifests as hypoxia in ARDS.

Damage-associated molecular patterns (DAMPs) are also released from kidney cells upon damage. They are not cytokines, but yet they can also activate immune cells and travel through the bloodstream to unleash distant injury. The consequences of mitochondrial DAMPs released in the context of kidney ischemia-reperfusion AKI convey the effects these molecules have on lung injury. It is known that the mitochondria plays an indispensable role in the cell's function and survival, and it has been proven that these particular DAMPs lead to metabolic alteration of lung epithelial cells, particularly the fatty-acid oxidation pathway. Furthermore, they promote neutrophil infiltration and pulmonary endothelial cell's apoptosis [22].

9.3.2 Immune Cells

The cytokines mentioned above are only part of a much bigger network. They are secreted by a number of specialized immune cells in the context of AKI as an inflammatory triggering event. Spreading distantly through the bloodstream, they act as chemokines attracting other immune cells to a specific organ, and activating them as well. In this reciprocal way, they perpetuate the inflammatory response and may potentially lead to organ injury.

Neutrophils are key mediators of lung injury in AKI. Infiltration of this type of cells have been studied in multiple animal models and were reported to be elevated in early phases of lung injury, mostly within the first 2 h after kidney injury [13, 19]. Chemoattraction leads to migration toward the vascular endothelium, and the accumulation likely leads to the formation of a plug, causing congestion and microvascular occlusion.

Once settled in the tissue, neutrophils release a series of enzymes, as well as oxygen reactive species, all which derive to cell and extracellular matrix damage, compromising tissue's structure and functionality [23]. A specific protease that merits special mention is the neutrophil elastase (NE), which acts primarily on collagen, proteoglycans, and elastin found in the pulmonary cell's membrane, and especially on the surrounding matrix. It has been studied that the NE activity increases substantially in AKI both systemically and in the lungs, demonstrating its implication in this crosstalk [18]. Sivelestat sodium hydrate is a specific NE inhibitor for clinical use in the context of ALI induced by systemic inflammation. It has been studied in mice models for specific AKI scenarios and evidenced reduced lung inflammation, furthermore enhancing its pathological role.

Methods that inhibit certain molecules can help elucidate its contribution to the pathology of a disease, as was seen with the neutralization of granulocyte colony-stimulating factor (G-CSF) that reduces lung damage in AKI. This is a cytokine involved in mature neutrophil activation and is also responsible for emergency granulopoiesis under stressful conditions, a situation that has been linked with lung injury [9].

Another emerging mechanism of damage proposed with neutrophil's involvement is necroinflammation, where necrotic renal tubular cells lead to the release of histones as damage-associated molecular patterns. The citrullination of these histones potentiates the signaling for the formation of neutrophils extracellular traps, also known as NETs and NETosis [24]. Due to the anatomical distribution, through the vena cava and given the lung's fine capillary network, they are likely to end up in the lungs. The NETs contain proinflammatory proteins, produce endothelial damage by itself, can activate the complement and coagulation cascade, and by auto-amplification induce other neutrophils to form more NETs. Studies revealed an increase in NET in ischemic and ischemia-reperfusion AKI models that can potentially be reduced by inhibitors such as anti-histone antibodies [19, 25].

Macrophages are another cellular lineage responsible for many of the pathological mechanisms of lung injury mentioned above. They come from monocytes that are recruited during inflammation and differentiate in order to secrete various cytokines that orchestrate the inflammatory response: IL-6, TNF-α, and G-CSF to name a few. This happens not only by the DAMPs exposed during AKI, but macrophages were evidenced to secrete G-CSF upon an increase of urea as well. They also up-regulate CXCL1 in the lungs, which as mentioned above causes neutrophil infiltration and activation [9, 26].

T-lymphocyte involvement reflects the bridge between innate and adaptive immunity. With regard to lung damage, T-cells are particularly implicated in lung cell apoptosis in AKI models. Cytotoxic CD8+ lymphocytes through the release of granzyme B, a serine protein present in its granules, and the Fas–Fas ligand interaction (two molecules involved in cell death regulation) cause caspase activation, which translates into cell death, vascular barrier dysfunction, and pulmonary edema [14, 27].

Cytokines are not the only products released by these immune cells. They are a major source of free radicals and oxygen reactive species that cause lipid peroxidation, mutations, and DNA damage which in turns leads to aberrant protein production for cell function and repair. It is furthermore aggravated in patients that require MV, as oxidative stress is related to high levels of oxygen administration. It is evidenced that antioxidant substances such as glutathione, beta-carotene, and vitamin C are reduced significantly in patients with ARDS [13, 23]. A constant environment of oxidative stress is also present in chronic kidney disease (CKD), and this can explain why there is evidence of DNA changes, fibrosis, cell apoptosis, and tissue damage in the lungs even when there is no objectifiable lung disease nor acute respiratory failure [28] (Table 9.3).

9.3.3 Ischemia Induced Damage

The role that an appropriate oxygen delivery has for suitable organ function and homeostasis cannot be put into question. In a kind of tendentious way, we usually attribute blood oxygenation merely to the lungs. Nevertheless, bearing the crosstalk mechanism in mind, it also depends on an adequate cardiac and kidney function. The kidneys are crucial for a proper vascular tone through renin secretion, maintaining a good preload by managing fluid balance, and for stimulating red blood cells formation via erythropoietin secretion [6]. An inadequate blood supply leads to organ stress, as it can happen in prerenal AKI, where hypovolemia causes ischemia; or after renal transplantation, as grafts undergo a period of ischemia and reperfusion.

The ischemia-reperfusion (IR) scenario causes cytokine production in the kidney, which as mentioned previously, evokes an inflammatory response and is accountable for the distant-organ damage. IR increases the mRNA expression of IL-6, TNF-α, and IL-1 not only in the kidney but in the lungs as well [29]. Another soluble mediator suggested to have a pathological role is osteopontin (OPN), a protein released from the immune cells activated in this context. It has a proinflammatory effect and can act synergistically with TNF-α in remote lung damage [30]. As inflammation itself is a solid explanation for distant organ dysfunction, studies are compelled to intervene in its progression. Anti-inflammatory effects of medications such as artesunate, or induction of heme oxygenase, which is normally up-regulated

Table 9.3 Cytokines and main immune cells involved in the inflammatory response

Cytokine	Effect	Immune cell	Effect
IL-6	Stimulates production of chemokines CXCL-1 and MIP-2, causing neutrophil infiltration. Stimulates lung endothelial cells to produce IL-8. IL-6 deficient mice have less lung inflammation and capillary leak.	Neutrophils	Accumulation may cause a microvascular plug leading to occlusion and congestion. Release of neutrophil elastase and other proteolytic enzymes that drive to extracellular matrix damage and tissue disruption. Necroinflammation: formation of NETs causing inflammation and endothelial damage.
IL-8	Increases lung neutrophil infiltration. Increased in bronchoalveolar fluid and related to prolonged mechanical ventilation and mortality.		
IL-10	Anti-inflammatory cytokine that limits the systemic inflammatory response. Prolonged and exaggerated increase may reflect an unbalanced and insufficient compensatory response.	Macrophages	Release of multiple cytokines that perpetuates inflammation and chemoattraction. Upregulation of CXCL1 in the lungs.
TNF-α	Neutrophil and lymphocyte migration and degranulation. Signals receptor TNRF1, triggering lung endothelial cell apoptosis leading to edema.	T-Lymphocytes	Involved in cell apoptosis: CD8+ lymphocytes release Granzyme B and through the Fas–FasL interaction cause caspase activation end programmed cell death.
G-CSF	Neutrophil activation and emergency granulopoiesis.		

in stressful conditions because its byproducts have cytoprotective effects, have been proven to reduce lung damage in IR models. Even though the exact mechanisms are far from being established, they furthermore highlight the importance that inflammation has as a common factor for multiple adverse outcomes of AKI [11, 31].

9.3.4 Pulmonary Edema

We have already seen that the systemic inflammation, oxidative stress, and soluble mediators cause increased capillary permeability, leakage, and epithelium-endothelium barrier dysfunction, leading to the formation of a non-hydrostatic edema. Cytokines also mediate their effects by binding to cell receptors and changing the levels of phosphorylated proteins [32]. It is believed that this explains why it has been seen that in early stages of AKI, there is a down-regulation of sodium and aquaporin channels in the lungs. In physiological conditions, these energy dependent channels create an osmotic gradient which drives water from the alveoli inside the cells. Without a suitable amount, water will accumulate and contribute to pulmonary edema [13, 23].

It has also been known for decades that uremia causes serositis and fluid effusion. This can also happen in the pericardium, which in serious conditions may lead to cardiac tamponade and fluid overload in the lungs; or as a pleural effusion itself. The edema is also present in the alveoli as well, manifesting as a reduced carbon dioxide diffusion capacity (DLCO). Pathology autopsies even described lung affectation as *"uremic pneumonitis,"* characterized by hyaline membrane formation and inflammatory exudates [33]. It is worth noticing that uremic toxins also have remote effects that can perpetuate AKI and furthermore complicate the clinical scenario. Symptoms usually present are nausea and vomiting, and a common condition in uremic patients is platelet dysfunction that can lead to hemorrhage. If any of these ends up in a significant volume depletion, prerenal AKI can be seriously aggravated, feeding the damage cycle [34, 35].

Nonetheless, this is not the only cause of water accumulation in alveolar space and lung interstitium that impairs gas exchange and respiratory mechanics. In kidney failure, most of the patients present oliguria or an important reduction in the GFR. With the subsequent water retention, the heart becomes unable to manage this excess. Bearing that the concomitant electrolyte and acid/base imbalances deteriorate its contractile function, the fluid overload ends up in the lungs, as they can hold a greater volume due to their extensive capillary network and characteristic compliance. This condition has long been recognized as an important cause of respiratory failure and is associated with increased mortality [33].

9.4 Lung-Induced Renal Damage

Considering the bidirectional nature of the organ crosstalk concept, we can now fairly imagine that when the lung is under stress, remote repercussions are always a possibility. The association of ARDS and AKI has been studied and proved [36]. Having the concepts of distant lung damage during AKI, similar mechanisms of distant kidney damage in lung injury can be proposed, always adjusting to the biological plausibility and clinical conditions that may lead to them. Organ dysfunction in the context of ARDS has been investigated and specifically AKI has been pinpointed as a need for attention, simply because, as both organs receive all of the cardiac output they have an extensive capillary network which is prone to be exposed to circulating mediators [37] (Fig. 9.2).

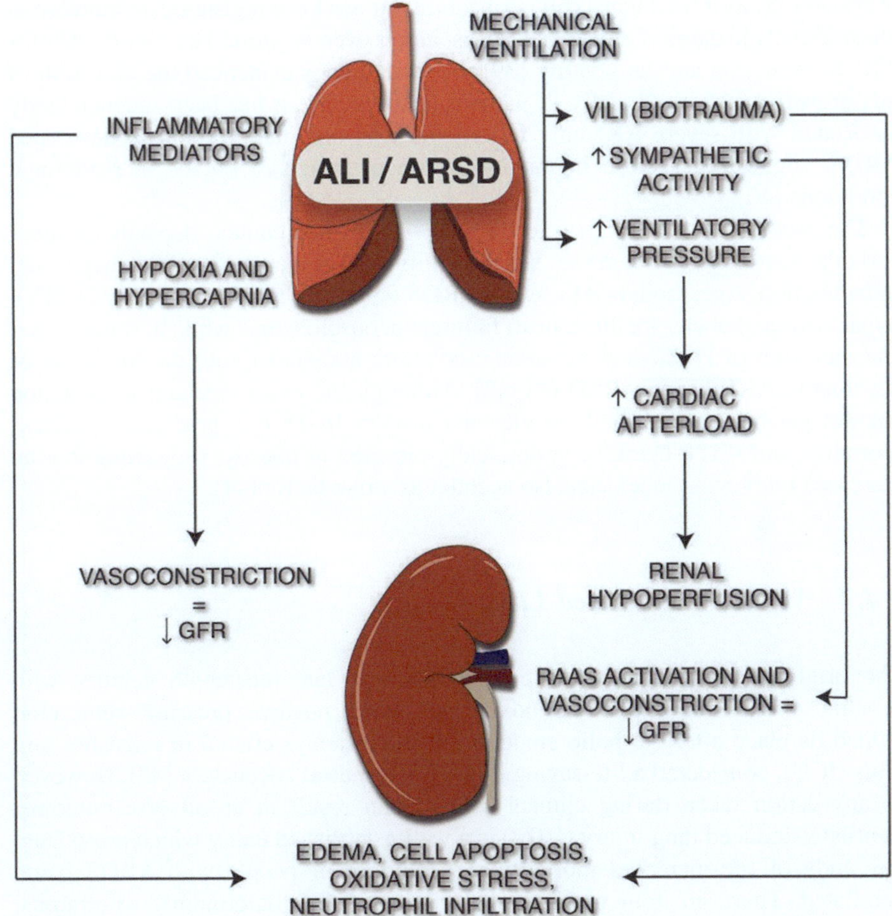

Fig. 9.2 Lung–kidney crosstalk during acute lung injury (ALI). *GFR* glomerular filtration rate, *RAS* renin-angiotensin system, *VILI* ventilator-induced lung injury, *ARDS* acute respiratory distress syndrome

9.4.1 Systemic Inflammation

IL-6, IL-1, IL-8, and TNF-α (mainly) together with the battery of immune cells mentioned in the renal-induced lung damage are not only limited to renal injury, but are the commanders of systemic inflammation arising from any injured organ. Proinflammatory mediators are also released during ALI and ARDS, affecting renal vascular tone by vasodilation of vessels and reducing perfusion pressure, as well as by activating apoptotic pathways in renal epithelial cells [6]. A particular mediator that promotes neutrophil infiltration and endothelial cell apoptosis, angiopoietin-2 (AGPT2) has been studied in ARDS pathogenesis. It acts as a marker of fluid overload [38] as it modulates cell permeability, it has been registered an increase in plasma levels in cases of shock and sepsis, and is even suggested as a biomarker for ARDS prediction and its severity [39]. Several studies evidenced the elevation of this growth factor in critically ill patients. Particularly, it has been independently associated with severe AKI only in patients who also had previously developed ARDS, suggesting a close interaction between these two organs in pathologic conditions [40].

The probability for a patient to develop AKI in this context depends on other variable factors that increase susceptibility to propagation of damage and inflammation. Age, moderate to severe ARDS (specially as it involves use of MV), hypertension, diabetes mellitus, heart failure, unconsciousness while hospitalization and elevation of D-dimer were some riskfactors associated with the likeliness of developing AKI during ARSD [41–43]. Although the exact mechanism of action has not yet been established, an elevated urinary IL-18 is a predictor of ARDS mortality, and it is a cytokine systemically elevated in obesity, suggesting that an increased body mass index can also account as a risk factor [44].

9.4.2 Ventilator-Induced Lung Injury

The origins of MV can be traced down to the late nineteenth century with subatmospheric body-enclosing boxes and when positive pressure ventilation gained its place after the polio epidemic. It is nowadays crucial in intensive care units (ICU), considered a life-saving therapy when used adequately [45]. However, as any action taken during clinical care, it can result in an adverse outcome. Ventilator-induced lung injury (VILI) is a well-established entity which arose from the study of the increased mortality in a number of people with ARDS being ventilated. There are four main mechanisms for VILI: barotrauma, volutrauma, atelectrauma, and biotrauma. Systematic reviews of invasive mechanical ventilation as a risk factor evidenced a distressing three-fold risk of developing AKI [46].

Reasonably if there is a notable trauma and/or atelectasis in the lungs that derives to a significant hypoxemia the kidneys will suffer in the context of a multiorgan dysfunction, specially being a highly metabolic organ susceptible to minimal changes in blood oxygen levels due to the amount of energy it requires to work. Anyhow, biotrauma deserves special attention when considering remote kidney injury during MV. It consists of a biological proinflammatory response of the lungs that can emerge from direct cell injury or indirectly by cell-signaling from the other three physical VILI mechanisms [47, 48]. Particular cytokines could be identified when scenarios of AKI during MV were replicated in animal models, as, for example, macrophage inflammatory protein (MIP-1α), NF-κB, VCAM-1 adhesion molecule, and vascular endothelial growth factor (VEGF) [7, 49]. The release of inflammatory mediators through the bloodstream reaches the kidneys, changing the expression of adhesion molecules, attracting immune cells, and even causing remote renal tubular cell apoptosis evidenced by increasing levels of circulating Fas–Fas ligand [50]. Using adequate levels of tidal volume (like the once adjusted by weight) has been studied as a protective ventilation strategy that reduces the AKI incidence during ARDS by creating a mild hypercapnic acidotic environment that acts as cytoprotective and anti-inflammatory [23].

Other mechanisms can be accounted for by the deterioration of ventilated patients, involving the decrease in the GFR. On the one hand, when high ventilatory pressures are used, this results in an increase of pressure that the right heart has to overcome. With a greater afterload, together with a reduced venous return, the cardiac output decreases, putting into danger an adequate renal perfusion. MV also activates the sympathetic nervous system and the RAAS, which drive to vasoconstriction, further decreasing the GFR [6].

9.4.3 Hypoxia and Hypercapnia

Hypercapnia has significant effects in the kidney by acting directly and indirectly in antagonistic ways with regard to changes of the vascular tone. Directly, high levels of CO_2 cause constriction of intrarenal vessels. Indirectly, it causes dilation of the systemic vasculature. The net effect is a reduction in the renal blood flow which leads to cell hypoxia and hence loss of functional and metabolic processes, and a reduction in the GFR which will lead to fluid retention and accumulation of toxic substances. This has been evidenced in patients with chronic obstructive pulmonary disease (COPD), as they may usually present with fluid retention and reduced urinary sodium excretion. In extreme emphysematous cases, where intra-abdominal pressure is extremely elevated, veins are compressed and hence with less venous drainage kidney edema can develop which will furthermore aggravate the cell's function [51].

Patients that present obstructive sleep apnea, another chronic condition, also show renal repercussions. Permanent nocturnal hypoxemia primarily induces a constant inflammatory state that is known to produce vascular disease such as atherosclerosis and is also related to hypertension [52]. The cytokines together with the vascular dysfunction, as already noted, can affect kidney function at various levels.

9.5 Conclusion

To only consider that organ communication involves a simple bidirectional cause and effect mechanism would be a reductionism. As it has been discussed, organ crosstalk is a vast network of simultaneous and consequent events, which are as complex in physiological conditions that aim to maintain homeostasis, as in a pathological state. AKI and ARDS are two everyday clinical conditions managed in hospitalization and intensive care units. When either of these major organs is injured first, we can think about the remote repercussions in two ways: functional and inflammatory. The first involves the direct effects of the loss of functionality of one organ; as it is in AKI, the accumulation of urea, fluid retention, and electrolyte imbalance will mainly lead to pulmonary edema; and in ARDS, the hypoxia will lead to renal ischemia and cell death. On the other hand, inflammation is elicited by most, if not all, of the damage mechanisms that lead to respiratory or kidney failure. Cytokines have the particularity of traveling through the bloodstream and being able to establish in distant organs, evoke inflammation, and immune cell activation. And even though here we focus specifically on the lungs and kidneys, the other organs also discussed in this book are as well-being altered, hence crosstalk comes from multiple directions.

The boundless communication pathways and mechanisms of remote organ damage in particular clinical conditions should not overwhelm when planning and delivering patient care. The objective of acknowledging this is being able to have a greater awareness of red flags and adapt to what to expect about each patient's evolution, anticipating the possible aggravating conditions. Curiosity upon organ crosstalk and its components guides studies to unfold each time more the complexity of these interactions, enlightening the pathophysiological understanding but also giving rise to novel and beneficial therapeutic approaches. The findings of these studies are clinically relevant and show the importance of an integrative approach in the management of critical patients.

References

1. Domenech P, Perez T, Saldarini A, Uad P, Musso CG. Kidney-lung pathophysiological crosstalk: its characteristics and importance. Int Urol Nephrol. 2017;49(7):1211–5.
2. Seeley EJ. Updates in the management of acute lung injury: a focus on the overlap between AKI and ARDS. Adv Chronic Kidney Dis. 2013;20(1):14–20.
3. Du J, Abdel-Razek O, Shi Q, Hu F, Ding G, Cooney RN, Wang G. Surfactant protein D attenuates acute lung and kidney injuries in pneumonia-induced sepsis through modulating apoptosis, inflammation and NF-κB signaling. Sci Rep. 2018;8(1):15393. https://doi.org/10.1038/s41598-018-33828-7.
4. Kinsey GR. The spleen as a bidirectional signal transducer in acute kidney injury. Kidney Int. 2017;91(5):1001–3.
5. Bhargava R, et al. Acute lung injury and acute kidney injury are established by four hours in experimental sepsis and are improved with pre, but not post, sepsis administration of TNF-α antibodies. PLoS One. 2013;8(11):e79037.
6. Basu RK, Wheeler DS. Kidney–lung cross-talk and acute kidney injury. Pediatr Nephrol. 2013;28(12):2239–48.
7. Hepokoski M, et al. Ventilator-induced lung injury increases expression of endothelial inflammatory mediators in the kidney. Am J Physiol Renal Physiol. 2017;312(4):F654–60.
8. Faubel S, Edelstein CL. Mechanisms and mediators of lung injury after acute kidney injury. Nat Rev Nephrol. 2016;12(1):48–60.
9. Jing W, et al. G-CSF mediates lung injury in mice with adenine-induced acute kidney injury. Int Immunopharmacol. 2018;63:1–8.
10. Costa ELV, Amato MBP. The new definition for acute lung injury and acute respiratory distress syndrome: is there room for improvement? Curr Opin Crit Care. 2013;19:16. https://journals.lww.com/co-criticalcare/fulltext/2013/02000/the_new_definition_for_acute_lung_injury_and_acute.4.aspx.

11. Rossi M, et al. HO-1 mitigates acute kidney injury and subsequent kidney-lung cross-talk. Free Radic Res. 2019;53(9–10):1035–43.
12. Goyal A, Daneshpajouhnejad P, Hashmi MF, Bashir K, John BK. Acute kidney injury (nursing). Treasure Island, FL: StatPearls Publishing; 2021.
13. Lee SA, Cozzi M, Bush EL, Rabb H. Distant organ dysfunction in acute kidney injury: a review. Am J Kidney Dis. 2018;72(6):846–56.
14. Andres-Hernando A, et al. Circulating IL-6 upregulates IL-10 production in splenic CD4+ T cells and limits acute kidney injury-induced lung inflammation. Kidney Int. 2017;91(5):1057–69.
15. Zhu M, et al. Erythropoietin ameliorates lung injury by accelerating pulmonary endothelium cell proliferation via Janus kinase-signal transducer and activator of transcription 3 pathway after kidney ischemia and reperfusion injury. Transplant Proc. 2019;51(3):972–8.
16. Ma T, Liu XW, Liu Z. Function of the p38MAPK-HSP27 pathway in rat lung injury induced by acute ischemic kidney injury. Biomed Res Int. 2013;2013:981235. https://doi.org/10.1155/2013/981235.
17. de Abreu KLS, et al. Acute kidney injury in critically ill patients with lung disease: kidney-lung crosstalk. Rev Bras Ter Intensiva. 2013;25(2):130–6.
18. Ishii T, et al. Neutrophil elastase contributes to acute lung injury induced by bilateral nephrectomy. Am J Pathol. 2010;177(4):1665–73.
19. Teixeira JP, Ambruso S, Griffin BR, Faubel S. Pulmonary consequences of acute kidney injury. Semin Nephrol. 2019;39(1):3–16.
20. Ahuja N, et al. Circulating IL-6 mediates lung injury via CXCL1 production after acute kidney injury in mice. Am J Physiol Renal Physiol. 2012;303(6):F864–72.
21. Andrés-Hernando A, et al. Splenectomy exacerbates lung injury after ischemic acute kidney injury in mice. Am J Physiol Renal Physiol. 2011;301(4):F907–16.
22. Hepokoski M, et al. Altered lung metabolism and mitochondrial DAMPs in lung injury due to acute kidney injury. Am J Physiol Lung Cell Mol Physiol. 2021;320(5):L821–31.
23. Malek M, Hassanshahi J, Fartootzadeh R, Azizi F, Shahidani S. Nephrogenic acute respiratory distress syndrome: a narrative review on pathophysiology and treatment. Chin J Traumatol. 2018;21(1):4–10.
24. Tsourouktsoglou T-D, Warnatsch A, Ioannou M, Hoving D, Wang Q, Papayannopoulos V. Histones, DNA, and citrullination promote neutrophil extracellular trap inflammation by regulating the localization and activation of TLR4. Cell Rep. 2020;31(5):107602. https://doi.org/10.1016/j.celrep.2020.107602.
25. Hayase N, et al. Recombinant thrombomodulin prevents acute lung injury induced by renal ischemia-reperfusion injury. Sci Rep. 2020;10(1):289. https://doi.org/10.1038/s41598-019-57205-0.
26. Altmann C, et al. Macrophages mediate lung inflammation in a mouse model of ischemic acute kidney injury. Am J Physiol Renal Physiol. 2012;302(4):F421–32. https://doi.org/10.1152/ajprenal.00559.2010.
27. Lie ML, White LE, Santora RJ, Park JM, Rabb H, Hassoun HT. Lung T lymphocyte trafficking and activation during ischemic acute kidney injury. J Immunol. 2012;189(6):2843–51. https://doi.org/10.4049/jimmunol.1103254.
28. Nemmar A, Karaca T, Beegam S, Yuvaraju P, Yasin J, Ali BH. Lung oxidative stress, DNA damage, apoptosis, and fibrosis in adenine-induced chronic kidney disease in mice. Front Physiol. 2017;8:896. https://doi.org/10.3389/fphys.2017.00896. eCollection 2017.
29. Tulafu M, et al. Atrial natriuretic peptide attenuates kidney-lung crosstalk in kidney injury. J Surg Res. 2014;186(1):217–25.
30. Zhao H, et al. Osteopontin mediates necroptosis in lung injury after transplantation of ischaemic renal allografts in rats. Br J Anaesth. 2019;123(4):519–30.
31. Liu Z, Qu M, Yu L, Song P, Chang Y. Artesunate inhibits renal ischemia-reperfusion-mediated remote lung inflammation through attenuating ROS-induced activation of NLRP3 inflammasome. Inflammation. 2018;41(4):1546–56. https://doi.org/10.1007/s10753-018-0801-z.

32. Ma T, Liu Z. Functions of aquaporin 1 and α-epithelial Na channel in rat acute lung injury induced by acute ischemic kidney injury. Int Urol Nephrol. 2013;45(4):1187–96. https://doi.org/10.1007/s11255-012-0355-1.
33. Doi K, Ishizu T, Fujita T, Noiri E. Lung injury following acute kidney injury: kidney–lung crosstalk. Clin Exp Nephrol. 2011;15(4):464–70.
34. Twardowski ZJ, Alpert MA, Gupta RC, Nolph KD, Madsen BT. Circulating immune complexes: possible toxins responsible for serositis (pericarditis, pleuritis, and peritonitis) in renal failure. Nephron. 1983;35(3):190–5.
35. Prezant DJ. Effect of uremia and its treatment on pulmonary function. Lung. 1990;168(1):1–14. https://doi.org/10.1007/bf02719668.
36. Darmon M, et al. Acute respiratory distress syndrome and risk of AKI among critically ill patients. Clin J Am Soc Nephrol. 2014;9(8):1347–53.
37. Kallet RH, Lipnick MS, Zhuo H, Pangilinan LP, Gomez A. Characteristics of nonpulmonary organ dysfunction at onset of ARDS based on the Berlin definition. Respir Care. 2019;64(5):493–501.
38. Fisher J, Douglas JJ, Linder A, Boyd JH, Walley KR, Russell JA. Elevated plasma angiopoietin-2 levels are associated with fluid overload, organ dysfunction, and mortality in human septic shock. Crit Care Med. 2016;44((11)):2018–27. https://doi.org/10.1097/ccm.0000000000001853.
39. van der Heijden M, van Nieuw Amerongen GP, Koolwijk P, van Hinsbergh VWM, Groeneveld ABJ. Angiopoietin-2, permeability oedema, occurrence and severity of ALI/ARDS in septic and non-septic critically ill patients. Thorax. 2008;63(10):903–9.
40. Araújo CB, et al. Angiopoietin-2 as a predictor of acute kidney injury in critically ill patients and association with ARDS. Respirology. 2019;24(4):345–51.
41. Han H, Li J, Chen D, Zhang F, Wan X, Cao C. A clinical risk scoring system of acute respiratory distress syndrome-induced acute kidney injury. Med Sci Monit. 2019;25:5606–12.
42. Kaushik S, Villacres S, Eisenberg R, Medar SS. Acute kidney injury in pediatric acute respiratory distress syndrome. J Intensive Care Med. 2020;36:1084. https://doi.org/10.1177/0885066620944042.
43. Panitchote A, et al. Factors associated with acute kidney injury in acute respiratory distress syndrome. Ann Intensive Care. 2019;9(1):74. https://doi.org/10.1186/s13613-019-0552-5.
44. Soto GJ, Frank AJ, Christiani DC, Gong MN. Body mass index and acute kidney injury in the acute respiratory distress syndrome. Crit Care Med. 2012;40(9):2601–8.
45. Slutsky AS. History of mechanical ventilation. From Vesalius to ventilator-induced lung injury. Am J Respir Crit Care Med. 2015;191((10)):1106–15.
46. van den Akker JPC, Egal M, Groeneveld ABJ. Invasive mechanical ventilation as a risk factor for acute kidney injury in the critically ill: a systematic review and meta-analysis. Crit Care. 2013;17(3):R98.
47. Beitler JR, Malhotra A, Thompson BT. Ventilator-induced lung injury. Clin. Chest Med. 2016;37(4):633–46.
48. Slutsky AS, Ranieri VM. Ventilator-induced lung injury. N Engl J Med. 2013;369((22)):2126–36.
49. Wu Y, Wang L, Meng L, Cao G-K, Zhang Y. MIP-1α and NF-κB as indicators of acute kidney injury secondary to acute lung injury in mechanically ventilated patients. Eur Rev Med Pharmacol Sci. 2016;20(18):3830–4.
50. Imai Y, et al. Injurious mechanical ventilation and end-organ epithelial cell apoptosis and organ dysfunction in an experimental model of acute respiratory distress syndrome. JAMA. 2003;289(16):2104–12.
51. Husain-Syed F, Slutsky AS, Ronco C. Lung–kidney cross-talk in the critically ill patient. Am J Respir Crit Care Med. 2016;194(4):402–14.
52. Nicholl DDM, et al. Declining kidney function increases the prevalence of sleep apnea and nocturnal hypoxia. Chest. 2012;141(6):1422–30.

Chapter 10
Kidney–Heart Crosstalk in Acute Kidney Injury

César Antonio Belziti

10.1 Introduction

Heart failure (HF) is a syndrome of high prevalence that affects over 26 million people worldwide; 15 million in Europe, 7 million in the United States of America, and 800,000 in Argentina. It has an elevated mortality rate with frequent exacerbations that cause hospitalizations. Both have human, social, and economic repercussions [1]. Acute kidney injury (AKI) is also a frequent entity that affects up to 70% of hospitalized patients in intensive care units. Some of these require renal replacement therapy, which has a mortality rate of 50% [2, 3].

The aging population and the increased prevalence of risk factors affecting both the heart and kidney, such as hypertension and diabetes mellitus, increase the rates of both heart disease and renal injury.

The heart and kidneys are closely related in such a manner that any modification in one of these organs has an effect on the other organ, establishing a bidirectional relationship. One component of this relationship is that responses generated in one organ tend to prevail and magnify in time. This generates a circuit of perpetuation that serves to maintain cardiovascular and renal homeostasis, such as arterial pressure and renal perfusion. Nevertheless, this circuit of perpetuation may lead to an inefficient adaptation, such as renal hypoxia or volume overload with HF. Therefore, the established relationship between the organs serves to maintain homeostasis still may lead to collateral organ damage.

From a pathophysiological point of view, hemodynamic mechanisms are not the only circuits that exist between heart and kidney diseases. Other mechanisms are neurohumoral responses, inflammatory responses, the development of anemia,

C. A. Belziti (✉)
Heart Failure Unit, Institute of Cardiovascular Medicine, Hospital Italiano de Buenos Aires, Buenos Aires, Argentina
e-mail: cesar.belziti@hospitalitaliano.org.ar

C. G. Musso, A. Covic (eds.), *Organ Crosstalk in Acute Kidney Injury*,
https://doi.org/10.1007/978-3-031-36789-2_10

modifications in the acid-base status and corporal fluids, as well as in bone metabolism and nutritional status disorders.

The kidney–heart relationship is even more complex because beyond the pathophysiological interactions, clinical aspects must be considered. Patients with HF and AKI have an isolated higher mortality rate than healthy individuals, this being higher if both diseases coexist.

10.2 Cardiorenal Syndrome

Cardiorenal syndrome (CRS) is a pathological condition in which both the heart and the kidneys are affected. This term has been used for years but in 2008 a consensus in which the entity was properly defined was made by the ADKI group. It was then stated that the CRS is the acute or chronic dysfunction of either the heart or kidneys that generates acute or chronic dysfunction in the other organ. It is classified into five types:

CRS type 1: acute CRS in which acute HF precipitates AKI.
CRS type 2: chronic CRS in which chronic HF progressively leads to chronic kidney disease (CKD).
CRS type 3: acute CRS in which AKI precipitates acute HF.
CRS type 4: chronic CRS in which chronic kidney disease progressively leads to structural and functional cardiac alterations and HF.
CRS type 5: secondary CRS due to a systemic cause that generates HF and AKI.

This classification is clearly based on recognizing which of the two organs has been primarily damaged, as well as the chronic or acute nature of its appearance [4].

CRS type 1 examples are acute myocardial infarction or acute cardiac failure secondary to a tachyarrhythmia or acute mitral insufficiency, which precipitates AKI.
CRS type 2 example is chronic dilated myocardiopathy that causes progressive and chronic kidney disease.

Acute pyelonephritis, glomerulopathies, and obstruction of the urinary tract are examples of CRS type 3. Examples of CRS type 4 are chronic kidney disease that generates volume overload, elevated arterial pressure, and anemia, which leads to chronic cardiac failure. Lastly, systemic pathologies such as sepsis, diabetes mellitus, and amyloidosis are causes of CRS type 5 [5].

This classification has great theoretical value that aids in the clinical interpretation of cases, still it is not always possible to place all patients into one of the CRS categories. Thus, it must be considered as a tool to firstly interpret the clinical case.

At the same time, the clinical difference between an acute HF from an exacerbation of a previous and unknown chronic HF is sometimes unclear. It may seem clearer in the case of a patient with no previous cardiac pathology that debuts with an acute coronary syndrome with ST segment elevation that causes extensive myocardial necrosis and HF with low cardiac output. Still, the previous case may not always be easily determined if the patient, for instance, had hypertension and left ventricular hypertrophy with ongoing chronic cardiac failure. This lack of recognition of the chronic pathology may result in inadequate patient treatment, and therefore, progressive aggravation of the consequential ongoing pathophysiological mechanisms established. Having presented this complex case and for the sake of this text, acute HF is considered a case of isolated acute HF, such as is the mentioned case of an acute coronary syndrome with ST segment elevation in a patient with no previous history of cardiac pathologies.

In acute HF and AKI, hemodynamic mechanisms, neurohumoral mechanisms, and inflammatory mechanisms that implicate both organs arise. The previously mentioned will be discussed in the present chapter.

10.3   Acute Cardiorenal Syndrome

10.3.1   Hemodynamic and Neurohumoral Response

Renal perfusion pressure (RPP) depends on the pressure gradient established between the median arterial pressure (MAP) and central venous pressure (CVP), RPP = MAP − CVP. MAP depends on the cardiac output (CO) and the systemic vascular resistance (SVR). CO depends on preload, afterload, contractility, and heart rate.

Acute HF usually coexists with reduced CO or an inadequate CO to fill the vascular bed (underfilling). This tends to diminish the pressure gradient that allows proper renal perfusion. In physiological conditions, the kidneys receive 20% of the CO and become affected if compensatory mechanisms cease to exist. As the CO drops, renal hypoperfusion stimulates aortic arch receptors, carotid sinus receptors, and juxtaglomerular apparatus receptors. The previously mentioned mechanism stimulates the sympathetic nervous system (SNS) which subsequently activates the renin-angiotensin-aldosterone system (RAAS) via neurohumoral pathways and non-osmotic release of antidiuretic hormone (ADH). Therefore, this phenomenon leads to retention of water and sodium but decreasing renal perfusion and excretory function. Angiotensin II increases the release of ADH that enhances neurohumoral responses and generates reactive oxygen molecules that may provoke hypertension, arrhythmia, and cell death [6].

Compensatory mechanisms allow the maintenance of the glomerular filtration rate (GFR). Still, if over stimulation of neural-hormonal responses and diminished glomerular perfusion persists over time, it leads to hypoxia and damage of the parenchymal structure. Neurohumoral response mechanisms intend to maintain homeostasis and renal perfusion pressure, however its persistence over time is harmful [7].

The second component of the RPP formula is the central venous pressure (CVP). Any mechanisms or etiology of HF produces increased diastolic pressure of the left ventricle. This transmits in a retrograde manner to the left atrium, pulmonary veins, pulmonary capillaries, and pulmonary artery. The overall increase of pulmonary pressures may cause right ventricular claudication and increase of the right auricular pressure and CVP causing renal congestion.

Renal congestion leads to decreased intrarenal pressure gradient and lower renal blood flow. Moreover, capillary leak from the intravascular space to the extravascular space generates decline in the effective blood volume. This is an effective RAAS stimulus with consequential hydro-saline retention. In addition to the renal congestion, more severe cases of right chamber failure also cause congestion of other abdominal organs and increase of intra-abdominal pressure that transmits to kidneys and affects renal perfusion [8].

The increase of renal venous pressure can be observed in numerous cases of acute HF and it is more notable in chronic congestive HF. More than 70% of admitted patients with HF and CVP greater than 24 mmHg have impaired renal function. Reduction in CO produces a drop in renal perfusion with maintenance of GFR, nevertheless, in severe cases in which CVP is also elevated, the GFR does decline [9, 10] (Fig. 10.1).

10.3.2 Inflammatory Response

The previously mentioned concepts refer to classic hemodynamic mechanisms that intervene in AKI, anterograde failure hypothesis, which causes low CO and retrograde failure hypothesis, which causes visceral congestion. Despite this, in the last years, inflammatory mechanisms have been further recognized as playing a relevant role in the aggravation and compromise of cardiac and renal function.

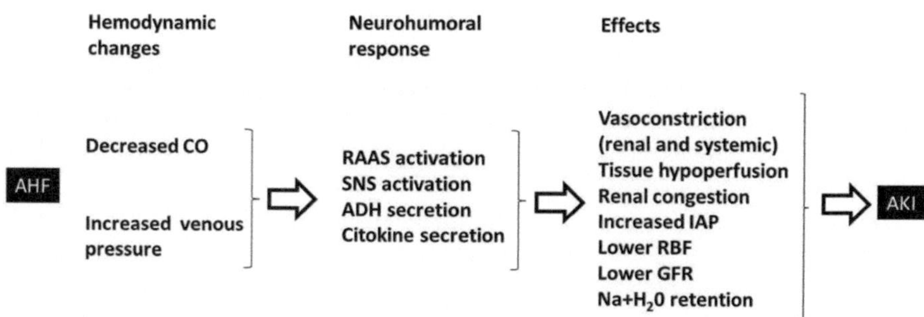

Fig. 10.1 Hemodynamic mechanisms and neurohumoral mechanisms that lead to acute kidney injury (AKI) in acute heart failure (AHF). *CO* cardiac output, *RAAS* renin-angiotensin-aldosterone system, *SNS* sympathetic nervous system, *ADH* antidiuretic hormone, *IAP* intra-abdominal pressure, *RBF* renal blood flow, *GFR* glomerular filtration rate, *Na* sodium, H_2O water

HF aggravation mechanisms provoked by inflammation are partially known. Still, there are hypotheses that explain this association via hemodynamic repercussions and structural repercussions in the heart. In HF, the RAAS and SNS activation increases pro-inflammatory molecules in the kidneys and heart, causing functional and structural repercussions in both organs. Liberation of pro-inflammatory cytokines, which is directly proportional to the severity of the HF, generates vasodilation and hypotension that aggravate the hemodynamic state and may cause fibrosis, remodeling and left ventricular function that worsens cardiac failure [11–13].

Inflammation is accepted as a prognostic factor for development and progression of HF, regardless of having a preserved or diminished systolic function [14, 15]. Cytokines more closely related to HF progression are interleukin (IL) 6 and tumoral necrosis factor α (TNFα), both having a pro-inflammatory action. Production of cytokines takes place predominantly in activated monocytes but also in damaged myocardial tissue and hypoperfused peripheral tissues. Moreover, activation of SNS with subsequent catecholamine liberation as a consequence of cardiac failure probably plays an important role. In addition, it has been proposed that intestinal edema due to HF promotes bacterial translocation and endotoxin production, which also stimulates the liberation of cytokines from monocytes [16]. IL-6 concentration becomes elevated in patients with cardiac failure and may induce myocardial hypertrophy and ventricular dysfunction. Additionally, IL-1 has been found in myocytes of patients with idiopathic dilated myocardiopathy, having a negative effect in contractility and favoring apoptosis and arrhythmias [17]. TNFα in the blood of patients with HF also becomes elevated, consequently generating ventricular dysfunction, apoptosis and playing a role in cardiac cachexia [18–20]. Within the multiple inflammatory markers associated with HF, C reactive protein (CPR) is probably one of the most studied ones. Its mechanism of action is monocyte stimulation for the release of pro-inflammatory cytokines [21]. Elevated CRP in chronic HF was associated with a worst prognosis. On the contrary, in acute HF results were contradictory; some authors concluded that CRP levels were independently associated with 6 months mortality rates, while a sub-analysis of ADHERE study did not show the aforementioned association [22–25]. Myeloperoxidase, an enzyme liberated by activated leukocytes during inflammatory processes, becomes elevated in patients with chronic HF and not in acute HF [26]. Intracellular adhesion molecules (ICAM) have also been associated with inflammatory response in HF as they intervene in the formation of nitric oxide (NO) [27]. In the latter years, the role of small molecules of non-coding RNA (ncRNA) in the modification of expression of cardiovascular genes has been further noticed; ncRNA intervenes in the expression of the development of fibrosis, ventricular remodeling, and in inflammatory response in HF [28].

Almost all studies that analyzed the relationship between inflammatory markers and the heart are retrospective and observational, thus clinical translation is difficult. Until the present moment and from a therapeutic point of view, drugs with anti-inflammatory effects, such as TNFα inhibitors, immunoglobulins corticoids, or statins, that have been tested in HF patients, have not yet proved clinical benefits [29].

10.4   Acute Renal-Cardiac Syndrome

Acute renal-cardiac syndrome occurs when an AKI triggers or aggravates HF. In AKI, cardiac compromise can be due to various mechanisms. Volume overload and electrolyte alterations, especially hyperkalemia and metabolic acidosis, are the main metabolic pathways that cause HF and arrhythmias. Furthermore, the increased inflammatory activity aggravates the condition.

Mechanisms by which AKI leads to cardiac dysfunction have more experimental support than clinical support. This is due to the difficulties in establishing the onset of the renal failure, still, it is accepted that the activation of the RAAS and the SNS, likewise in acute HF, leads to cardiac damage. Activation of the SNS, in addition to stimulating the RAAS, has a direct effect on the myocardium, causing increased oxygen consumption with consequential ventricular hypertrophy and myocyte apoptosis [30].

As previously mentioned, RAAS activation generates vasoconstriction and salt and water retention, hence provoking HF.

Inflammatory activity in AKI also plays an important role in the communication between the heart and kidneys. Renal injury in animal models activates renal inflammatory cells that increase production and liberation of proinflammatory cytokines, such as TNFα interleukins and interferons; all have negative impact on ventricular function [31, 32].

Furthermore, the increase of proinflammatory peptides in blood and the increase of TWEAK (tumor necrosis factor like weak) have been described in AKI. TWEAK provokes apoptosis and its inhibition diminished fibrosis, myocardial hypertrophy, and tubular damage [33].

Cardiac failure, as well as renal failure, conduces to an overstimulation of SNS, RAAS, and proinflammatory mechanisms that potentiate and perpetuate each other, leading to an alteration of the structure and function of the heart. Moreover, in AKI, metabolic acidosis greatly contributes in the reduction of contractility and ionic flow alteration causing arrhythmias [34].

AKI in animal models has been found to cause a reduction in mitochondrial activity and, consequently, reduction in the capacity to generate high energy phosphates with less myocardial contractility and higher apoptosis. In addition, urea and toxin retention in AKI provoke endothelial dysfunction, vascular damage and activate proinflammatory mechanisms [35, 36]. The previously mentioned communication mechanisms, compensatory mechanisms, and damage mechanisms persist and exacerbate over time. In addition, aggravating factors such as anemia, iron deficit, and the presence of risk factors, such as diabetes and hypertension, worsen renal and cardiac structure and function (Fig. 10.2).

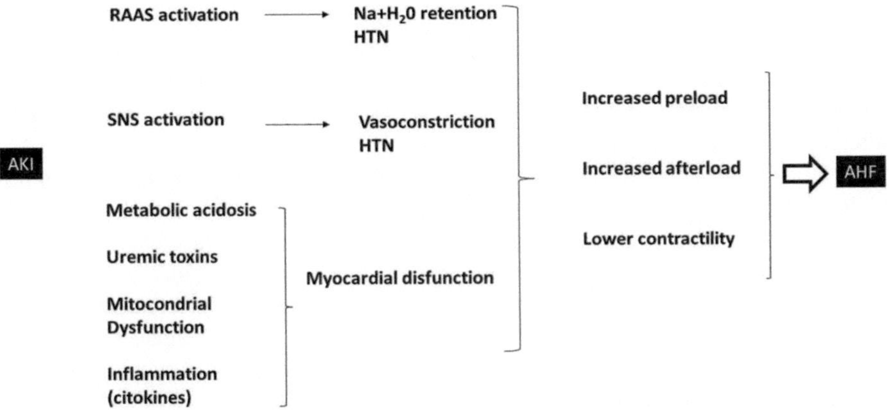

Fig. 10.2 Mechanism of cardiac damage in acute kidney injury (AKI). *RAAS* renin-angiotensin-aldosterone system, *SNS* sympathetic nervous system, *Na* sodium, *H₂O* water, *HTN* high blood arterial pressure, *AHF* acute heart failure

10.5   Acute HF Treatment and Its Relationship with Renal Function

Despite not being this chapter's aim, the treatment of acute HF and its relationship with the kidneys is going to be briefly described. Treatment of newly installed HF is comparable to the one of chronic HF exacerbations. Treatment should be initiated to ensure adequate oxygenation and tissue perfusion and simultaneously initiate the search of the cause of HF [37].

The clinical presentation of AHF can be as three different forms:

1. Predominantly pulmonary congestion, such as acute pulmonary edema.
2. Predominantly right HF with volume overload.
3. Low cardiac output, with its most severe form the cardiogenic shock.

Each of the aforementioned mechanisms requires different treatments [38]. Management of acute pulmonary edema requires oxygen supply via mask or invasive or non-invasive mechanical ventilation since hemoglobin oxygen saturation maintenance is fundamental. Likewise, tissue perfusion must be maintained by avoiding arterial hypotension with the use of loop diuretics and vasodilators, such as nitroglycerine and sodium nitroprusside, especially when the patient has hypertension [39, 40].

Systemic congestion in patients with acute pulmonary edema is uncommon, especially in flash pulmonary edema, a condition where lung congestion is predominantly due to arterial and venous peripheral vasoconstriction, rather than volume overload. Therefore, while treating this condition, an excess in negative balance will lead to unnecessary water loss and worsening of renal function. Patients with this form of acute HF usually have comorbidities such as arterial hypertension, advanced age, and preserved systolic function.

Patients with predominantly right HF and volume overload present signs such as elevated CVP, jugular ingurgitation, edemas, ascites, hepatomegaly and may have altered hepatic and renal function.

From a renal point of view, the elevation of renal venous pressure and intra-abdominal pressure diminished renal blood flow and GFR plays an important role as previously mentioned. In this group of patients achieving a negative salt and water balance must be prioritized in the treatment. This may be obtained by the use of intravenous loop diuretics sometimes associated with aldosterone antagonists and/or thiazides. Ultrafiltration is indicated in cases with inadequate response to diuretics. Renal perfusion and GFR improve with the reduction of renal congestion and intra-abdominal pressure [41].

The characteristics of the patient with volume overload are different from the patient with acute pulmonary edema, they commonly have chronic HF, and reduced ($\leq$40%) or slightly reduced (41–49%) ejection fraction. Cardiogenic shock is the most severe form of presentation of acute HF. It could also be seen as the final form of presentation of the evolution of chronic HF and the consequence of a non-ST segment elevation acute coronary syndrome or ST segment elevation acute coronary syndromes, tachyarrhythmias, acute valve disease, or complications of prosthetic valves. Moreover, on top of treating congestion, inotropes, vasoactive drugs, and eventually ventricular assist device are required [42–44].

AKI is expected in the progression of cardiogenic shock and it is due to multiple mechanisms, hemodynamic compromise, inflammatory response, and specific mechanisms of the etiology of the shock, such as septic embolisms and immune deposits in infective endocarditis or thromboembolisms in valvular complications.

10.6 Conclusion

Heart failure insufficiency and acute kidney injury are prevalent and increasing entities that entail great sanitary and economic implications. The association of both pathologies leads to further risks than they would as isolated entities. Bidirectional relationship between heart and kidneys is established at the hemodynamic and neurohumoral level with the participation of multiple mechanisms that enhance and perpetuate it, such as the inflammatory and metabolic response. The better understanding of intervening processes may allow a better approximation to the pathophysiology and, therefore, to a better treatment of both conditions.

References

1. Ponikowski P, Anker SD, AlHabib KF, et al. Heart failure: preventing disease and death worldwide. ESC Heart Failure. 2014;1:4–25.
2. McCullough PA. Cardiorenal syndromes: pathophysiology to prevention. Int J Nephrol. 2010;2011:762590. https://doi.org/10.4061/2011/762590.
3. Di Lullo L, Bronson Reeves P, Bellasi A, Ronco C. Cardiorenal syndrome in acute kidney injury. Semin Nephrol. 2019;39:31–40.
4. Ronco C, McCullough P, Anker SD, et al. Cardio-renal syndromes: report from the consensus conference of the acute dialysis quality initiative. Eur Heart J. 2010;31(6):703–71.
5. Monkowski M, Lombi F, Trimarchi H. Revisión Sistemática Síndrome Cardiorenal: Manejo Actual y Nuevas Perspectiva. Revista Nefrología Argentina. 2020;18(2):3–43.
6. Wen H, Gwathmey JK, Xie LH. Oxidative stress-mediated effects of angiotensin II in the cardiovascular system. World J Hypertens. 2012;2(4):34–44.
7. Schrier RW, Abraham WT. Hormones and hemodynamics in heart failure. N Engl J Med. 1999;341:577–85.
8. Mullens W, Abrahams Z, Francis GS, Taylor DO, Starling RC, Tang WH. Prompt reduction in intraabdominal pressure following large volume mechanical fluid removal improves renal insufficiency in refractory decompensated heart failure. J Card Fail. 2008;14:508–14.
9. Mullens W, Abrahams Z, Francis GS, Sokos G, Taylor DO, Starling RC, Young JB, et al. Importance of venous congestion for worsening of renal function in advanced decompensated heart failure. J Am Coll Cardiol. 2009;53(7):589–96.
10. Ichikawa I, Pfeffer JM, Pfeffer MA, Hostetter TH, Brenner BM. Role of angiotensin II in the altered renal function of congestive heart failure. Circ Res. 1984;55(5):669–75.
11. Jones DP, Jyoti Patel J. Therapeutic approaches targeting inflammation in cardiovascular disorders. Biology. 2018;7(49):1–14.
12. Katayama T. Significance of acute-phase inflammatory reactants as an indicator of prognosis after acute myocardial infarction: which is the most useful predictor? J Cardiol. 2003;42:49–56.
13. Pearson TA, Mensah GA, Wayne RA, Anderson JL, Cannon RO, et al. Markers of inflammation and cardiovascular disease application to clinical and public health practice: a statement for healthcare professionals from the Centers for Disease Control and Prevention and the American Heart Association. Circulation. 2003;107:499–511.
14. Dick SA, Epelman S. Chronic heart failure and inflammation: what do we really know? Circ Res. 2016;119(1):159–76.
15. Van Linthout S, Tschope C. Inflammation - cause or consequence of heart failure or both? Curr Heart Fail Rep. 2017;14(4):251–65.
16. Anker SD, von Haehling S. Inflammatory mediators in chronic heart failure: an overview. Heart. 2004;90:464–70.
17. Thaik CM, Calderone A, Takahashi N, Colucci WS. Interleukin-1 beta modulates the growth and phenotype of neonatal rat cardiac myocytes. J Clin Invest. 1995;96(2):1093–9.
18. Mann DL. Inflammatory mediators and the failing heart: past, present, and the foreseeable future. Circ Res. 2002;91:988–98.
19. Bolger AP, Anker SD. Tumour necrosis factor in chronic heart failure: a peripheral view on pathogenesis, clinical manifestations and therapeutic implications. Drugs. 2000;60:1245–57.
20. von Haehling S, Jankowska EA, Anker SD. Tumour necrosis factor-alpha and the failing heart: pathophysiology and therapeutic implications. Basic Res Cardiol. 2004;99:18–28.
21. Wrigley BJ, Lip GYH, Shantsila E. The role of monocytes and inflammation in the pathophysiology of heart failure. Eur J Heart Fail. 2015;13:1161–71.
22. Anand IS, Latini R, Florea VG, Kuskowski MA, Rector T, Masson S, et al. C-reactive protein in heart failure: prognostic value and the effect of valsartan. Circulation. 2005;112(10):1428–34.

23. Lamblin N, Mouquet F, Hennache B, Dagorn J, Susen S, Bauters C, et al. High-sensitivity C reactive protein: potential adjunct for risk stratification in patients with stable congestive heart failure. Eur Heart J. 2005;26(21):2245–50.
24. Minami Y, Kajimoto K, Sato N, Hagiwara N. Effect of elevated C-reactive protein level at discharge on long-term outcome in patients hospitalized for acute heart failure. Am J Cardiol. 2018;121(8):961–8.
25. Kalogeropoulos AP, Tang WH, Hsu A, Felker GM, Hernandez AF, Troughton RW, et al. High sensitivity C-reactive protein in acute heart failure: insights from the ASCEND-HF trial. J Card Fail. 2014;20(5):319–26.
26. Tang WH, Brennan ML, Philip K, Tong W, Mann S, Van Lente F, et al. Plasma myeloperoxidase levels in patients with chronic heart failure. Am J Cardiol. 2006;98(6):796–9.
27. Tsutamoto T, Hisanaga T, Fukai D, et al. Prognostic value of plasma soluble intercellular adhesion molecule-1 and endothelin-1 concentration in patients with chronic congestive heart failure. Am J Cardiol. 1995;76:803–8.
28. Condorelli G, Latronico MV, Dorn GW. MicroRNAs in heart disease: putative novel therapeutic targets? Eur Heart J. 2010;31:649–58.
29. Dutka M, Bobiński R, Ulman-Włodarz I, Hajduga M, Bujok J, Pająk C, Ćwiertnia M. Various aspects of inflammation in heart failure. Heart Fail Rev. 2020;25:537–48.
30. Cumming AD, Driedger AA, McDonald JW, Lindsay RM, Solez K, Linton AL. Vasoactive hormones in the renal response to systemic sepsis. Am J Kidney Dis. 1988;11:23–32.
31. Goes N, Urmson J, Ramassar V, Halloran PF. Ischemic acute tubular necrosis induces an extensive local cytokine response. Evidence for induction of interferon-gamma, transforming growth factor-beta 1, granulocyte-macrophage colony-stimulating factor, interleukin-2, and interleukin-10. Transplantation. 1995;59:565–72.
32. Kadiroglu AK, Sit D, Atay AE, Kayabasi H, Altintas A, Yilmaz ME. The evaluation of effects of demographic features, biochemical parameters, and cytokines on clinical outcomes in patients with acute renal failure. Ren Fail. 2007;29:503–8.
33. Sanz AB, Ruiz-Andres O, Sanchez-Niño MD, Ruiz-Ortega M, Ramos AM, Ortiz A. Out of the TWEAK light: elucidating the role of Fn14 and TWEAK in acute kidney injury. Semin Nephrol. 2016;36:189–98.
34. Stengl M, Ledvinova L, Chvojka J, Benes J, Jarkovska D, Holas J, Soukup P, Sviglerova J, Matejovic M. Effects of clinically relevant acute hypercapnic and metabolic acidosis on the cardiovascular system: an experimental porcine study. Crit Care. 2013;17:R303.
35. Sumida M, Doi K, Ogasawara E, Yamashita T, Hamasaki Y, Kariya T, Takimoto E, Yahagi N, Nangaku M, Noiri E. Regulation of mitochondrial dynamics by dynamin-related protein-1 in acute cardiorenal syndrome. J Am Soc Nephrol. 2015;26:2378–87.
36. Schepers E, Glorieux G, Dhondt A, Leybaert L, Vanholder R. Role of symmetric dimethylarginine in vascular damage by increasing ROS via store-operated calcium influx in monocytes. Nephrol Dial Transpl. 2009;24:1429–35.
37. McDonagh TA, Metra M, Adamo M, et al. 2021 ESC guidelines for the diagnosis and treatment of acute and chronic heart failure. Eur Heart J. 2021;42(36):3599–726. https://doi.org/10.1093/eurheartj/ehab368.
38. Belziti C, Garagoli F, Favini A, et al. Prognostic value of clinical presentation in acute heart failure syndromes. Rev Argent Cardiol. 2019;87:33–9.
39. Felker GM, Ellison DH, Mullens W, Cox ZL, Testani JM. Diuretic therapy for patients with heart failure: JACC state-of-the-art review. J Am Coll Cardiol. 2020;75:1178–95.
40. Brisco MA, Zile MR, Hanberg JS, Wilson FP, Parikh CR, Coca SG, Tang WH, Testani JM. Relevance of changes in serum creatinine during a heart failure trial of decongestive strategies: insights from the DOSE trial. J Card Fail. 2016;22:753–60.
41. Damman K, Kjekshus J, Wikstrand J, et al. Loop diuretics, renal function and clinical outcome in patients with heart failure and reduced ejection fraction. Eur J Heart Fail. 2016;18:328–36.

42. Tehrani BN, Truesdell AG, Sherwood MW, et al. Standardized team-based care for cardiogenic shock. J Am Coll Cardiol. 2019;73:16591669.
43. Thiele H, Zeymer U, Thelemann N, et al. IABPSHOCK II Trial Investigators. Intraaortic balloon pump in cardiogenic shock complicating acute myocardial infarction: long-term 6-year outcome of the randomized IABP-SHOCK II Trial. Circulation. 2019;139:395–403.
44. Combes A, Price S, Slutsky AS, et al. Temporary circulatory support for cardiogenic shock. Lancet. 2020;396:199–212.

Chapter 11
Kidney–Gut Crosstalk in Acute Kidney Injury

Ramiro Cruz Gonzalez-Sueyro

11.1 Introduction

Acute kidney injury (AKI) is defined as an abrupt decrease in kidney function, which encompasses structural damage and impairment of renal function. This syndrome has a mix of etiologic factors that include sepsis, ischemia, and nephrotoxicity [1]. The mortality rate associated with AKI remains high despite better understanding of its pathogenesis.

Crosstalk or intercommunication among different organs is a concept that, based on the biosemiotic perspective, understands the organism as a dynamic structure generated and maintained by a continuous flow of information from and to cells, tissues, organs, and organ systems [2]. Under this perspective, the kidney–gut crosstalk is one of the most complex forms of organic intercommunication in the economy since it involves not only these organs but also the gut microbiota [2]. This community of at least 1000 species of mostly bacteria but also viruses, fungi, and protozoa plays a key role in maintaining homeostasis of the gastrointestinal tract in regard to immunity and nutrient metabolism [3].

R. C. Gonzalez-Sueyro (✉)
Human Physiology Department, Instituto Universitario del Hospital Italiano de Buenos Aires, Buenos Aires, Argentina

Physiology Department, Medicine Faculty, Universidad de Buenos Aires, Buenos Aires, Argentina

Gastroenterology Service, Hospital Italiano de Buenos Aires, Buenos Aires, Argentina
e-mail: ramiro.gonzalez@hospitalitaliano.org.ar

11.1.1 Gut Barrier

The intestinal epithelial barrier has three components: a physical barrier, a biological barrier, and an immune barrier. The first one is composed of a contiguous layer of cells joined together by tight junctions (TJs) that limits interactions between luminal contents and the remainder of the organism, while supporting vectorial transport of nutrients, electrolytes, water, and waste products. Changes in TJs can lead to increased gut permeability. The biological barrier is composed of (predominantly) bacterial symbionts that are closely attached to the intestinal mucosal surface and avoid pathogenic bacteria, endotoxins, and macromolecules to enter the circulatory system. The immune barrier is the third system for maintaining microbial homeostasis which includes compounds of both adaptive and innate immune response [4]. The first one is driven by dendritic cells in the lamina propria who activate T cells, the second one driven by innate lymphoid cells that produce immune-activating cytokines (IL-22, interferon-gamma, IL-1beta, IL12, and IL-23) [3].

The composition of the gut microbiota is in constant flow under the influence of different factors such as diet, drugs (antibiotics), intestinal mucosa, immune system, and microbiota itself. Colonization resistance is the mechanism by how symbionts are closely attached to the intestinal mucosal surface and compete with pathogenic bacteria avoiding colonization and excessive growth of pathogens [5]. Alteration in the composition of the gut microbiota is called dysbiosis. Plenty of studies suggest that dysbiosis can lead to disrupted homeostasis and contribute to the pathogenesis of various diseases, including inflammatory bowel disease, obesity, diabetes, cancer, Alzheimer disease, non-alcoholic fatty liver disease, and chronic obstructive pulmonary disease [4]. It has been proposed that one of the mechanisms linked to crosstalk between gut microbiota and distant organs might be mediated by altering the function of the intestinal barrier, modifying local and systemic inflammation, controlling the production of metabolites, and affecting immune responses. Increasing interest has been made on the gut-kidney and the potential relationship between both systems in health and under pathological scenarios such as AKI and chronic kidney disease (CKD).

11.1.2 Metabolites Derived from Microbiota

Part of the communication between microbiota and cells is a consequence of the interaction between microbiota-derived metabolites and cells located in other parts of the economy. Short-chain fatty acids (SCFAs) are a subset of fatty acids produced from fermentation of non-digestible carbohydrates by the gut microbiota. In germ-free mice, SCFA detection is abruptly reduced suggesting that SCFA production requires the presence of bacteria [6]. SCFAs (including acetate, propionate, and butyrate) are proposed to contribute in immune modulation (locally and systemically), maintenance of barrier integrity, pH reduction in the intestinal tract, colonic blood flow, dictating colonic mobility, induction of regulatory T cells, and serving as energy for colonocytes [7]. SCFAs bind G-protein coupled receptors (GPCR) activating internal signal transduction pathways in cells of organs like colon, kidney, sympathetic nervous system, and blood vessels. Another mechanism of action of SCFA involves the direct inhibition of histone deacetylases (HDACs) regulating gene expressions. This last mechanism is particularly characteristic of butyrate and propionate but it is not perfectly known the exact mechanism of HDACs inhibition. Some information suggests that SCFAs might either act directly on HDACs by entering into the cells via transporters or indirectly through the activation of GPCRs [7] (Fig. 11.1).

Humans cannot metabolize some nutrients such as choline, an essential nutrient that forms the headgroup of the phospholipid phosphatidylcholine, and carnitine. Gut microbiota can also metabolize these nutrients, and trimethylamine-*N*-oxide (TMAO) is the final product [3]. Some recent data in mouse models suggest that higher levels of TMAO are associated with renal interstitial fibrosis [8]. Reduced survival rates in CKD and higher risk of sudden cardiac and all-cause mortality rates in hemodiálysis patients have been associated with high TMAO levels [9, 10]. Very poor data is available in relation to TMAO levels and AKI.

11.1.3 Microbiota and Immunity

It seems pretty clear that microbiota play a key role in immunity but plenty of mechanisms have been described. By stimulation with lumen-derived antigens, dendritic cells (DCs) induce differentiation of gut-resident naive T cells into intestinal Tregs in the intestinal lamina propria. These intestinal Tregs likely regulate effector T-cell responses to gut bacteria, including the expression of cell surface

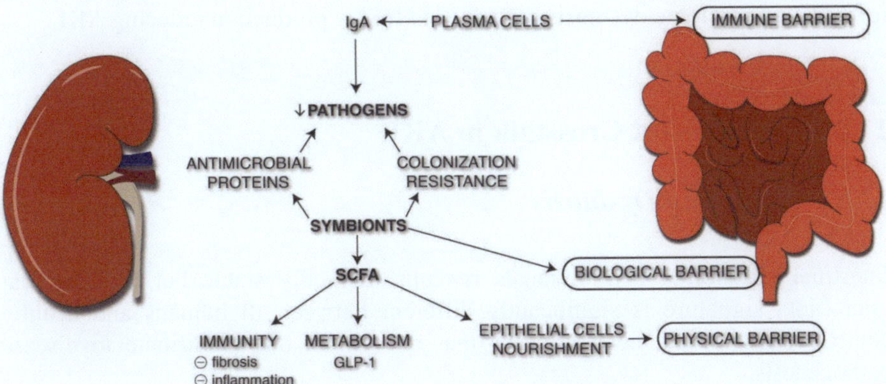

Fig. 11.1 Gut–kidney crosstalk in physiological state

proteins and cytokine production. Tregs participate in maintaining tolerance to intestinal antigens [11]. Increasing evidence further shows that the development of colonic Tregs occurs in response to species-specific bacterial antigens. It appears that Treg induction serves as a strategy to establish commensalism, not only by helping the microorganisms to colonize their niche, but also by protecting the host from inflammation.

It is largely known that in the steady state IgA is secreted by plasma cells in the gut wall by a mechanism that is independent of the presence of exogenous antigens, and microbiota as well as dietary antigens acting as natural polyreactive antibodies. IgA plays a key role in the human immune system including neutralizing toxins and viruses, clearing unwanted macromolecular structures at the epithelial surface, reducing excessive live bacterial adherence or translocation, and directed sampling of luminal antigen [12]. Ig A is also essential for maintaining the balance between the intestinal bacterial community and the host immune system. In one study, depletion of Tregs reduced the intestinal IgA level, suggesting that Tregs may directly induce IgA via secretion of transforming growth factor and also suggesting that there is an important Treg/IgA pathway at the host–microbiota interface [13] (Fig. 11.1).

11.1.4 Microbiome and Uremic Toxins

Gut bacteria can generate uremic toxins as part of the metabolism of dietary protein. These toxins are absorbed and then cleared by the kidney. Toxins amounts can be increased in the context of microbiome composition changes, leading to damage in renal tubular cells. As mentioned before, increased TMAO serum levels and related metabolites are associated with CKD and increased risk of mortality [9, 10]. *P*-cresol and indoxyl sulfate (IS) are also uremic toxins generated by colon bacteria that can increase mortality in hemodialysis patients.

Under the hypothesis that microbiome changes occur as part of renal disease, reversing microbiome dysbiosis may prevent toxins production reducing AKI.

11.2 Kidney–Gut Crosstalk in AKI

11.2.1 AKI and Dysbiosis

Intestinal microbiota in individuals remains markedly stable but the fact that microbiota signature is significantly different between ill humans and healthy controls have led to the hypothesis that microbiota may contribute to disease pathogenesis.

In the AKI scenery, only limited studies have studied this association but some data suggest that intestinal microbiota may affect outcomes in AKI. Kidney ischemia/reperfusion injury (IRI) mouse models have contributed to the hypothesis that microbiota is markedly different from that in control mice showing an increase of Escherichia, Enterobacter, and decrease in Lactobacillus amounts. This finding was associated with significantly reduced fecal levels of short-chain fatty acids (SCFAs) on day 1 of IRI, suggesting a metabolic change in the intestine under these circumstances [14].

It has been proposed that AKI induces intestinal dysbiosis and barrier disruption ("leaky gut") which leads to accumulation of neutrophils and proinflammatory macrophages and activation of the Th17 pathway. All these situations induce a proinflammatory status that can worsen kidney injury and systemic inflammation. On the other side, restoring the intestinal microbiota and gut barrier may contribute to regaining a renal normal function [4] (Fig. 11.2).

11.2.2 AKI and Barrier Integrity

Li et al. demonstrated a marked intestinal integrity disruption and increase in intestinal permeability in IRI rats compared to sham-operated ones. They also observed low grade of endotoxemia as well as increased bacterial load in the liver. Apart from that, in a pretreated with norfloxacin group they showed significant attenuation of the increase in serum urea. However, norfloxacin pretreatment did not produce any protective effects on renal tubular integrity [15]. A few more studies suggest the same observation in IRI models [14, 16] (Fig. 11.2).

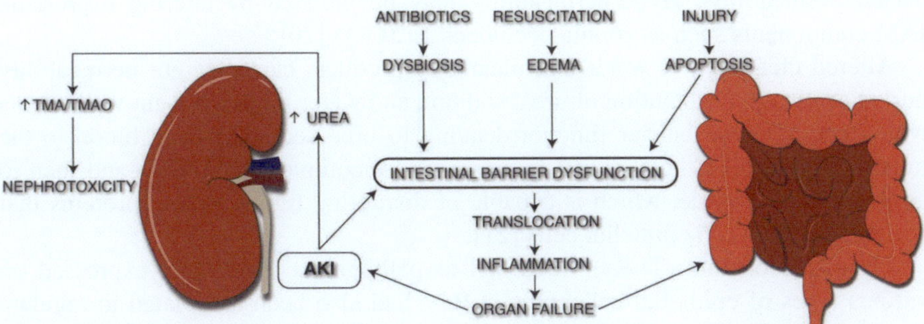

Fig. 11.2 Gut–kidney crosstalk in acute kidney injury (AKI)

11.2.3 AKI and Altered Immunity

After IRI, cells of the innate immune system in the intestine are activated. Neutrophils quickly appear in the lamina propria of the colon and then disappear by day 3 [17]. Macrophages, another effector cell type involved in innate immunity, show phenotypic changes.

Accumulation of neutrophils and proinflammatory macrophages after kidney IRI is thought to contribute to intestinal inflammation, leaky gut, and bacterial translocation, which could then potentiate systemic inflammation via multiple inflammatory mediators.

After AKI, IL17A+CD4+ cells increase in the small and large intestine. The activation of these cells of the adaptive immune system results in an induction of the Th17 pathway [17]. It is not clear if this Th17 activation directly induces kidney injury. What is known is that some cytokines such as TGF-beta and IL-6, as well as specific microbes (*Escherichia coli* and *Staphylococcus aureus*) can induce intestinal Th17 cells. In one recent study in a mouse model of ANCA-associated GN, Krebs et al. showed the egress of Th17 cells from the intestine to injured kidneys [18] (Fig. 11.2).

11.2.4 Crosstalk in Septic AKI

About half of AKI cases in the intensive care unit are caused by sepsis [19]. As already mentioned, the gut barrier is a continuous layer of cells joined together by TJs composed by junctional adhesion molecules (JAM). During septic AKI, increased levels of cytokines can act on these junctional complexes, altering the barrier permeability. Hyperpermeability may be induced by altering expression JAM components such as zonula occludens 1 (ZO-1) [20].

Altered clearance of water and metabolic products can alter gut permeability during septic AKI. Retention of urea, sodium, and water may cause gut wall edema which can alter the barrier function leading to urea secretion from blood to the lumen. Urea can be metabolized to ammonia by commensal bacteria and then to ammonium hydroxide, which is capable of disrupting tight junction proteins that seal the gap between epithelial cells [21].

Toll-like receptors (TLRs) which act as pathogen receptors are expressed on various types of epithelial cells. Gut TLR4s, had also been associated to regulate apoptosis/proliferation rates [22]. Moreover, in septic AKI, increased cytokine levels can impair gut cell regeneration and promote apoptosis in a TLR4-dependent manner contributing to the gut barrier alteration [16].

Gut injury due to hypoperfusion during sepsis results in translocation of bacteria and toxins from the intestinal lumen to the mesenteric lymph and systemic circulation inducing immune cells. This situation will cause an amplified inflammation in septic AKI that shifts metabolism toward aerobic glycolysis leading to decreased levels of intracellular adenosine triphosphate (ATP) and consecuent mitochondrial injury in the kidney, main causes of kidney dysfunction and injury [23].

In summary, AKI can compromise barrier integrity by different mechanisms which can result in bacterial and toxins translocation to the circulation, promoting an increase in systemic inflammatory response, deeper alteration of kidney function, and other organs failures [16] (Fig. 11.2).

11.3 Therapeutic Targets

Considering all the evidence above mentioned, it seems very tempting to introduce some therapeutic strategies against barrier dysfunction and gut microbiome alteration. Strategies under investigation include intake of live microbiota, addition of nutrients for microbiota regeneration, and administration of exogenous supplements such as SCFAs.

11.3.1 Selective Decontamination of the Digestive Tract (SDD)

SDD consists of prevention of secondary colonization with gram-negative bacteria, *Staphylococcus aureus* and yeasts by administering non-absorbable antimicrobial agents in the oropharynx and gastrointestinal tract, preserving the anaerobic microbiota, thereby preventing excess infectious disease in critically ill patients [24, 25].

Since nearly all the normal anaerobic flora is lost after sepsis, the addition of SDD to a septic AKI patient is promising to regain gut's barrier integrity, microbiome, and immune function, breaking down the continuous cycle of injury followed by amplification of inflammation [24].

A comprehensive systematic review and network meta-analysis suggested that SDD can prevent nosocomial infections and reduce overall mortality rates in the subset of general intensive care units. But SDD in the field of AKI is not well studied yet.

11.3.2 Probiotics

Some studies in animal models have tried to elucidate the impact of probiotics in the gut–kidney axis. It has been observed that treatment with *Bifidobacterium bifidum* BGN4 (BGN4) before inducing AKI in IRI mice significantly reduced the severity of renal IRI and distant organ (liver) injury. Moreover, these findings were associated with expansion of regulatory T cells and reduced interleukin-17A expression in the colon, mesenteric lymph nodes, and kidney [17]. Lee et al. have observed that

Lactobacillus salivarius BP121 attenuated cisplatin induced kidney injury by decreasing inflammation, oxidative stress, and serum levels of uremic toxins, and by modulating the gut environment [26].

In cirrhotic patients, two studies have evaluated the role of long-term use of rifaximin, an oral broad-spectrum antibiotic that concentrates in the gastrointestinal tract, in renal function. They found that the intervention increased glomerular filtration rate and natriuresis, thus improving systemic hemodynamics and renal function in patients with advanced cirrhosis (ascitis) and hepatorenal syndrome [27, 28].

In another study, *L. casei Zhang* showed a protective effect on renal injury induced by IRI, including reduction of inflammatory infiltration, promoting renal repair, and alleviating chronic renal interstitial fibrosis. *L. casei Zhang also* improves intestinal dysregulation, reduces intestinal inflammation, and repairs intestinal epithelial tight junction disruption [29].

Fecal microbiota transplantation (from selected donors) had shown to be more effective in recurrent *Clostridium difficile* infection than standard antibiotics regimen and has become the elective therapy for refractory pseudomembranous colitis. Many other sceneries such as inflammatory bowel disease are being explored for this therapy [30]. This intervention in the AKI context has not been studied yet.

It seems that probiotics have a potential role in AKI treatment but since evidence is still limited to animal models, no conclusions can be made about the possible benefit of using them in humans.

11.3.3   Short-Chain Fatty Acids (SCFAs)

Also in IRI mouse model, some authors observed that therapy with the three main SCFAs (acetate, propionate, and butyrate) improved renal dysfunction caused by injury. This protection was associated with low levels of local and systemic inflammation, oxidative cellular stress, cell infiltration/activation, and apoptosis. These findings suggest that SCFAs may improve organ function and viability after an injury through modulation of the inflammatory process [31, 32].

In the same direction, in a rat model of contrasts-induced nephropathy, the administration of sodium butyrate decreased IL6 levels in kidney tissue, preventing the translocation of NF-kB into the nucleus, and reducing inflammation and oxidative damage.

All these animal models findings seem to indicate that modulation of SCFAs in the gut could be a novel therapeutic approach against AKI.

11.4 Conclusions

Accumulating evidence in favor of the existence of a close communication between the gut and the kidney, during the physiological and pathological state is available nowadays. Acute kidney injury can induce gut barrier permeability modifications as well as microbiota alteration. On the other hand, barrier permeability alteration associated with increased bacterial and gut toxins translocation can aggravate acute kidney injury. However, proposed molecular and intervening mechanisms are so wide that it becomes unclear what is the real relevance of each one of them.

Future studies are needed to clarify the role of the intestinal microbiota in acute kidney injury and to explore whether modification of the gut microbiota using probiotics or supplementation with their metabolites or any other intervention are potential effective therapeutic options.

References

1. Makris K, Spanou L. Acute kidney injury: definition, pathophysiology and clinical phenotypes. Clin Biochem Rev. 2016;37:85–98.
2. Colombo I, Aiello-Battan F, Elena R, Ruiz A, Petraglia L, Musso CG. Kidney-gut crosstalk in renal disease. Ir J Med Sci. 2021;190:1205–12.
3. Gong J, Noel S, Pluznick JL, Hamad ARA, Rabb H. Gut microbiota-kidney cross-talk in acute kidney injury. Semin Nephrol. 2019;39:107–16.
4. Kim CH, Moon SJ. The role of the gut microbiota in acute kidney injury: a new therapeutic candidate? Kidney Res Clin Pract. 2021;40:505–7.
5. Kranich J, Maslowski KM, Mackay CR. Commensal flora and the regulation of inflammatory and autoimmune responses. Semin Immunol. 2011;23:139–45.
6. Høverstad T, Midtvedt T. Short-chain fatty acids in germfree mice and rats. J Nutr. 1986;116:1772–6.
7. Tan J, McKenzie C, Potamitis M, Thorburn AN, Mackay CR, Macia L. The role of short-chain fatty acids in health and disease. Adv Immunol. 2014;121:91–119.
8. Sun G, Yin Z, Liu N, Bian X, Yu R, Su X, et al. Gut microbial metabolite TMAO contributes to renal dysfunction in a mouse model of diet-induced obesity. Biochem Biophys Res Commun. 2017;493:964–70.
9. Mafune A, Iwamoto T, Tsutsumi Y, Nakashima A, Yamamoto I, Yokoyama K, et al. Associations among serum trimethylamine-N-oxide (TMAO) levels, kidney function and infarcted coronary artery number in patients undergoing cardiovascular surgery: a cross-sectional study. Clin Exp Nephrol. 2016;20:731–9. https://doi.org/10.1007/s10157-015-1207-y.
10. Shafi T, Powe NR, Meyer TW, Hwang S, Hai X, Melamed ML, et al. Trimethylamine N-oxide and cardiovascular events in hemodialysis patients. J Am Soc Nephrol. 2017;28:321–31.
11. Cebula A, Seweryn M, Rempala GA, Pabla SS, McIndoe RA, Denning TL, et al. Thymus-derived regulatory T cells contribute to tolerance to commensal microbiota. Nature. 2013;497:258–62.
12. Strugnell RA, Wijburg OLC. The role of secretory antibodies in infection immunity. Nat Rev Microbiol. 2010;8:656–67.

13. Alexander KL, Katz J, Elson CO. CBirTox is a selective antigen-specific agonist of the Treg-IgA-microbiota homeostatic pathway. PLoS One. 2017;12:e0181866.
14. Yang J, Kim CJ, Go YS, Lee HY, Kim M-G, Oh SW, et al. Intestinal microbiota control acute kidney injury severity by immune modulation. Kidney Int. 2020;98:932–46.
15. Li J, Moturi KR, Wang L, Zhang K, Yu C. Gut derived-endotoxin contributes to inflammation in severe ischemic acute kidney injury. BMC Nephrol. 2019;20(1):16. https://doi.org/10.1186/s12882-018-1199-4.
16. Zhang J, Ankawi G, Sun J, Digvijay K, Yin Y, Rosner MH, et al. Gut–kidney crosstalk in septic acute kidney injury. Crit Care. 2018;22(1):117. https://doi.org/10.1186/s13054-018-2040-y.
17. Yang J, Ji GE, Park MS, Seong YJ, Go YS. Probiotics partially attenuate the severity of acute kidney injury through an immunomodulatory effect. Kidney Res. 2021. https://www.ncbi.nlm.nih.gov/pmc/articles/pmc8685362/;40:620.
18. Krebs CF, Paust H-J, Krohn S, Koyro T, Brix SR, Riedel J-H, et al. Autoimmune renal disease is exacerbated by S1P-receptor-1-dependent intestinal Th17 cell migration to the kidney. Immunity. 2016;45:1078–92. https://doi.org/10.1016/j.immuni.2016.10.020.
19. Uchino S, Kellum JA, Bellomo R, Doig GS, Morimatsu H, Morgera S, et al. Acute renal failure in critically ill patients: a multinational, multicenter study. JAMA. 2005;294:813–8.
20. Turner JR. Intestinal mucosal barrier function in health and disease. Nat Rev Immunol. 2009;9:799–809.
21. Vaziri ND, Yuan J, Norris K. Role of urea in intestinal barrier dysfunction and disruption of epithelial tight junction in chronic kidney disease. Am J Nephrol. 2013;37:1–6.
22. El-Achkar TM, Huang X, Plotkin Z, Sandoval RM, Rhodes GJ, Dagher PC. Sepsis induces changes in the expression and distribution of Toll-like receptor 4 in the rat kidney. Am J Physiol Renal Physiol. 2006;290:F1034–43.
23. Gómez H, Kellum JA, Ronco C. Metabolic reprogramming and tolerance during sepsis-induced AKI. Nat Rev Nephrol. 2017;13:143–51.
24. de Smet AMGA. Selective decontamination of the oropharynx and the digestive tract in ICU patients. Utrecht University; 2009.
25. Price R, MacLennan G, Glen J, on behalf of the SuDDICU collaboration. Selective digestive or oropharyngeal decontamination and topical oropharyngeal chlorhexidine for prevention of death in general intensive care: systematic review and network meta-analysis. BMJ. 2014;348:g2197. https://doi.org/10.1136/bmj.g2197.
26. Lee T-H, Park D, Kim YJ, Lee I, Kim S, Oh C-T, et al. Lactobacillus salivarius BP121 prevents cisplatin-induced acute kidney injury by inhibition of uremic toxins such as indoxyl sulfate and p-cresol sulfate via alleviating dysbiosis. Int J Mol Med. 2020;45:1130–40.
27. Kalambokis GN, Mouzaki A, Rodi M, Pappas K, Fotopoulos A, Xourgia X, et al. Rifaximin improves systemic hemodynamics and renal function in patients with alcohol-related cirrhosis and ascites. Clin Gastroenterol Hepatol. 2012;10:815–8.
28. Dong T, Aronsohn A, Gautham Reddy K, Te HS. Rifaximin decreases the incidence and severity of acute kidney injury and hepatorenal syndrome in cirrhosis. Dig Dis Sci. 2016;61:3621–6.
29. Zhu H, Cao C, Wu Z, Zhang H, Sun Z, Wang M, et al. The probiotic L. casei Zhang slows the progression of acute and chronic kidney disease. Cell Metab. 2021;33:1926–1942.e8. https://doi.org/10.1016/j.cmet.2021.06.014.
30. Kim KO, Gluck M. Fecal microbiota transplantation: an update on clinical practice. Clin Endosc. 2019;52:137–43.
31. Andrade-Oliveira V, Amano MT, Correa-Costa M, Castoldi A, Felizardo RJF, de Almeida DC, et al. Gut bacteria products prevent AKI induced by ischemia-reperfusion. J Am Soc Nephrol. 2015;26:1877–88. https://doi.org/10.1681/asn.2014030288.
32. Beker BM, Colombo I, Gonzalez-Torres H, Musso CG. Decreasing microbiota-derived uremic toxins to improve CKD outcomes. Clin Kidney J. 2022;15(12):2214–9. https://doi.org/10.1093/ckj/sfac154.

Chapter 12
Kidney–Liver Crosstalk in Acute Kidney Injury

Adrian Gadano, Malena Colombo, and Victoria Paula Musso-Enz

12.1 Introduction

The definition of "organ crosstalk" establishes that signals are passed from organ to organ via neural pathways, paracrine interactions within cells of the same tissue, and through the endocrine system. In this way, it reinforces the concept that neurons and bloodstream allow perfect interaction between the organs for maintaining an adequate homeostasis. However, this communication also facilitates the spread of damage mediators [1]. Crosstalk between liver and kidney has aroused great interest in recent years.

Acute kidney injury (AKI), defined as an absolute increase in serum creatinine $\geq$0.3 mg/dL ($\geq$26.4 mol/L) in less than 48 h, or as a percentage increase in serum creatinine $\geq$50% (1.5-fold from baseline) in less than 7 days, can per se lead to multiorgan dysfunction (MOF) or be one of the initial manifestations of a severe clinical condition [2].

Advanced cirrhosis is a condition characterized by impaired liver function, portal hypertension, increased splanchnic blood volume, hyperdynamic state with increased cardiac output, systemic vasodilation, a state of decreased central blood volume, and systemic inflammatory response. AKI is one of the most severe complications of cirrhosis, occurring in up to 50% of hospitalized patients, and has been associated with higher mortality, which increases with severity of AKI [2, 3]. Hepatorenal syndrome is one of the phenotypes of AKI that occurs in patients with

A. Gadano (✉)
Research Department, Hospital Italiano de Buenos Aires, Buenos Aires, Argentina
e-mail: adrian.gadano@hospitalitaliano.org.ar

M. Colombo · V. P. Musso-Enz
Physiology Department, Instituto Universitario del Hospital Italiano de Buenos Aires, Buenos Aires, Argentina
e-mail: malena.colombo@hospitalitaliano.org.ar; victoria.musso@hospitalitaliano.org.ar

C. G. Musso, A. Covic (eds.), *Organ Crosstalk in Acute Kidney Injury*,
https://doi.org/10.1007/978-3-031-36789-2_12

advanced cirrhosis and is characterized by decreased kidney blood flow that is unresponsive to volume expansion [4–6].

12.2 Definitions

Acute deterioration of renal function, determined by an increase in serum creatinine, is a prevalent condition (19–26%) in hospitalized patients with cirrhosis [7–10]. Despite its wide use, it is known that creatinine has serious limitations in patients with decompensated cirrhosis. The synthesis of creatinine is reduced in patients with cirrhosis, either because of a lower muscle mass or because of a lower protein intake. Moreover, there is a gender bias [10]. Therefore, creatinine is a sub-optimal biomarker for risk stratification in this population. In this setting, new alternative biomarkers with greater precision in patients with cirrhosis, such as cystatin C (CysC), are gaining ground not only because of their early diagnostic capacity, but also because of their ability to establish prognosis [11]. Despite its limitations, serum creatinine continues to be the most affordable and available biomarker for estimated glomerular filtration rate (eGFR) and consequently, the definition of acute renal failure has evolved over the last two decades based on the variability of this serological biomarker. The recent modifications of the International Club of Ascites (ICA) in terms of the diagnostic criteria for AKI in patients with cirrhosis, based on an absolute increase in serum creatinine of at least 0.3 mg/dL or 50% from baseline have shown a greater ability for the early detection of patients at higher risk of longer hospital stay, multiple organ failure, admission to intensive care units, in-hospital mortality, and mortality at 90 days [12–14] (Table 12.1).

Recently, the ICA also updated the definition of type 1 HRS, now called HRS-AKI. Among the main implications of the recent modification, the 2-week interval required to double the serum creatinine stipulated in the previous definition was modified given the risk of delay in the start of treatment for hepatorenal syndrome. In line with this, it has been shown that the higher the creatinine at the start of

Table 12.1 Definition of AKI according to International Club of Ascites (ICA)

ICA AKI in cirrhosis	Increase in sCr ≥ 0.3 mg/dL (26.5 μmol/L) within 48 h *OR* sCr percentage increase ≥50% × baseline, which is known or presumed to have occurred within the prior 7 days
ICA Determining baseline sCr in cirrhosis	SCr value obtained in the previous 3 months should be used, when available if multiple sCr values within previous 3 months, value closest to admission sCr should be used. If no previous sCr available, admission sCr serves as baseline value
ICA AKI staging in cirrhosis	Stage 1: Increase in sCr ≥ 0.3 mg/dL (26.5 umol/L) within 48 h *OR* increase in sCr 1.5–2 × baseline
	Stage 2: Increase in sCr 2–3 × baseline Stage 3: Increase in sCr > 3 × baseline *OR* sCr >4 mg/dL (353.6 μmol/L) with an acute rise >0.5 mg/dL (44 μmol/L) *OR* initiation of RRT

vasoconstrictor treatment, the lower the probability of HRS reversal [15], and therefore this new definition has eliminated the need to establish a minimum creatinine cut-off for the diagnosis of HRS-AKI. In contrast, the new definition established by ICA establishes that functional kidney injury that does not meet the HRS-AKI criteria is called HRS-NAKI (that is, not AKI) and is defined by eGFR instead of serum creatinine. The presence of NAKI is divided into HRS acute kidney disease (HRS-AKD) if the eGFR is less than 60 mL/min/1.73 m^2 for less than 3 months and HRS Chronic Kidney Disease (HRS-CKD) if it is less than this for more than 3 months.

12.3   Pathogenesis of Hepatorenal Syndrome

12.3.1   Circulatory Dysfunction

The main driver involved in the development of complications of cirrhosis is represented by the development of clinically significant portal hypertension (CSPH). The consequent splanchnic arteriolar vasodilation is a key factor for the pathophysiology of HRS-AKI [3]. In an early stage of cirrhosis, there is a modest increase in intraportal hypertension along with a decrease in systemic resistance caused by vasodilation. This vasodilation, which is the main cause of HRS, is triggered by the overproduction of vasodilator substances (nitric oxide, carbon monoxide, and endocannabinoids) and their low degradation due to increased portal hypertension and the leakage of these substances by portosystemic searches to general circulation. As a compensatory physiological measure, an increase in cardiac output, heart rate, and activation of powerful vasoconstrictor systems and the renin-angiotensin-aldosterone system are triggered. In the same direction, the development of liver complications implies that these measures, which were initially adaptive, are not efficient enough, thus causing deterioration of renal blood flow [16]. The aforementioned consequences are associated with the retention of sodium and free water with the accumulation of ascites and edema [17]. Later on there is an even more pronounced renal vasoconstriction, decreased eGFR, and the eventual development of HRS. Finally, if extreme renal vasoconstriction is not corrected in time, it could lead to the development of acute tubular necrosis, although this evolution at the moment remains controversial [6, 7] (Figs. 12.1 and 12.2).

12.3.2   Systemic Inflammation

In almost half of the patients with HRS-AKI, the presence of systemic inflammatory response syndrome was evidenced, even independently of the presence of infection [18]. Systemic inflammation occurs as a result of increased intestinal permeability

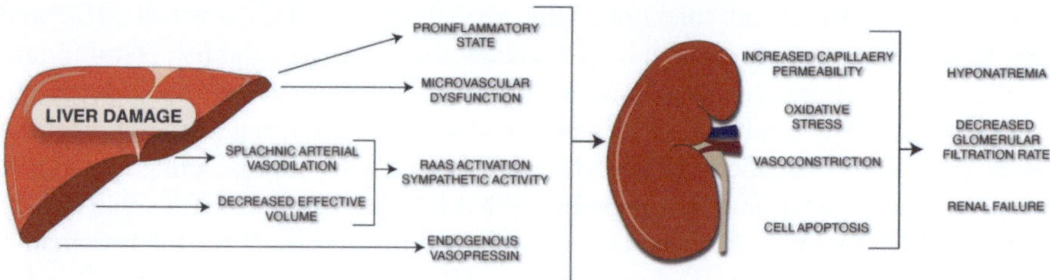

Fig. 12.1 Pathophysiology of hepatorenal syndrome

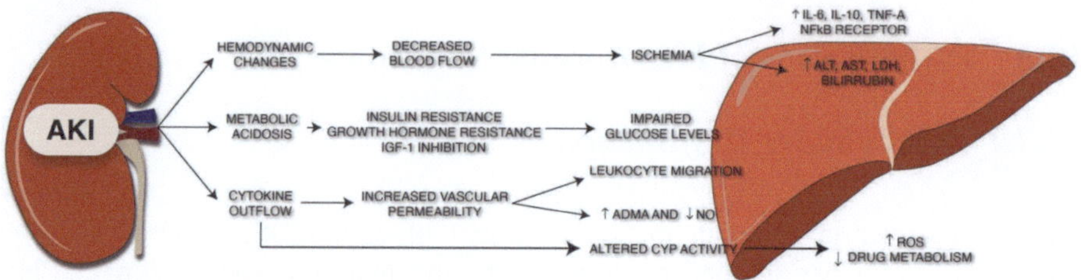

Fig. 12.2 Pathophysiology of renal-hepatic syndrome. *AKI* acute kidney injury, *ALT* alanine transaminase, *AST* aspartate transaminase, *LDH* lactate dehydrogenase, *ADMA* asymmetric dimethylarginine, *NO* nitric oxide, *ROS* oxygen reactive species, *CYP* cytochrome p450, *IL-6* interleukin 6, *IL-10* interleukin 10, *TNF-a* tumor necrosis factor alpha, *NF-kB* nuclear factor KB

which leads to pathological bacterial translocation from the intestine to the systemic circulation and changes in the quantity and quality of the microbiome and immune dysfunction associated with cirrhosis [19]. Bacterial translocation induces a broad spectrum of genes that encode molecules responsible for triggering an inflammatory response through specific receptors called pattern recognition receptors [20]. The toll-like receptor 4 (TLR4) is the main pattern recognition receptor that has been studied in this context. Tubular TLR4 overexpression has been described in patients with cirrhosis and renal dysfunction [21]. A subset of patients diagnosed with HRS showed TLR4 overexpression in tubular cells and evidence of tubular cell damage, suggesting an overlap in the pattern of kidney damage and not a pure form of HRS-AKI [22]. The inflammatory components can spread to the systemic circulation and peripheral organs, conditioning the development of dysfunction of extrahepatic organs, including the kidney. Immune dysfunction and changes in systemic inflammation can contribute to systemic circulatory changes associated with the development of HRS. Clear evidence of this situation is represented by high levels of pro-inflammatory cytokines (TNF-a, and IL-6) [22] (Figs. 12.1 and 12.2).

12.3.3 Cirrhotic Cardiomyopathy

Cirrhotic cardiomyopathy (CCM) is a silent condition that is difficult to identify in a stable setting but can become symptomatic under a decompensating event, and clearly is involved in the pathophysiology of HRS, mainly because it greatly alters renal perfusion. Recent studies have shown that the presence of CCM, either based on echocardiographic parameters or biomarkers such as NT-proBNP, is entirely related to the development of HRS, with said relationship being direct in the dynamics and decreased cardiac output [23] (Fig. 12.1).

12.3.4 Cytokines

In pro-inflammatory liver processes, there is an increase in hepatic vascular permeability which affects liver flow, and ends up favoring neutrophil and lymphocyte migration, stimulating an inflammatory cascade on liver cells. Moreover, during AKI there are several cytokines released (IL-6, IL-17A, and TNF-α) that also affect hepatic blood supply, liver intrinsic clearance, and unbound drug fraction, all ending in the modification of hepatic clearance. A new theory suggests that this increase of circulating levels of pro-inflammatory cytokines and chemokines directly stimulates the development of HRS [1] (Fig. 12.2).

12.4 Clinical Application of Kidney Biomarkers

Despite the multiple limitations of creatinine as a renal biomarker, it continues to be the most widely accepted parameter worldwide. However, the development of new renal biomarkers that could be of clinical utility is promising [10]. One of the main utilities of urinary biomarkers is the ability to elucidate the etiology of renal failure, more specifically in being able to differentiate ATN from HRS-AKI. In this context, the most investigated biomarker has been neutrophil gelatinase-associated lipocalin (N-GAL), which has demonstrated robustness in differentiate ATN from HRS-AKI and thus be able to guide vasoconstrictor therapy [8]. The power of the N-GAL in the diagnostic capacity of ATN has been established from the cut-off of 220 µg/g, showing that about 86% of the diagnosis of ATN presented values above the mentioned threshold, while those with HRS-AKI or prerenal-AKI in 88% and 93%, respectively, had values below said cut-off [24, 25]. However, despite its discriminative capacity, the availability of said urinary biomarkers in daily practice is scarce worldwide, which is why there is a need for simpler tools with greater availability.

The use of the fractional excretion of sodium (FENa) continues to be a useful tool for differentiating between functional and structural damage. In the case of functional damage, the tubules are usually intact, conditioning greater sodium reabsorption due to renal hypoperfusion. However, circulatory disorders, especially in the setting of advanced cirrhosis, could condition chronic renal hypoperfusion and therefore estimate values of FENa <1%. Despite this, different studies in HRS-AKI have been able to demonstrate values that FENa values <0.2% have adequate capacity to differentiate HRS-AKI from ATN [24–28]. In the same direction, recent studies have been able to demonstrate a similar capacity in the diagnosis of ATN, based on high levels of albuminuria.

Finally, the use of serum CysC has recently taken on greater relevance not only for its ability to identify patients at risk of developing renal events independent of muscle mass or sex but also for its predictive value in the development of acute on chronic liver failure (ACLF) and mortality on the waiting list (WL) for liver transplant [18].

12.5 Prevention of Hepatorenal Syndrome

12.5.1 Prevention of Circulatory Dysfunction

Multiple predictors of the development of HRS have been described: hyponatremia, high plasma renin activity [29], degree of ascites [30], and elevated CysC values [31]. However, the main factors related to HRS-AKI are the acute hemodynamic changes associated with infections and large-volume paracentesis without albumin administration, and the development of AKI without a clear triggering factor being very rare (1.8%) [32].

The prevalence of HRS-AKI in the setting of spontaneous bacterial peritonitis (SBP) or other bacterial infections is 30%, determining a worse short-term prognosis [33–35].

Post-paracentesis circulatory dysfunction occurs after large-volume paracentesis (≥5 L) and is associated with hypotension, hyponatremia, and increased risk of HRS-AKI. Albumin administration after large-volume paracentesis significantly reduces this risk and improves overall survival in these patients. This protective effect appears to be unique to albumin, compared to other volume expanders, suggesting an additional benefit of albumin other than its ability as a plasma expander [36].

In the same direction, the development of HRS-AKI can be prevented by the administration of intravenous albumin in addition to the early initiation of effective antibiotic treatment in the context of SBP (8.3% vs. 30.6% with antibiotics alone; $p = 0.01$), leading to a reduction in overall mortality (16% vs. 35.4%; OR: 0.34) [33–37]. In contrast, although the administration of albumin in patients with non-spontaneous bacterial peritonitis (SBP) infections may improve circulatory function and delay the development of renal dysfunction [38], it has not been shown to prevent the development of HRS-AKI or benefit survival [39].

Regarding the prolonged use of albumin as a preventive strategy in the context of decompensated cirrhosis, the evidence is controversial. This hypothesis has been evaluated in a recent RCT, compared with standard treatment, adding weekly albumin administration for 18 months improved overall survival (77% vs. 66%; $p = 0.028$), reducing the incidence of HRS-AKI (OR: 0.39) [40]. In contrast, a similar trial evaluating the long-term use of albumin and midodrine in 196 patients with decompensated cirrhosis on the WL for liver transplantation failed to show a one-year survival benefit, nor in the prevention of complications of cirrhosis [41]. In conclusion, although there is a biological plausibility in its use, future trials such as PRECIOSA12 or ATTIRE trial are expected to shed light on long-term albumin use in this population.

12.5.2 Antibiotic Prophylaxis

Prophylactic antibiotics to prevent SBP and after gastrointestinal bleeding have been shown to decrease the incidence of HRS-AKI. The risk of SBP is determined by a lower concentration of protein in ascites fluid (<1.5 mg/dL) associated with liver and/or kidney dysfunction (bilirubin >3 mg/dL, serum sodium <130 mmol/L, Child Pugh score >10, and/or serum creatinine >1.2 mg/dL), and it is in this setting that antibiotic prophylaxis not only prevents the development of SBP but also significantly reduces the risk of HRS-AKI and overall mortality [42, 43].

12.6 Management and Treatment of Hepatorenal Syndrome

At current time, vasoconstrictor agents in combination with albumin represent the first-line treatment for HRS-AKI [44–48]. Terlipressin, a vasopressin analog, is the most commonly used drug. The efficacy of terlipressin plus albumin in the treatment of hepatorenal syndrome has been evaluated in a large number of patients, with a response rate that ranges from 25% to 75%. Treatment should be maintained until complete response or for a maximum of 14 days. Side effects of terlipressin are related to vasoconstriction with a risk of myocardial infarction and intestinal or peripheral ischemia.

Continuous infusion of terlipressin at a dose of 2–12 mg/day has been shown to have similar effects as bolus administration but with lower rates of adverse events in a single study [49]. Baseline serum creatinine and the degree of ACLF (the higher the degree, the greater the inflammation) are inversely associated with the response to terlipressin [46–50]. Other vasoconstrictive agents in combination with albumin have been proposed. Norepinephrine is an alternative treatment that has been shown in small studies to be effective [51–53]; however, a recent controlled trial suggests that norepinephrine is inferior to terlipressin in reversal of HRS-AKI, renal replacement therapy (RRT) requirement, and overall survival in the setting of ACLF

[49]. The combination of midodrine plus octreotide, used in countries where terlipressin is not yet available, has been shown in a single-center study to be less effective than terlipressin [44]. The role of RRT in HRS is described in Chap. 16.

12.7 Conclusion

There is a significant kidney–liver crosstalk in acute kidney injury. Ischemia, reperfusion, cytokine outflow, pro-inflammatory cascades, oxidative stress, and changes in enzymatic and metabolic pathways provide the bases for this bidirectional kidney-liver damage.

Disclosures Dr. Adrian Gadano is speaker for Gilead, Novartis, Novo Nordisk. Additionally, he received educational grants from Gilead, and research grants from MSD, Novartis and Novo Nordisk.

Compliance with Ethical Standards *Conflict of Interest*: No conflict of interest.

References

1. Capalbo O, Giuliani S, Ferrero-Fernández A, Casciato P, Musso CG. Kidney-liver pathophysiological crosstalk: its characteristics and importance. Int Urol Nephrol. 2019;51(12):2203–7. https://doi.org/10.1007/s11255-019-02288-x.
2. Tandon P, James MT, Abraldes JG, Karvellas CJ, Ye F, Pannu N. Relevance of new definitions to incidence and prognosis of acute kidney injury in hospitalized patients with cirrhosis: a retrospective population-based cohort study. PLoS One. 2016;11(8):e0160394. https://doi.org/10.1371/journal.pone.0160394.
3. Simonetto DA, Gines P, Kamath PS. State of the art review. Hepatorenal syndrome: pathophysiology, diagnosis, and management. BMJ. 2020;370:2687. https://doi.org/10.1136/bmj.m2687.
4. Francoz C, Durand F, Kahn JA, Genyk YS, Nadim MK. Hepatorenal syndrome. Clin J Am Soc Nephrol. 2019;14(5):774–81. https://doi.org/10.2215/CJN.12451018.
5. Angeli P, Garcia-Tsao G, Nadim MK, Parikh CR. News in pathophysiology, definition and classification of hepatorenal syndrome: a step beyond the International Club of Ascites (ICA) consensus document. J Hepatol. 2019;71(4):811–22. https://doi.org/10.1016/j.jhep.2019.07.002.
6. Tonon M, Rosi S, Gambino CG, et al. Natural history of acute kidney disease in patients with cirrhosis. J Hepatol. 2020;74:578. https://doi.org/10.1016/j.jhep.2020.08.037.
7. Solé C, Solà E, Kamath PS, Ginès P. Lack of evidence for a continuum between hepatorenal syndrome and acute tubular necrosis. J Hepatol. 2020;72(3):581–2. https://doi.org/10.1016/j.jhep.2019.09.016.
8. Garcia-Tsao G, Angeli P, Nadim MK, Parikh CR. Reply to: "Lack of evidence for a continuum between hepatorenal syndrome and acute tubular necrosis". J Hepatol. 2020;72(3):582–3. https://doi.org/10.1016/j.jhep.2019.11.005.

9. Wohlauer MV, Sauaia A, Moore EE, Burlew CC, Banerjee A, Johnson J. Acute kidney injury and posttrauma multiple organ failure: the canary in the coal mine. J Trauma Acute Care Surg. 2012;72(2):373–8; discussion 379–80. https://doi.org/10.1097/TA.0b013e318244869b.

10. Piano S, Romano A, Di Pascoli M, Angeli P. Why and how to measure renal function in patients with liver disease. Liver Int. 2017;37:116–22. https://doi.org/10.1111/liv.13305.

11. Mauro E, Crespo G, Martinez-Garmendia A, et al. Cystatin C and sarcopenia predict acute on chronic liver failure development and mortality in patients on the liver transplant waiting list. Transplantation. 2020;104(7):e188–98. https://doi.org/10.1097/TP.0000000000003222.

12. Belcher JM, Garcia-Tsao G, Sanyal AJ, et al. Association of AKI with mortality and complications in hospitalized patients with cirrhosis. Hepatology. 2013;57(2):753–62. https://doi.org/10.1002/hep.25735.

13. Angeli P, Ginès P, Wong F, et al. Diagnosis and management of acute kidney injury in patients with cirrhosis: revised consensus recommendations of the International Club of Ascites. J Hepatol. 2015;62(4):968–74. https://doi.org/10.1016/j.jhep.2014.12.029.

14. Fagundes C, Barreto R, Guevara M, et al. A modified acute kidney injury classification for diagnosis and risk stratification of impairment of kidney function in cirrhosis. J Hepatol. 2013;59(3):474–81. https://doi.org/10.1016/j.jhep.2013.04.036.

15. Piano S, Brocca A, Angeli P. Renal function in cirrhosis: a critical review of available tools. Semin Liver Dis. 2018;38(3):230–41. https://doi.org/10.1055/s-0038-1661372.

16. Ojeda-Yuren AS, Cerda-Reyes E, Herrero-Maceda MR, Castro-Narro G, Piano S. An integrated review of hepatorenal syndrome. Ann Hepatol. 2020;22:100236. https://doi.org/10.1016/j.aohep.2020.07.008.

17. Solé C, Solà E, Huelin P, et al. Characterization of inflammatory response in hepatorenal syndrome: relationship with kidney outcome and survival. Liver Int. 2019;39(7):1246–55. https://doi.org/10.1111/liv.14037.

18. Thabut D, Massard J, Gangloff A, et al. Model for end-stage liver disease score and systemic inflammatory response are major prognostic factors in patients with cirrhosis and acute functional renal failure. Hepatology. 2007;46(6):1872–82. https://doi.org/10.1002/hep.21920.

19. Bajaj JS, Reddy KR, O'Leary JG, et al. Serum levels of metabolites produced by intestinal microbes and lipid moieties independently associated with acute-on-chronic liver failure and death in patients with cirrhosis. Gastroenterology. 2020;159:1715. https://doi.org/10.1053/j.gastro.2020.07.019.

20. Albillos A, Lario M, Álvarez-Mon M. Cirrhosis-associated immune dysfunction: distinctive features and clinical relevance. J Hepatol. 2014;61(6):1385–96. https://doi.org/10.1016/j.jhep.2014.08.010.

21. Shah N, Mohamed FE, Jover-Cobos M, et al. Increased renal expression and urinary excretion of TLR4 in acute kidney injury associated with cirrhosis. Liver Int. 2013;33(3):398–409. https://doi.org/10.1111/liv.12047.

22. Du Plessis J, Vanheel H, Janssen CEI, et al. Activated intestinal macrophages in patients with cirrhosis release NO and IL-6 that may disrupt intestinal barrier function. J Hepatol. 2013;58(6):1125–32. https://doi.org/10.1016/j.jhep.2013.01.038.

23. Izzy M, VanWagner LB, Lin G, et al. Redefining cirrhotic cardiomyopathy for the modern era. Hepatology. 2020;71(1):334–45. https://doi.org/10.1002/hep.30875.

24. Belcher JM, Garcia-Tsao G, Sanyal AJ, et al. Urinary biomarkers and progression of AKI in patients with cirrhosis. Clin J Am Soc Nephrol. 2014;9(11):1857–67. https://doi.org/10.2215/CJN.09430913.

25. Huelin P, Solà E, Elia C, et al. Neutrophil gelatinase-associated lipocalin for assessment of acute kidney injury in cirrhosis: a prospective study. Hepatology. 2019;70(1):319–33. https://doi.org/10.1002/hep.30592.

26. Ariza X, Solà E, Elia C, et al. Analysis of a urinary biomarker panel for clinical outcomes assessment in cirrhosis. PLoS One. 2015;10(6):e0128145. https://doi.org/10.1371/journal.pone.0128145.

27. Benozzi P, Vallecillo B, Musso CG. Urinary indices: their diagnostic value in current nephrology. Front Med Health Res. 2017;102(1):1–5.
28. Aiello F, Bajo M, Marti F, Musso CG. How to evaluate renal function in stable cirrhotic patients. Postgrad Med. 2017;129(8):866–71. https://doi.org/10.1080/00325481.2017.1365569.
29. Ginès A, Escorsell A, Ginès P, et al. Incidence, predictive factors, and prognosis of hepatorenal syndrome in cirrhosis with ascites. Gastroenterology. 1993;105(1):229–36. https://doi.org/10.1016/0016-5085(93)90031-7.
30. Wong F, Jepsen P, Watson H, Vilstrup H. Un-precipitated acute kidney injury is uncommon among stable patients with cirrhosis and ascites. Liver Int. 2018;38(10):1785–92. https://doi.org/10.1111/liv.13738.
31. Markwardt D, Holdt L, Steib C, et al. Plasma cystatin C is a predictor of renal dysfunction, acute-on-chronic liver failure, and mortality in patients with acutely decompensated liver cirrhosis. Hepatology. 2017;66(4):1232–41. https://doi.org/10.1002/hep.29290.
32. Sort P, Navasa M, Arroyo V, et al. Effect of intravenous albumin on renal impairment and mortality in patients with cirrhosis and spontaneous bacterial peritonitis. N Engl J Med. 1999;341(6):403–9. https://doi.org/10.1056/NEJM199908053410603.
33. Navasa M, Follo A, Filella X, et al. Tumor necrosis factor and interleukin-6 in spontaneous bacterial peritonitis in cirrhosis: relationship with the development of renal impairment and mortality. Hepatology. 1998;27(5):1227–32. https://doi.org/10.1002/hep.510270507.
34. Follo A, Llovet JM, Navasa M, et al. Renal impairment after spontaneous bacterial peritonitis in cirrhosis: incidence, clinical course, predictive factors and prognosis. Hepatology. 1994;20(6):1495–501.
35. Barreto R, Fagundes C, Guevara M, et al. Type-1 hepatorenal syndrome associated with infections in cirrhosis: natural history, outcome of kidney function, and survival. Hepatology. 2014;59(4):1505–13. https://doi.org/10.1002/hep.26687.
36. Fernández J, Monteagudo J, Bargallo X, et al. A randomized unblinded pilot study comparing albumin versus hydroxyethyl starch in spontaneous bacterial peritonitis. Hepatology. 2005;42(3):627–34. https://doi.org/10.1002/hep.20829.
37. Salerno F, Navickis RJ, Wilkes MM. Albumin infusion improves outcomes of patients with spontaneous bacterial peritonitis: a meta-analysis of randomized trials. Clin Gastroenterol Hepatol. 2013;11(2):123–30.e1. https://doi.org/10.1016/j.cgh.2012.11.007.
38. Thévenot T, Bureau C, Oberti F, et al. Effect of albumin in cirrhotic patients with infection other than spontaneous bacterial peritonitis. A randomized trial. J Hepatol. 2015;62(4):822–30. https://doi.org/10.1016/j.jhep.2014.11.017.
39. Fernández J, Angeli P, Trebicka J, et al. Efficacy of albumin treatment for patients with cirrhosis and infections unrelated to spontaneous bacterial peritonitis. Clin Gastroenterol Hepatol. 2020;18(4):963–973.e14. https://doi.org/10.1016/j.cgh.2019.07.055.
40. Caraceni P, Riggio O, Angeli P, et al. Long-term albumin administration in decompensated cirrhosis (ANSWER): an open-label randomised trial. Lancet (London, England). 2018;391(10138):2417–29. https://doi.org/10.1016/S0140-6736(18)30840-7.
41. Solà E, Solé C, Simón-Talero M, et al. Midodrine and albumin for prevention of complications in patients with cirrhosis awaiting liver transplantation. A randomized placebo-controlled trial. J Hepatol. 2018;69(6):1250–9. https://doi.org/10.1016/j.jhep.2018.08.006.
42. Fernández J, Navasa M, Planas R, et al. Primary prophylaxis of spontaneous bacterial peritonitis delays hepatorenal syndrome and improves survival in cirrhosis. Gastroenterology. 2007;133(3):818–24. https://doi.org/10.1053/j.gastro.2007.06.065.
43. Aiello FI, Bajo M, Marti F, Gadano A, Musso CG. Model for end-stage liver disease (MELD) score and liver transplant: benefits and concerns. AME Med J. 2017;2:168–70.
44. Cavallin M, Kamath PS, Merli M, et al. Terlipressin plus albumin versus midodrine and octreotide plus albumin in the treatment of hepatorenal syndrome: a randomized trial. Hepatology. 2015;62(2):567–74. https://doi.org/10.1002/hep.27709.

45. Martín-Llahí M, Pépin M-N, Guevara M, et al. Terlipressin and albumin vs albumin in patients with cirrhosis and hepatorenal syndrome: a randomized study. Gastroenterology. 2008;134(5):1352–9. https://doi.org/10.1053/j.gastro.2008.02.024.
46. Boyer TD, Sanyal AJ, Garcia-Tsao G, et al. Predictors of response to terlipressin plus albumin in hepatorenal syndrome (HRS) type 1: relationship of serum creatinine to hemodynamics. J Hepatol. 2011;55(2):315–21. https://doi.org/10.1016/j.jhep.2010.11.020.
47. Boyer TD, Sanyal AJ, Wong F, et al. Terlipressin plus albumin is more effective than albumin alone in improving renal function in patients with cirrhosis and hepatorenal syndrome type 1. Gastroenterology. 2016;150:1579. https://doi.org/10.1053/j.gastro.2016.02.026.
48. Arora V, Maiwall R, Rajan V, et al. Terlipressin is superior to noradrenaline in the management of acute kidney injury in acute on chronic liver failure. Hepatology. 2020;71(2):600–10. https://doi.org/10.1002/hep.30208.
49. Cavallin M, Piano S, Romano A, et al. Terlipressin given by continuous intravenous infusion versus intravenous boluses in the treatment of hepatorenal syndrome: a randomized controlled study. Hepatology. 2016;63(3):983–92. https://doi.org/10.1002/hep.28396.
50. Piano S, Schmidt HH, Ariza X, et al. Association between grade of acute on chronic liver failure and response to terlipressin and albumin in patients with hepatorenal syndrome. Clin Gastroenterol Hepatol. 2018;16(11):1792–1800.e3. https://doi.org/10.1016/j.cgh.2018.01.035.
51. Alessandria C, Ottobrelli A, Debernardi-Venon W, et al. Noradrenalin vs terlipressin in patients with hepatorenal syndrome: a prospective, randomized, unblinded, pilot study. J Hepatol. 2007;47(4):499–505. https://doi.org/10.1016/j.jhep.2007.04.010.
52. Sharma P, Kumar A, Shrama BC, Sarin SK. An open label, pilot, randomized controlled trial of noradrenaline versus terlipressin in the treatment of type 1 hepatorenal syndrome and predictors of response. Am J Gastroenterol. 2008;103(7):1689–97. https://doi.org/10.1111/j.1572-0241.2008.01828.
53. Singh V, Ghosh S, Singh B, et al. Noradrenaline vs. terlipressin in the treatment of hepatorenal syndrome: a randomized study. J Hepatol. 2012;56(6):1293–8. https://doi.org/10.1016/j.jhep.2012.01.012.

Chapter 13
Kidney–Muscle Crosstalk in Acute Kidney Injury

Titus Adriean and Adrian Covic

13.1 Acute Kidney Injury Definition Based on Creatinine and Creatinine Metabolism

According to the current AKI KDIGO Guidelines published in 2012, acute kidney injury (AKI) is defined as any of the following: an increase in serum levels of creatinine by 0.3 mg/dL (26.5 mol/L) within 48 h, an increase in SCr to 1.5 times baseline, which is known or presumed to have occurred within the prior 7 days, or the urine output definition: urine volume 0.5 mL/kg/h for 6 h [1]. Serum creatinine represents at this moment the most important and commonly used biomarker of kidney function.

Creatinine is an organic acid of nitrogenous nature that is the result of a complex metabolic pathway of creatine and creatine phosphate. Creatine is stored in muscle tissues where it is transformed to creatine phosphate by phosphorylation by the actions of CK (creatine kinase). Creatine phosphate is used as an energy source. Creatinine is the result of spontaneous dehydration of creatine in the muscle tissue. Production occurs at a constant rate but increases with temperature and lower pH [2].

Creatinine has a renal elimination. It is a free low-weight molecule, and it has a free glomerular filtration. However, proximal tubular cells have the ability to secrete creatinine and this is why clearance is about 10% more than the golden standard inulin clearance (eliminated only by glomerular filtration). Certain molecules can compete with tubular creatinine transport, inhibiting secretion (trimethoprim, cimetidine, salicylates, antiretrovirals, chemotherapeutic drugs) [3].

Recently, the intestinal microbiome has been considered as a possible clearance way as an extrarenal way of elimination of serum creatinine, which is mainly relevant in the CKD patients. Chronically increased serum creatinine is associated with higher stool enzymatic activity and more important creatinine degradation [4].

T. Adriean · A. Covic (✉)
IAOSR, University of Medicine "Grigore T Popa" Iasi, Iasi, Romania

C. G. Musso, A. Covic (eds.), *Organ Crosstalk in Acute Kidney Injury*,
https://doi.org/10.1007/978-3-031-36789-2_13

Creatinine is used as a marker in clinical medicine because its serum levels vary with glomerular filtration rate. One of the pitfalls in its use is the dependency on muscular mass (because it is a product of muscle catabolism). False judgment occurs mainly in patients with very low or high muscular mass [5, 6].

Certain limitations have been underlined in the AKI setting when GFR estimation depends on serum creatinine. Critical illness alters production of creatinine in paradoxal ways—catabolic status increases production and sepsis may be associated with decreased production. Therapeutic measures such as parenteral hydration may result in serum creatinine dilution, and other medication used in this setting may interfere with its metabolism and measurement.

Caution is warranted in the acute setting when clinicians need to interpret kidney function based on creatinine. However, this biomarker remains the most important tool at this moment due to its availability, easy use, and low cost.

13.2 Rhabdomyolysis

Acute kidney injury is the main distant complication of rhabdomyolysis in terms of frequency and importance of prognosis. Rhabdomyolysis comprises the destruction of skeletal muscle tissue and secondary leakage of cellular toxic contents into the circulation that cause systemic damage. Classic muscle-derived molecules that have been incriminated for their potential harm are mainly represented by creatine kinase, lactate dehydrogenase, aminotransferases, and myoglobin. There is a substantial elevation of the creatine kinase (CK) serum levels—more than five to ten times the superior laboratory normal levels [7].

Clinically patients present with muscle pain and dark urine (pigmenturia). Modern classification considers rhabdomyolysis due to acquired and inherited causes (Table 13.1) [8].

Table 13.1 Common rhabdomyolysis causes. Adapted from [8]

Type	Cause	Examples
Acquired	Trauma	"Crush syndrome"
	Exertion	Muscular activity, electrolyte disturbance
	Ischemia	Immobilizations, compression, thrombosis
	Illicit drugs	Cocaine, heroin, LSD, alcohol consumption
	Drugs	Statins, neuroleptics
	Infections	Bacterial, viral, parasitic
	Extreme weather	Hyperthermia, hypothermia
	Endocrine disorders	Hyper/hypothyroidism, diabetic complications
	Toxins	Spider bites, wasp stings, venom
Inherited	Metabolic myopathies	Glycogen storage, fatty acid, mitochondrial disorders
	Structural myopathies	Dystrophinopathy, dysferlinopathy
	Others	Lipin-1 gene mutation, sickle-cell disease

Three important pathways are involved in causing kidney injury: intrarenal vasoconstriction, tubular injury (direct or ischemic), tubular obstruction. Vasoconstriction manifests as a result of several pathogenic alterations: volume depletion by "third spacing" within affected muscular tissue, secondary activation of renin-angiotensin system, secretion of vasopressin and sympathetic nervous system, reduction of renal blood flow by known mediators (endothelin-1, thromboxane A, TNF-α), deficit in vasodilators (nitric oxide that is scavenged by myoglobin) [7].

Renal involvement in rhabdomyolysis may exhibit particular and characteristic findings: pigmented granular casts, myoglobinuria, more rapid increase in plasma creatinine (creatine and creatinine leak from damaged muscles), low ratio of blood urea nitrogen to creatinine, frequent oliguria and anuria, acute tubular necrosis with low fractional excretion of sodium (paramount importance of renal vasoconstriction and tubular occlusion, and delayed tubular necrosis), severe electrolyte derangements (rapid hyperkalemia, hyperphosphatemia, hyperuricemia, high anion-gap metabolic acidosis and hypermagnesemia), calcium-phosphate complex deposition in tissues, hypocalcemia (avid calcium deposition in injured muscular tissue), and hypercalcemia in the recovery phase (mobilization of calcium from preformed deposits) (Fig. 13.1) [9].

Treatment implies a central measure: i.v. fluid therapy and additional measures. Also, addressing the origin of the muscular damage is important by cessation of the offending drug, temperature control, infection treatment, hormonal control, and others [10]. Aggressive fluid administration will increase renal blood flow and the secretion of the damaging toxins. Due to the heterogeneity of studies conducted addressing which type of i.v. fluid to use, no evidence-based recommendations can be offered in this selection. Signs of benefit were obtained with early initiation of fluid resuscitation while obtaining a 300 mL/h urine output [11]. Isolated or combination therapy can be used with employment of 5% dextrose, 0.9% normal saline, Ringer's lactated solution, bicarbonate. Bicarbonate represents still an attractive therapeutic measure explained by some pathophysiological mechanistic explanations: acidic milieu increases toxicity of myoglobin, increases tubular precipitation of uric acid and myoglobin, promotes electrolyte derangements, and sustains redox-production and lipid peroxidation. Alkali therapy has its pitfalls: paradoxical intracellular acidosis may increase the risk of overhydration [12].

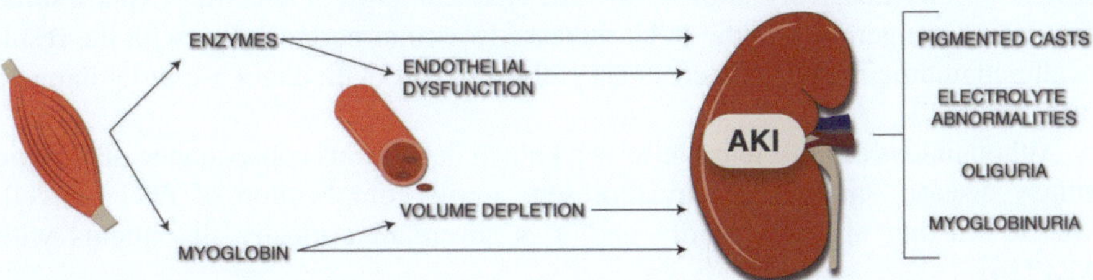

Fig. 13.1 Rhabdomyolysis

The electrolyte abnormalities need to be addressed promptly due to their severity: metabolic acidosis and hyperkalemia may lead to life-threatening complications. Calcium supplementation should be avoided as it could lead to further muscle damage.

Mannitol, although a diuretic, may exhibit some benefits in rhabdomyolysis. Theoretically, it improves diuresis and excretes excess myoglobin and may have a direct antioxidant mechanism. However it could provoke further volume depletion.

If failure in preventing life-threatening AKI has occurred and there are indications in starting renal replacement therapies, continuous renal replacement therapy (CRRT) has been postulated to possess some advantages. A systematic review of the potential benefits of CRRT has been conducted and included three studies with few patients ($n = 101$). Increased clearance of myoglobin, creatinine and improved electrolyte homeostasis were all obtained. However survival rates were not different. CRRT remains in this setting the renal replacement therapy to choose when life-threatening electrolyte derangements do not respond to initial therapies [13].

13.3 AKI and Muscular Damage

Acute kidney injury is associated with excess mortality and morbidity. It seldom occurs as an isolated entity and is frequently associated with remote organ dysfunction. AKI induces systemic organ dysfunction, particularly in the intensive care unit (ICU) setting. Several damaging pathways have been elucidated in experimental and clinical settings: dysfunctional inflammatory responses, cytokine release, oxidative stress, proapoptotic mechanisms, differential molecular expression, leukocyte trafficking, endothelial injury, increased vascular permeability [14].

AKI is frequently hospitalized in the ICU setting, because of the severity of the presentation. Critically ill patients exhibit muscle damage that has been recently characterized as the muscle weakness of ICU. Impaired muscular function due to prolonged ICU stay and critical illness has serious consequences both short and long term: inability to perform usual activity after discharge for as long as 2 years, delayed weaning from mechanical ventilation, increased mortality rate.

Disturbances in the structure and function of the musculoskeletal system in AKI have not been extensively studied. Specific characteristics of AKI may explain some muscular derangements in the ICU: increased vascular permeability with the result of altered microcirculation, increased cytokine release with direct muscular damage (Fig. 13.2) [15].

Although loss of muscle proteins is a known deleterious consequence of chronic kidney disease, sarcopenia may represent a true complication of AKI as well. Muscle wasting appears rapidly and it is severe in critically ill patients with AKI [16].

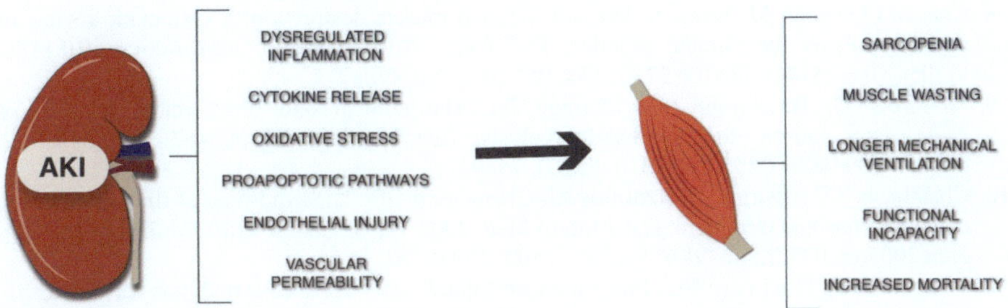

Fig. 13.2 Musculoskeletal consequences of AKI

13.4 Conclusion

Muscle-kidney crosstalk in acute kidney injury represents a bidirectional axis implying several pathological entities and processes: rhabdomyolysis as the paradigm of musculoskeletal damage and leakage of nephrotoxic intracellular compounds, and the important and lesser known consequences of acute kidney injury on muscle structure and metabolism: long functional incapacity, ventilator dependence in the ICU, muscle wasting, and higher mortality rates.

References

1. Kellum JA, Lameire N, KDIGO AKI Guideline Work Group. Diagnosis, evaluation, and management of acute kidney injury: a KDIGO summary (Part 1). Crit Care. 2013;17(1):204. https://doi.org/10.1186/cc11454. PMID: 23394211; PMCID: PMC4057151.
2. Kashani K, Rosner MH, Ostermann M. Creatinine: from physiology to clinical application. Eur J Intern Med. 2020;72:9–14. https://doi.org/10.1016/j.ejim.2019.10.025. Epub 2019 Nov 8. PMID: 31708357.
3. Andreev E, Koopman M, Arisz L. A rise in plasma creatinine that is not a sign of renal failure: which drugs can be responsible? J Intern Med. 1999;246(3):247–52. https://doi.org/10.1046/j.1365-2796.1999.00515.x. PMID: 10475992.
4. Chen YY, Chen DQ, Chen L, Liu JR, Vaziri ND, Guo Y, Zhao YY. Microbiome-metabolome reveals the contribution of gut-kidney axis on kidney disease. J Transl Med. 2019;17(1):5. https://doi.org/10.1186/s12967-018-1756-4. PMID: 30602367; PMCID: PMC6317198.
5. Delanaye P, Cavalier E, Pottel H. Serum creatinine: not so simple! Nephron. 2017;136(4):302–8. https://doi.org/10.1159/000469669. Epub 2017 Apr 26. PMID: 28441651.
6. Bouquegneau A, Vidal-Petiot E, Vrtovsnik F, Cavalier E, Rorive M, Krzesinski JM, Delanaye P, Flamant M. Modification of Diet in Renal Disease versus Chronic Kidney Disease Epidemiology Collaboration equation to estimate glomerular filtration rate in obese patients. Nephrol Dial Transplant. 2013;28 Suppl 4:iv122–30. https://doi.org/10.1093/ndt/gft329. Epub 2013 Sep 11. PMID: 24026245.
7. Bosch X, Poch E, Grau JM. Rhabdomyolysis and acute kidney injury. N Engl J Med. 2009;361(1):62–72. https://doi.org/10.1056/NEJMra0801327. Erratum in: N Engl J Med. 2011 May 19;364(20):1982. PMID: 19571284.

8. Chavez LO, Leon M, Einav S, Varon J. Beyond muscle destruction: a systematic review of rhabdomyolysis for clinical practice. Crit Care. 2016;20(1):135. https://doi.org/10.1186/s13054-016-1314-5. PMID: 27301374; PMCID: PMC4908773.

9. Woodrow G, Brownjohn AM, Turney JH. The clinical and biochemical features of acute renal failure due to rhabdomyolysis. Ren Fail. 1995;17(4):467–74. https://doi.org/10.3109/08860229509037610. PMID: 7569117.

10. Chatzizisis YS, Misirli G, Hatzitolios AI, Giannoglou GD. The syndrome of rhabdomyolysis: complications and treatment. Eur J Intern Med. 2008;19(8):568–74. https://doi.org/10.1016/j.ejim.2007.06.037. Epub 2008 Apr 28. PMID: 19046720.

11. Scharman EJ, Troutman WG. Prevention of kidney injury following rhabdomyolysis: a systematic review. Ann Pharmacother. 2013;47(1):90–105. https://doi.org/10.1345/aph.1R215. Epub 2013 Jan 16. PMID: 23324509.

12. Berend K, de Vries AP, Gans RO. Physiological approach to assessment of acid-base disturbances. N Engl J Med. 2015;372(2):195. https://doi.org/10.1056/NEJMc1413880. PMID: 25564913.

13. Zeng X, Zhang L, Wu T, Fu P. Continuous renal replacement therapy (CRRT) for rhabdomyolysis. Cochrane Database Syst Rev. 2014;(6):CD008566. https://doi.org/10.1002/14651858.CD008566.pub2. PMID: 24929959.

14. Kellum JA, Romagnani P, Ashuntantang G, Ronco C, Zarbock A, Anders HJ. Acute kidney injury. Nat Rev Dis Primers. 2021;7(1):52. https://doi.org/10.1038/s41572-021-00284-z. PMID: 34267223.

15. Koukourikos K, Tsaloglidou A, Kourkouta L. Muscle atrophy in intensive care unit patients. Acta Inform Med. 2014;22(6):406–10. https://doi.org/10.5455/aim.2014.22.406-410. Epub 2014 Dec 19. PMID: 25684851; PMCID: PMC4315632.

16. Wang XH, Mitch WE, Price SR. Pathophysiological mechanisms leading to muscle loss in chronic kidney disease. Nat Rev Nephrol. 2022;18(3):138–52. https://doi.org/10.1038/s41581-021-00498-0. Epub 2021 Nov 8. PMID: 34750550.

Chapter 14
Kidney–Placenta Crosstalk in Acute Kidney Injury

Amelia Bernasconi, Ricardo M. Heguilen, Liliana S. Voto, Olivia Maria Capalbo, and Omar Cabarcas

14.1 Introduction

Neuron and bloodstream signaling via hormones, transmitters, chemical mediators, and paracrine interactions within the same tissue provide communication pathways within and between organs, allowing the orchestration of body functions to maintain homeostasis. This crosstalk allows coordination and adaptation to a constantly changing environment, but its bidirectional or multidirectional nature also enables the exchange of inflammatory mediators, and consequently the extension of injury from one organ to others [1].

The process of placentation and the new hormonal milieu during pregnancy trigger a series of physiological changes. The kidney plays a key role in maintaining and managing the plasma volume expansion necessary for an optimal maternal and fetal perfusion, as well as to control an adequate blood pressure. Hence, a diseased

A. Bernasconi
Departamento de Medicina, Hospital Juan A. Fernández, Buenos Aires, Argentina

R. M. Heguilen
Nephrology, Hospital Juan A. Fernández, Buenos Aires, Argentina

L. S. Voto
Departamento Materno Infantil Juvenil, Hospital Juan A. Fernández, Buenos Aires, Argentina
e-mail: lvoto@intramed.net

O. M. Capalbo
Fisiologia, Instituto Universitario del Hospital Italiano de Buenos Aires,
Buenos Aires, Argentina
e-mail: olivia.capalbo@hospitalitaliano.org.ar

O. Cabarcas (✉)
Facultad de Ciencias de la Salud, Universidad Simón Bolivar, Barranquilla, Colombia

C. G. Musso, A. Covic (eds.), *Organ Crosstalk in Acute Kidney Injury*,
https://doi.org/10.1007/978-3-031-36789-2_14

kidney will undergo a poor adaptation and provide an adverse scenario increasing the risks of complications during pregnancy and delivery. On the other hand, gestational disease will also impact the kidney, which will break down, feeding the loop of damage [2].

Preeclampsia, acute fatty liver of pregnancy, HELLP syndrome (hemolysis, elevated liver enzymes and low platelet count), and thrombotic microangiopathies (TMAs) and atypical uremic syndrome (aUHS) are considered pregnancy-related disorders. Diagnosis is often difficult, especially in patients with overlying symptoms from other diseases [2, 3].

The risk of adverse outcomes is further increased if acute kidney injury (AKI) develops in these conditions and pregnancy-related disorders are the most common cause of AKI in pregnancy [4, 5].

Hypertensive disorders of pregnancy constitute one of the leading causes of maternal and perinatal mortality worldwide. It has been estimated that preeclampsia complicates 2–8% of pregnancies globally. In Latin America and the Caribbean, hypertensive disorders are responsible for almost 26% of maternal deaths, whereas in Africa and Asia they contribute to 9% of deaths. Although maternal mortality is much lower in high-income countries than in developing countries, 16% of maternal deaths can be attributed to hypertensive disorder. Moreover, in comparison with women giving birth in 1980, those giving birth in 2003 were at 6.7-fold increased risk of severe preeclampsia (PE) [6, 7].

In a systematic review and meta-analysis of 11 studies, women suffering from pregnancy-AKI had a greater probability of cesarean section, hemorrhage, placenta abruption, maternal death, longer intensive care unit (ICU) stays, and stillbirth [8].

Women in childbearing age with chronic kidney disease (CKD) have an increased risk of adverse pregnancy-related outcomes, including increased perinatal death and prematurity, which further increase with worsening CKD. CKD also increases the risk of developing PE and other pregnancy-related disorders that may aggravate the kidney condition [9].

In this chapter, we describe first the pathological mechanisms of pregnancy-related diseases that adversely impact the kidney and secondly, the pathological mechanisms of kidney disease, and how the physiological stress of pregnancy adversely interacts with pregnancy-related diseases. The use of this knowledge optimizes care during gestation and eventually reduces the risk of pregnancy-related disorders, AKI and associated adverse outcomes. Pre-conception and pregnancy management can change the outcome. General measures to treat pregnancy-related AKI include identification of the underlying cause of kidney injury, intravenous fluid resuscitation, timely initiation of dialysis if needed, and prompt fetal delivery, if necessary.

Specific treatment includes steroid and immunosuppressive therapy for glomerulonephritis; prompt delivery for severe preeclampsia, hemolysis, elevated liver enzymes and low platelet count syndrome, and acute fatty liver of pregnancy; as well as plasmapheresis and eculizumab for thrombotic microangiopathies such as thrombotic thrombocytopenic purpura and atypical hemolytic uremic syndrome.

14.2 Placenta-Kidney Perspective

From the placenta to kidney point of view, we should understand the physiological kidney changes during pregnancy, the pathogenesis of pregnancy-related diseases and impact on healthy kidneys, and pregnancy effects on kidney disease. There are long-term effects of PE on both maternal and fetal health, but this remains an area of active research with many unknowns. PE is a risk factor for the future development of CKD and ESRD in the mother. The reasons are not fully understood; podocyte loss is a hallmark of PE, suggesting permanent glomerular damage. Endotheliosis, associated with PE, but also found in normal pregnancies, may herald glomerulosclerosis; tubular and vascular damage may coexist [10].

14.3 Physiological Adaptation to Pregnancy

A state of vasodilatation makes vasculature sensitive to an array of vasoactive mediators, vasodilators as nitric oxide, prostacyclin, bradykinin, and relaxin. The renal hemodynamic driven by increased cardiac output increases renal blood flow and decreases blood pressure due to hormonal and anatomic changes during pregnancy. This result in an approximately 40–50% increase renal plasma flow and hence in glomerular filtration rate (GFR), which peaks during the first trimester and results in altered tubular reabsorption of protein, glucose, amino acids, uric acid, and bicarbonate [11].

Vasodilation in the first stages of gestation is mainly related to relaxin, a hormone produced by the decidua, placenta, and corpus luteum. The actions of relaxin are mediated by relaxin family peptide receptor 1 (Rxfp1). Activated relaxin exerts both rapid (minutes) and sustained (hours to days) vasodilatory actions through different molecular mechanisms that have increased endothelial nitric oxide (N_3O) availability as a final common pathway [12]. Thus, it leads to generalized renal vasodilation, decreased renal afferent and efferent arteriolar resistance, and a subsequent increase in renal blood flow and GFR [13]. Relaxin administration to male and female non-pregnant rats reproduced hemodynamic changes observed in pregnancy [14].

The renin-angiotensin-aldosterone system (RAAS) regulates blood pressure, volume status, and vascular remodeling during pregnancy. Because the placenta has no autonomic innervation, it relies on angiotensin II (AII) to regulate vascular resistance. The system is upregulated, and estrogens increase angiotensinogen synthesis by the liver. Aldosterone and deoxycorticosterone from progesterone conversion promote sodium retention. On the other hand, progesterone competes with tubular mineralocorticoid receptors agonists to limit sodium retention [15].

The expansion of plasma volume is due to the increased total body sodium by 3–4 mmol/day (net balance 900–1000 mmol), and water retention with a net excess of water resulting in decreased osmolality. There is an interaction between natriuretic and anti-natriuretic factors. The increase in natriuretic peptides and the higher GFR promote salt excretion. The decrease in the set point for thirst and ADH release favors water gain that reduces the oncotic pressure, intensifying the increase in GFR [16]. Paradoxically, vascular insensitivity to AII infusion has been demonstrated in normal pregnant women. There is a sustained decline in blood pressure in normal women. We suggest closely watching patients whose systolic blood pressure in the first trimester is higher than 120 mmHg, and diastolic blood pressure above 70 mmHg. Physiological hydronephrosis in pregnancy is mainly explained by anatomic compressive factors. The prevalence of right-kidney hydronephrosis supports this as the right ureter crosses the pelvis and iliac vessels in a more acute angle than the left ureter, which descends parallel to the vessels [16]. Progesterone also reduces the ureteral tone and may contribute to hydronephrosis· Even though this hydronephrosis constitutes a normal state, it is worth noting that urine stasis can increase the risk of pyelonephritis, thus the importance of detecting and treating asymptomatic bacteriuria [17].

14.4 Pathogenesis of Pregnancy-Related Diseases and its Impact on Healthy Kidneys

PE is a disorder of pregnancy associated with new-onset hypertension, which occurs most often after 20 weeks of gestation and frequently near term. PE is generally accompanied by new-onset proteinuria, hypertension, and other signs or symptoms of PE may present in some women in the absence of proteinuria. We must take into account that PE is more than hypertension with proteinuria, since PE implies risk of eclampsia, stroke, AKI, and pulmonary edema. Worldwide PE leads to 30,000 maternal deaths/year and 250,000 fetal and neonatal deaths. Dramatically 99% of those deaths are mainly attributed to missed or delayed diagnosis, and lack of derivation to complex care facilities [18] (Table 14.1).

Even though, a certain degree of glomerular endotheliosis may not be uncommon even in healthy pregnant women. Women with PE show signs of severe endothelial dysfunction in glomeruli. These changes manifest in expression of podocyte associated proteins, and possibly even podocyte injury and loss. Women with PE can develop AKI in the absence of other kidney disease, thrombocytopenia

Table 14.1 Preeclampsia (PE): main clinical characteristics

1	"De novo" hypertension ($\geq$ systolic BP 140 mmHg or diastolic $\geq$BP 90 mmHg on two occasions) after 20 weeks' gestation frequently accompanied by proteinuria and/or evidence of maternal AKI, liver dysfunction, neurological features, hemolysis or thrombocytopenia, or fetal growth restriction
2	Proteinuria is not mandatory for a diagnosis of PE
3	PE may develop or be recognized for the first time intrapartum or early postpartum in some cases
4	Watch if patient is 120/80 in the first trimester

BP blood pressure, *AKI* acute kidney injury

($<100,000 \times 10^9$/L) or increased liver transaminases ($\geq$two-fold over the upper limit of the normal concentrations). Pulmonary edema or new-onset and persistent headache, unresponsive to usual doses of analgesics, and/or accompanied with visual symptoms (blurred vision, flashing lights or sparks, scotomata) are common to find in PE severe forms. In summary, PE is diagnosed by the presence of "de novo" hypertension after 20 weeks' gestation frequently accompanied by proteinuria and/or evidence of maternal AKI, liver dysfunction, neurological features, hemolysis, thrombocytopenia, or fetal growth restriction [19].

For more than 100 years, proteinuria was necessary for the diagnosis of preeclampsia, but recent guidelines recommend that proteinuria is sufficient but not necessary for the diagnosis. It is important to remark that proteinuria is not mandatory for a diagnosis of PE. In recent years, the pathobiology of renal damage in preeclampsia has shifted from the glomerular endothelial cells to the podocytes. Current data suggest that the number of urinary podocytes in women with preeclampsia is higher than in women with gestational hypertension or normal pregnancies. In the kidney, podocytes produce vascular endothelial growth factor (VEGF), and VEGF receptors have been found in endothelial cells and podocytes themselves. Thus, paracrine and autocrine pathways could affect the integrity of the glomerular filtration barrier with tight regulation of VEGF signaling to maintain a healthy glomeruli [20].

In addition, PE may develop or be recognized for the first time intrapartum or early postpartum in some cases [21].

The placenta and, specifically, impaired placentation play a key role in the pathogenesis of PE.

A two-stage model was proposed in which deficient uterine spiral artery remodeling leads to placental ischemia (stage 1), and the consequent release of antiangiogenic factors, such soluble fms-like tyrosine kinase 1 (sFlt-1 or sVEGFR-1), and soluble endoglin (sEng), which lead to generalized endothelial dysfunction (stage 2). Defective trophoblast invasion of the spiral arteries may be favored by defective cytotrophoblast differentiation from an epithelial phenotype to an endothelial one that prevents the development of lower resistance vessels, and consequently the increased blood flow that nourishes the fetus [22].

Immunological and environmental factors together with genetic predisposition may also contribute [23]. Diverse immune abnormalities have been described from agonistic antibodies to the angiotensin AT-1 receptor to immunologic abnormalities, similar to those observed in organ rejection [24].

The heme oxygenase enzyme is usually upregulated in hypoxia as it generates the vasodilatory product carbon monoxide. However, heme oxygenase 1 (HO-1) gene expression was decreased in chorionic villus samples from 11 weeks pregnant women who would develop preeclampsia [25].

Inflammatory and angiogenic factors are thought to play a considerable role in this disease. Among antiangiogenic factors, released by the hypoxic placenta, sFlt-1 is a decoy receptor that prevents VEGF binding to receptors on podocytes and renal endothelial cells. The resultant endothelial dysfunction causes cell ballooning with consequent capillary obstruction (glomerular endotheliosis), mesangiolysis, reduced nitric oxide (NO) and prostacyclin production, and consequently glomerular filtration barrier dysfunction. The normal paracrine signaling of VEGF released from podocytes is also impaired [26].

Pregnancy is a condition associated with higher levels of antiangiogenic and pro-inflammatory factors than the non-pregnant state. PE is associated with an imbalance of these factors in maternal circulation. Endothelial dysfunction results in the release of thromboxane A [2], complement activation and an imbalance of anti- and procoagulant regulators which leads to disseminated coagulation in glomerular vessels, and AKI [27]. Angiotensin AT1 receptor agonistic autoantibodies increase oxidative stress, and the secretion of endothelin 1 (ET1), which is a powerful vasoconstrictor that contributes to hypertension [28].

Endoglin (Eng), or CD105, is a homodimeric transmembrane glycoprotein localized on cell surfaces that functions as a co-receptor for transforming growth factor (TGF)-β1 and TGF-β3 isoforms. sEng might play an antiangiogenic effect in PE through binding to circulating TGF-β1, thus preventing its interaction with the cell membrane, and consequently the pro-angiogenic and vasodilator effects of TGF-β1 in the normal endothelium [29].

Placental hypoxia promotes placental cell death resulting in the release of cell-free DNA and other danger-associated molecular patterns (DAMPs) into the maternal circulation that may interact with increased expression of receptors such as toll-like receptor 4 to exacerbate inflammatory responses [30].

The renal lesion of PE has always been considered predominantly endothelial in nature. "Glomerular endotheliosis" is cited as characteristic of this disease, although the glomerular foot-processes depicted in electron micrographs of biopsy specimens of preeclamptic women appear relatively well-preserved. Karumanchi suggests that there may be subtle pathologic evidence in the podocytes as well PE's effect on foot-process health might even be the primary event as the epithelial podocyte secretes VEGF. Additionally, at least certain VEGF receptors such as neuropilins are expressed in podocytes [31].

Although most cases of PE occur in healthy nulliparous women with no obvious risk factors, it is more frequent in CKD population (superimposed PE). Even though the precise role of genetic–environmental interactions on the risk and incidence of PE is unclear, emerging data suggest the tendency to develop PE may have some genetic component [32].

Currently, there is no clear consensus on the practical use of angiogenic biomarkers in the detection and management of PE in routine clinical practice. While major international clinical guidelines exist, they do not define which specific parameters signal patient admission, or outpatient evaluation of suspected PE, and most clinicians follow local practices.

HELLP syndrome is considered a severe form of PE and not a separate disorder, as it has a higher maternal morbimortality. It is defined as elevated lactate dehydrogenase (LDH) (>600 IU/L), aspartate and alanine aminotransferases twice the normal upper limit, and thrombocytopenia (<100,000 × 10^9/L). The abnormal placentation pathway is also responsible, leading to endothelial dysfunction and antiangiogenic factors release. RAAS regulates blood pressure, volume status, and vascular remodeling during pregnancy. Because the placenta has no autonomic innervation, it relies on Angiotensin II (Ang II) to regulate vascular resistance. It has been demonstrated vascular insensitivity to Ang II in pregnant normal women [33].

Elevated titers of Angiotensin receptor AT1 agonistic autoantibodies and ET1 in plasma were registered in HELLP patients, and AT1 receptor 1 agonistic autoantibodies administration in rats elicited typical HELLP features [34]. Activation of the alternative complement pathway was also evidenced. Around 50% of women with HELLP developed AKI and AKI was associated with higher maternal mortality [35].

TMAs involve endothelial dysfunction leading to platelet aggregation in small vessels which cause mechanical hemolytic anemia, thrombocytopenia, and tissue ischemia, with predominant kidney and neurological disease. Thrombotic thrombocytopenic purpura (TTP) and atypical hemolytic uremic syndrome (aHUS) may be observed in pregnancy. Gestation itself is a procoagulant state and a trigger for complement activation (as for PE and HELLP that may be considered as a form of TMA) that cause endothelial cell injury. TTP may be triggered by pregnancy in persons with congenital ADAMTS-13 deficiency or acquired anti-ADAMTS-13 IgG antibodies [36].

aHUS may be triggered by pregnancy in persons with complement dysregulation resulting from genetics (mutations in genes encoding for factor H, factor I, C3) or acquired cause. Besides, it may also come out after delivery, when inflammation, hemorrhage, and circulating fetal cells activate the alternative complement pathway [37].

When confronted with liver abnormalities during the third trimester of pregnancy, acute fatty liver of pregnancy should be considered. Pregnancy related liver diseases include intrahepatic cholestasis of pregnancy (ICP), acute fatty liver of pregnancy (AFLP), and HELLP. The differential diagnosis with PE and HELLP syndrome is sometimes difficult because acute fatty liver of pregnancy shares features with both. This pathology is characterized by microvesicular steatosis in the hepatocytes of zone 3 (centrilobular), rapid loss of liver function, jaundice, and coagulopathy requiring maternal supportive care. AFLP may be caused by a fetal deficiency of mitochondrial beta-oxidation of fatty acids, thus leading to accumulation of free fatty acids and intermediate products of metabolism. Increased accumulation of placental free fatty acids and 3-hydroxy fatty acyl-CoA causes oxidative stress, mitochondrial dysfunction, and placental lipotoxicity. Further, lipolysis induced in the third trimester of pregnancy would also trigger the accumulation of fatty acid intermediates. Finally, these are shunted from the placenta to maternal circulation, where they can promote oxidative and nitrosative stress, inducing catastrophic acute maternal liver injury resulting in microvesicular steatosis, hepatic mitochondrial dysfunction, and hepatocyte lipo-apoptosis. The timing of the occurrence of clinical manifestations and abnormal liver function tests (LFTs) are critical for determining diagnosis and treatment strategies, to avoid the development of AKI [38].

Overall, these entities can cause AKI through different mechanisms, ranging from direct effects on the kidney (thrombotic microangiopathy, glomerular

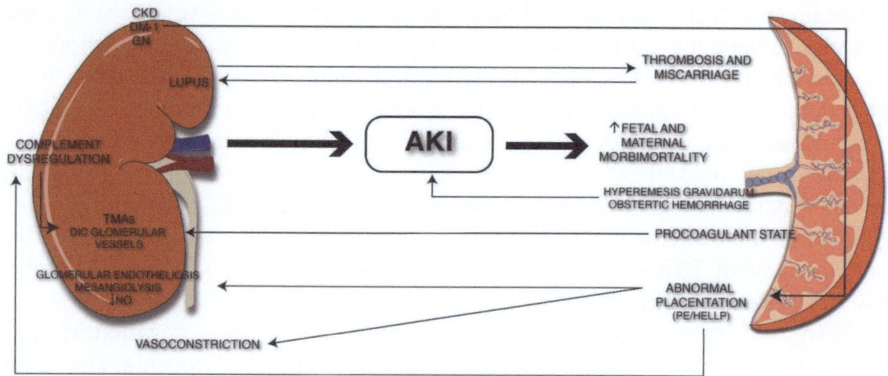

Fig. 14.1 Kidney–placenta crosstalk. *AKI* acute kidney injury, *PE* preeclampsia, *NO* nitric oxide, *DM-1* Diabetes mellitus type 1, *GN* glomerulonephritis, *CKD* Chronic kidney disease, *TMAs* thrombotic microangiopathies, *DIC* disseminated intravascular coagulation, *ET-1* endothelin 1, *AT1-AA* agonistic angiotensin receptor 1 autoantibodies, *sFlt-1* soluble fms-like tyrosine kinase, *sEng* soluble endoglin

endotheliosis, mesangiolysis, vasoconstriction) to prerenal AKI due to hemorrhage, hypovolemia, or edema leading to acute tubular necrosis and/or acute renal cortical necrosis that increases perinatal mortality by three-fold and may lead to CKD [39] (Fig. 14.1).

14.5 Pregnancy Effects on Kidney Disease

Pregnancy is the most common cause of AKI in women of childbearing age. Several diseases and conditions, besides PE, hypertensive disorders of pregnancy, and CKD, can lead to pregnancy-related AKI. PE and hypertensive disorders of pregnancy occur in 5–10% of all pregnancies. In these disorders, the kidney is the main target of an unbalanced pro-angiogenic and antiangiogenic derangement, leading to hypertension, proteinuria, and widespread endothelial damage [40].

Kidney diseases increase both the risk of adverse pregnancy outcomes and the risk of loss of kidney function. The pathogenesis may be disease specific. The physiologic compensatory hyperfiltration may increase signs of renovascular stress. As more women with reduced nephron numbers become pregnant, there is an increased risk of adverse pregnancy outcomes in this population. Whether congenital or acquired from low birth weight and prematurity and/or advanced maternal age, small kidney and renal transplantation make a model in which to study severely decreased nephron numbers, specially in those patients with mild renal dysfunction, even in the absence of hypertension, proteinuria, or systemic disease [41].

Although clearly important, kidney function alone does not uniformly predict pregnancy outcomes. There are likely to be additional contributing factors to pregnancy outcomes, such as active systemic disease or endothelial injury. Specific diseases, such as systemic lupus erythematosus (SLE), may exert a greater adverse effect on the pregnancy, making it impossible to isolate the role of kidney function per se on outcomes. Around 3–5% of women with SLE develop severe flares after pregnancy [42]. Suggested mechanisms include high estrogen levels that interact with regulatory T cells and an upregulation of placenta-expressed interferon-alpha [43–46].

The incidence of preterm delivery and development of proteinuria and hypertension was higher in women with glomerulonephritis (GN) than in controls. Women with IgA nephropathy were at higher risk for development of preeclampsia.

Women with renal-relevant pregnancy complications had a shorter latency time to a diagnosis of GN than those with uncomplicated pregnancy. However, it is still unclear whether pre-existent undiagnosed GN may have favored pregnancy complications. GN may also be misdiagnosed as PE or there could be pathogenic links between both conditions [47, 48].

14.6 Renal Damage: Kidney-Placenta Perspective

From the kidney to placenta perspective, we should understand the impact of both AKI and CKD on pregnancy.

AKI is a common, costly, and increasingly frequent complication of hospitalization worldwide. The incidence of AKI ranges from 10–30% of all medical and surgical hospital admissions and its risk rises substantially in association with patient age, preexisting comorbidities, and exposure to major surgical and diagnostic imaging procedures [49].

Standardized criteria, based on serum creatinine changes, are routinely measured to identify AKI. Unfortunately, AKI can go unrecognized in its initial stages and these relatively simple interventions can be neglected. When not recognized, AKI may progress to more advanced stages of kidney failure, requiring specialized care, dialysis treatment, a lengthy hospital stay, and high costs. Although the true incidence of AKI is possibly underestimated, it is appreciated that AKI affects 10–20% of hospitalized adults and up to 60% of the critically ill patients. AKI is associated in non-pregnant and probably in pregnant women with an increased risk of CKD and further end-organ complications. Moreover, it remains one of the major pathological factors in clinical practice worldwide, with rates of mortality as high as 20–40% [4, 38, 50–52].

The uncertainty regarding AKI definition is demonstrated by the current variation in diagnostic criteria in the literature, with a recent systematic review and meta-analysis of pregnancy outcomes in AKI reporting studies using varying definitions of AKI including the RIFLE (Risk, Injury, Failure, Loss of kidney function and End-stage kidney disease) classification, AKIN (Acute Kidney Injury Network) definition, absolute serum creatinine cut-offs, and oliguria AKI effects on pregnancy. While a validated definition of AKI in pregnancy has not been determined yet, the

KDIGO (Kidney Disease: Improving Global Outcomes) definition of AKI which has merged RIFLE and AKIN criteria has been validated outside of pregnancy and has gained international consensus as a useful guideline and could be useful during pregnancy [52].

Pregnant women may develop AKI from multiple causes beyond the pregnancy-related disorders. With the premise of organ crosstalk in mind, both AKI arising from abnormal placentation or AKI from unrelated conditions are associated with adverse outcomes and increased perinatal and maternal morbimortality. In the past, AKI was mainly related to complications from septic abortions and postpartum hemorrhages. Nowadays, PE is a leading cause of AKI mainly in developed countries while in developing countries where abortion is illegal, septic abortion is a frequent cause of AKI [53].

Prerenal AKI can also result from heart failure, hyperemesis gravidarum, hemorrhage while sepsis may complicate pyelonephritis or post-obstructive causes. Drugs such as diuretics and nonsteroidal anti-inflammatory drugs that can cause prerenal AKI are not generally used during pregnancy. Additionally, the most prevalent causes change according to the gestational period. In the first trimester, these are septic abortions and hyperemesis gravidarum and for the second and third trimesters, hypertensive disorders of pregnancy, acute liver disease, thrombotic microangiopathies, and autoimmune diseases· The most characteristic histological lesion in pregnancy hypertensive disorders associated with AKI is glomeruloendotheliosis, although tubular injury also occurs [47, 54].

The equations used to calculate GFR in pregnancy are inaccurate, with the Modification of Diet in Renal Disease (MDRD) shown to underestimate, and the Cockcroft-Gault formula overestimate, the true GFR value, leaving 24-h urinary creatinine clearance as the gold standard method [55, 56].

Additionally, perfusion of the fetus-placental circulation can be affected by the hemodynamic changes associated with kidney replacement therapy [57]. Moreover, systematic reviews have reported that pregnant women with AKI have a higher risk of postpartum hemorrhage (OR 1.2; CI 1.02–1.56), HELLP syndrome (OR 1.86; CI 1, 4–2.46), placental abruption (OR 3.13; 1.96–5.02), perinatal death (OR 3.39; CI 2.76–4.18), and low birth weight [58].

Hypertensive disorders during pregnancy by themselves can be associated with a risk of preterm delivery and consequently a decrease in nephron mass, making this a risk factor for developing CKD in adulthood· Guidelines and recommendations for management of hypertension in pregnancy are typically written for implementation in an ideal setting. It is acknowledged that in many parts of the world, it will not be possible to adopt all these recommendations; for this reason, options for the management in less-resourced settings are discussed separately in relation to diagnosis, evaluation, and treatment. Although current evidence is limited, some studies suggest that episodes of AKI are associated with an increased risk of CKD and the development of PE in the mother [59].

14.7 AKI in CKD Pregnant Woman

It is estimated that women with CKD are ten times more likely to develop preeclampsia than women without CKD, with preeclampsia affecting up to 40% of pregnancies in women with CKD. However, the shared phenotype of hypertension, proteinuria, and impaired excretory kidney function complicates the diagnosis of superimposed preeclampsia in women with CKD who have hypertension and/or proteinuria that predates pregnancy [59, 60].

CKD prevalence increases with age. Thus, the overall prevalence of CKD among pregnant women is low. However, CKD increases the risk of adverse maternal and fetal outcomes, in proportion to the stage and severity of the disease. Accordingly, the physiological hyperfiltration of pregnancy on existent renal scarring can be unsafe [52, 59].

The renal functional reserve represents the capacity of the intact nephron mass to increase GFR from "baseline" in response to physiologic or pathologic stimuli and can be clinically elicited by administering a protein load and measuring creatinine/inulin clearance. It essentially replaces the lost function by increasing the GFR of residual nephrons and thereby maintains the whole organ's GFR [38, 59]. Normal pregnant women have a progressive increase in baseline GFR and a parallel reduction in renal functional reserve due to its progressive utilization. Women with preexisting renal dysfunction will not be able to keep up with the increased filtration needs of pregnancy, and therefore will be at increased risk of adverse maternal and fetal outcomes. Therefore, it is conceivable that patients with preexisting renal dysfunction will not be able to keep up with their increased filtration needs, and therefore will be at increased risk of adverse maternal and fetal outcomes. Estimating functional renal reserve before and during pregnancy in selected women could be useful to establish prognosis of pregnancy outcomes [53, 59].

Among CKD pregnant women, 40% presented PE, 48% anemia and fetal growth reduction, and 56% chronic hypertension. Additionally, women suffering from glomerulopathies with moderate-severe CKD showed preterm deliveries [54, 59].

In addition, women suffering from type 1 diabetes mellitus, one of the main causes of CKD, are at increased risk of developing PE, independently from the baseline proteinuria. This appears to be dependent on diabetic vascular dysfunction that increases the susceptibility to placental hypoperfusion [55, 59].

In a prospective follow-up of 83 pregnant patients with long-standing type 1 diabetes mellitus, it was assessed whether vascular dysfunction in the early stages of pregnancy predicted the risk of developing preeclampsia. There were no significant differences in vascular dysfunction parameters, VCAM-1 and ICAM-1 serum levels between patients who developed PE and those who did not (p: 0.77). Diabetes mellitus has been associated with fetal growth impairment, stillbirths, preterm delivery, and malformations, and this risk is increased in diabetic nephropathy [56, 59].

Since SLE affects mostly women of childbearing age, the risk of developing lupus nephritis and subsequent pregnancy-AKI is a concern. Complications of lupus during pregnancy include lupus flares, preeclampsia, thrombotic events, and/or fetal complications, such as miscarriage, preterm birth, intrauterine growth restriction, and neonatal lupus. The most frequent maternal complications include relapse of lupus (25.6%), hypertension (16.3%), lupus nephritis (16.1%), and preeclampsia (7.6%). Patients with established lupus nephritis had a higher risk of hypertension and premature birth. Antiphospholipid antibodies were associated with arterial hypertension, premature delivery, and abortion [57, 59].

Since kidney development is completed in the last phases of pregnancy, an insufficient kidney growth, resulting in low nephron number, is probably the basis of an increased CKD and hypertension risk in preterm babies. Additionally, inherited kidney diseases are likely underdiagnosed, as is the case of autosomal dominant conditions such as Alport syndrome, MYH9-associated disease, or autosomal dominant tubule-interstitial kidney disease. In these cases, any adverse impact on placentation or the fetus may occur on a background of fetal genetic predisposition to kidney disease [58, 59].

The timing of pregnancy should be carefully planned especially in kidney transplant receptors. Timing of birth for women with CKD is determined by obstetric indications, with consideration of renal factors including deteriorating renal function, symptomatic hypoalbuminemia, pulmonary edema, and refractory hypertension. It is important to remark that the level of proteinuria should not guide management, the variables, such as status of blood pressure control, evidence of increasing organ damage in the liver and hematological systems, evidence of falling GFR, and signs of neurological involvement, are more reliable indicators of the severity of PE [59, 60].

14.8 Post-Renal Pregnancy-Related Acute Kidney Injury (Pr-AKI)

The combination of urinary stasis and lithogenic factors of pregnancy (increased urinary calcium, oxalate, uric acid, and sodium concentration) may contribute to renal calculi formation. Bilateral renal calculi, although a rare cause of Pr-AKI, will almost always require a surgical intervention, such as ureteroscopy, placement of ureteral stents, or nephrostomy tubes. Iatrogenic injuries to the bladder and ureters are exceptionally rare causes of Pr-AKI and are usually a result of emergent cesarean deliveries, especially in women with altered urologic anatomy, such as ectopic kidneys or duplication of ureters. The etiologies ranged from multiple gestations, solitary kidney, polyhydramnios, and nephrolithiasis, and treatment was directed at the underlying cause. Ultimately, despite the infrequent occurrence, obstructive uropathy can result in high morbidity [17, 18].

14.9 Conclusion

The placenta and kidneys are two metabolically active organs that during pregnancy have a complex relationship with the aim of maintaining homeostasis. Given this bidirectional nature, the acute or chronic dysfunction of one organ can lead to compromise of the other. The process of placentation and hormonal release during pregnancy leads to multiple physiological changes in the kidney that induce volume retention, and they modulate acid-base balance, and the excretion of metabolic waste products. An imbalance between antiangiogenic and angiogenic factors in placentation disorders such as preeclampsia and HELLP syndrome results in hypertension that may cause kidney injury. By contrast, prior kidney injury or even causes of kidney injury may increase the risk of placentation disorders and adverse maternal and fetal outcomes. Understanding the bidirectional potential for compromise from the placenta to kidney and vice versa provides a better framework to limit damage to both organs and improve maternal and fetal outcomes.Compliance with Ethical StandardsConflict of Interest: All the authors declare that they have no conflict of interest.

References

1. Prakash J, Ganiger VC, Prakash S, Iqbal M, Kar DP, Singh U, et al. Acute kidney injury in pregnancy with special reference to pregnancy-specific disorders: a hospital based study (2014–2016). J Nephrol. 2018;31(1):79–85.
2. Liu Y, Ma X, Zheng J, Liu X, Yan T. Pregnancy outcomes in patients with acute kidney injury during pregnancy: a systematic review and meta-analysis. BMC Pregnancy Childbirth. 2017;17(1):235. https://doi.org/10.1186/s12884-017-1402-9.
3. Mehrabadi A, Liu S, Bartholomew S, Hutcheon JA, Magee LA, Kramer MS, et al. Hypertensive disorders of pregnancy and the recent increase in obstetric acute renal failure in Canada: population based retrospective cohort study. BMJ. 2014;349:g4731.
4. Liu Y, Ma X, Zheng J, et al. Pregnancy outcomes in patients with acute kidney injury during pregnancy: a systematic review and meta-analysis. BMC Pregnancy Childbirth. 2017;17(1):235. https://doi.org/10.1186/s12884-017-1402-9.
5. Cooke WR, Hemmilä UK, Craik AL, Mandula CJ, Mvula P, Msusa A, et al. Incidence, aetiology and outcomes of obstetric-related acute kidney injury in Malawi: a prospective observational study. BMC Nephrol. 2018;19(1):1–8.
6. Theilen LH, Fraser A, Hollingshaus MS, Schliep KC, Varner MW, Smith KR, et al. All-cause and cause-specific mortality after hypertensive disease of pregnancy. Obstet Gynecol. 2016;128(2):238–44.
7. Gonzalez Suarez ML, Kattah A, Grande JP, Garovic V. Renal disorders in pregnancy: core curriculum 2019. Am J Kidney Dis. 2019;73(1):119–30.
8. Marshall SA, Ng L, Unemori EN, et al. Relaxin deficiency results in increased expression of angiogenesis- and remodelling-related genes in the uterus of early pregnant mice but does not affect endometrial angiogenesis prior to implantation. Reprod Biol Endocrinol. 2016;14:11. https://doi.org/10.1186/s12958-016-0148-y.
9. Cabiddu G, Castellino S, Gernone G, Santoro D, Moroni G, Giannattasio M, et al. A best practice position statement on pregnancy in chronic kidney disease: the Italian study group on kidney and pregnancy. J Nephrol. 2016;29:277–303.

10. Conrad KP, Davison JM. The renal circulation in normal pregnancy and preeclampsia: is there a place for relaxin? Am J Physiol Ren Physiol. 2014;306(10):F1121–35.
11. Odutayo A, Hladunewich M. Obstetric nephrology: renal hemodynamic and metabolic physiology in normal pregnancy. Clin J Am Soc Nephrol. 2012;7(12):2073–80.
12. Lopes van Balen VA, van Gansewinkel TAGG, de Haas S, Spaan JJ, Ghossein-Doha C, van Kuijk SMJJ, et al. Maternal kidney function during pregnancy: systematic review and meta-analysis. Ultrasound Obstet Gynecol. 2019;54(3):297–307.
13. Voto L. (Hypertension and pregnancy). Buenos Aires. Ascune. 2020.
14. Brown MA, Magee LA, Kenny LC, Ananth Karumanchi S, McCarthy FP, Saito S, Hall DR, Warren CE, Doyi G, Ishaku S. Hypertensive disorders of Pregnancy: ISSHP classification, diagnosis, and management recommendations for International Practice. Hypertension. 2018;72:24–43.
15. Wiles K, Bramham K, Seed PT, Nelson-Piercy C, Lightstone L, Chappell LC. Serum creatinine in pregnancy: a systematic review. Kidney Int Rep. 2019;4(3):408–19.
16. Michal FB, et al. Proteinuria during pregnancy: definition, pathophysiology, methodology, and clinical significance. Am J Obstet Gynecol. 2022;226(2):S819–34.
17. Levine RJ, Maynard SE, Qian C, Lim KH, England LJ, Yu KF, Schisterman EF, Thadhani R, Sachs BP, Epstein FH, Sibai BM, Sukhatme VP, Karumanchi SA. Circulating angiogenic factors and the risk of preeclampsia. N Engl J Med. 2004;350(7):672–83. https://doi.org/10.1056/NEJMoa031884.
18. Haram K, Mortensen JH, Nagy B. Genetic aspects of preeclampsia and the HELLP syndrome. J Pregnancy. 2014;2014:1–13.
19. Phipps E, Prasanna D, Brima W, Jim B. Preeclampsia: updates in pathogenesis, definitions, and guidelines. Clin J Am Soc Nephrol. 2016;11(6):1102–13.
20. George EM, Warrington JP, Spradley FT, Palei AC, Granger JP. The heme oxygenases: important regulators of pregnancy and preeclampsia. Am J Phys Regul Integr Comp Phys. 2014;307(7):R769–77. https://doi.org/10.1152/ajpregu.00132.2014.
21. Bartlett CS, Jeansson M, Quaggin SE. Vascular growth factors and glomerular disease. Annu Rev Physiol. 2016;78:437–61. https://doi.org/10.1146/annurev-physiol-021115-105412.
22. Perucci LO, Gomes KB, Freitas LG, Godoi LC, Alpoim PN, Pinheiro MB, Miranda AS, Teixeira AL, Dusse LM, Sousa LP. Soluble endoglin, transforming growth factor-Beta 1 and soluble tumor necrosis factor alpha receptors in different clinical manifestations of preeclampsia. Plos One. 2014;9(5):e97632. https://doi.org/10.1371/journal.pone.0097632.
23. LaMarca B, Parrish MR, Wallace K. Agonistic autoantibodies to the angiotensin II type I receptor cause pathophysiologic characteristics of preeclampsia. Gend Med. 2012;9(3):139–46. https://doi.org/10.1016/j.genm.2012.03.001.
24. Perucci LO, Gomes KB, Freitas LG, Godoi LC, Alpoim PN, et al. Soluble Endoglin, transforming growth factor-Beta 1 and soluble tumor necrosis factor alpha receptors in different clinical manifestations of preeclampsia. PLoS One. 2014;9(5):e97632. https://doi.org/10.1371/journal.pone.0097632.
25. Phipps EA, Thadhani R, Benzing T, Karumanchi SA. Pre-eclampsia: pathogenesis, novel diagnostics and therapies. Nat Rev Nephrol. 2019;15(5):275–89.
26. Karumanchi SA, Lindheimer MD. Preeclampsia and the kidney: footprints in the urine. Am J Obstet Gynecol. 2007;196(4):287–8. https://doi.org/10.1016/j.ajog.2007.02.013.
27. Gestational hypertension and preeclampsia. Obstet Gynecol. 2020;135(6):e237–60. https://doi.org/10.1097/AOG.0000000000003891.
28. Bu S, Wang Y, Sun S, Zheng Y, Jin Z, Zhi J. Role and mechanism of AT1-AA in the pathogenesis of HELLP syndrome. Sci Rep. 2018;8(1):279. https://doi.org/10.1038/s41598-017-18553-x.
29. Ye W, Shu H, Yu Y, Li H, Chen L, Liu J, et al. Acute kidney injury in patients with HELLP syndrome. Int Urol Nephrol. 2019;51(7):1199–206.
30. Sarig G. ADAMTS-13 in the diagnosis and management of thrombotic microangiopathies. Rambam Maimonides Med J. 2014;5(4):e0026. https://doi.org/10.5041/RMMJ.10160.

31. Cadet B, Meshoyrer D, Kim Z. Atypical hemolytic uremic syndrome: when pregnancy leads to lifelong dialysis: a case report and literature review. Cardiovasc Endocrinol Metab. 2021;10(4):225–30. https://doi.org/10.1097/XCE.0000000000000247.

32. Naoum EE, Leffert LR, Chitilian HV, Gray KJ, Bateman BT. Acute fatty liver of pregnancy: pathophysiology, anesthetic implications, and obstetrical management. Anesthesiology. 2019;130(3):446–61. https://doi.org/10.1097/ALN.0000000000002597.

33. Ibdah JA, Yang Z, Bennett MJ. Liver disease in pregnancy and fetal fatty acid oxidation defects. Mol Genet Metab. 2000;71(1–2):182–9.

34. Monterrosa Robles M, Rico Fontalvo J, Daza Arnedo R, Pérez Olivo J, Cardona Blanco M, Pájaro Galvis NE, Pérez Calvo C, Caparroso Ramos L, Leal Martínez V, Abuabara Franco E, Uparella Gulfo I, Mendoza García M, Correa GJ. Acute kidney injury in pregnant women. Rev Colomb Nefrol. 2020;8(1):e513.

35. Han X, Kambham N, Linda M, Shortliffe D. Pregnancy and severely reduced renal mass: a stress model showing renal hyperfiltration. Pregnancy hypertens. 2022;28:41–3. https://doi.org/10.1016/j.preghy.2022.02.004.

36. Piccoli GB, Attini R, Cabiddu G, Kooij I, Fassio F, Gerbino M, et al. Maternal-foetal outcomes in pregnant women with glomerulonephritides. Are all glomerulonephritides alike in pregnancy? J Autoimmun. 2017;79:91–8.

37. Lightstone L, Hladunewich MA. Lupus nephritis and pregnancy: concerns and management. Semin Nephrol. 2017;37(4):347–53. https://doi.org/10.1016/j.semnephrol.2017.05.006. ISSN02709295.

38. Oliverio AL, Zee J, Mariani LH, Reynolds ML, O'Shaughnessy M, Hendren EM, et al. Renal complications in pregnancy preceding glomerulonephropathy diagnosis. Kidney Int Rep. 2019;4(1):159–62.

39. Torra R, Furlano M, Ortiz A, Ars E. Genetic kidney diseases as an underrecognized cause of chronic kidney disease: the key role of international registry reports. Clin Kidney J. 2021;14(8):1879–85.

40. Prakash J, Pant P, Prakash S, Sivasankar M, Vohra R, Doley PK, et al. Changing picture of acute kidney injury in pregnancy: study of 259 cases over a period of 33 years. Indian J Nephrol. 2016;26(4):262–7.

41. Taber-Hight E, Shah S. Acute kidney injury in pregnancy. Adv Chronic Kidney Dis. 2020;27(6):455–60. https://doi.org/10.1053/j.ackd.2020.06.002. https://www.sciencedirect.com/science/article/pii/S1548559520300902. ISSN15485595.

42. KDIGO. Clinical practice guideline for acute kidney injury. Kidney Int Off J Int Soc Nephrol. 2012;2(1):1–138. i-iv, http://www.kdigo.org/index.php

43. Piccoli GB, Zakharova E, Attini R, Ibarra Hernandez M, Covella B, Alrukhaimi M, Liu ZH, Ashuntantang G, Orozco Guillen A, Cabiddu G, Li P, Garcia-Garcia G, Levin A. Acute kidney injury in pregnancy: the need for higher awareness. A pragmatic review focused on what could be improved in the prevention and care of pregnancy-related AKI, in the year dedicated to women and kidney diseases. J Clin Med. 2018;7(10):318. https://doi.org/10.3390/jcm7100318.

44. Mahesh E, Puri S, Varma V, Madhyastha PR, Bande S, Gurudev KC. Pregnancy-related acute kidney injury: an analysis of 165 cases. Indian J Nephrol. 2017;27(2):113–7.

45. Tangren JS, Powe CE, Ankers E, Ecker J, Bramham K, Hladunewich MA, et al. Pregnancy outcomes after clinical recovery from AKI. J Am Soc Nephrol. 2017;28(5):1566–74.

46. Kao CC, Yang WS, Fang JT, Liu KD, Wu VC. Remote organ failure in acute kidney injury. J Formos Med Assoc. 2019;118(5):859–66.

47. Rao S, Jim B. Acute kidney injury in pregnancy: the changing landscape for the 21st century. Kidney Int Rep. 2018;3(2):247–57.

48. Moghaddas Sani H, Zununi Vahed S, Ardalan M. Preeclampsia: a close look at renal dysfunction. Biomed Pharmacother. 2019;109:408–16.

49. Luyckx VA, Bertram JF, Brenner BM, Fall C, Hoy WE, Ozanne SE, et al. Effect of fetal and child health on kidney development and long-term risk of hypertension and kidney disease. Lancet. 2013;382:273–83.

50. Wiles K, Chappell L, Lightstone L, Bramham K. Updates in diagnosis and management of preeclampsia in women with CKD. Clin J Am Soc Nephrol. 2020;15(9):1371–80. https://doi.org/10.2215/CJN.15121219.

51. Piccoli GB, Cabiddu G, Attini R, Neve Vigotti F, Maxia S, Lepori N, Tuveri M, Massidda M, Marchi C, Mura S, Coscia A, Biolcati M, Gaglioti P, Nichelatti M, Pibiri L, Chessa G, Pani A, Todros T. Risk of adverse pregnancy outcomes in women with CKD. J Am Soc Nephrol. 2015;26(8):2011–22. https://doi.org/10.1681/ASN.2014050459.

52. Heguilén R, Liste A, Bellusci A, Lapidus A, Bernasconi A. Renal response to an acute protein challenge in pregnant women with borderline hypertension. Nephrology. 2007;12:254–60. https://doi.org/10.1111/j.1440-1797.2007.00790.

53. Clausen P, Ekbom P, Damm P, Feldt-Rasmussen U, Nielsen B, Mathiesen ER, et al. Signs of maternal vascular dysfunction precede preeclampsia in women with type 1 diabetes. J Diabetes Complicat. 2007;21(5):288–93.

54. Siddiqui K, George TP, Nawaz SS, Joy SS. VCAM-1, ICAM-1 and selectins in gestational diabetes mellitus and the risk for vascular disorders. Futur Cardiol. 2019;15(5):339–46. https://doi.org/10.2217/fca-2018-0042.

55. Lapolla A, Dalfrà MG, Di Cianni G, Bonomo M, Parretti E, Mello G. Scientific committee of the GISOGD group. Nutr Metab Cardiovasc Dis. 2008;18(4):291–7.

56. LI J, et al. Maternal and neonatal outcomes of pregnancy complicated with Systemic Lupus Erythematosus. Food Sci Technol. 2022;42:e56921. https://doi.org/10.1590/fst.56921. [Accessed 7 March 2022].

57. Piccoli G, Alrukhaimi M, Liu Z-H, Zakharov E, Levin A. What we do and do not know about women and kidney diseases; questions unanswered and answers unquestioned: reflection on world kidney day and international Woman's day. Rev Colomb Nefrol. 2022;5(1):74–89.

58. Abibzadeh N, Fleury D, Labatut D, Bridoux F, Lionet A, Jourde-Chiche N, et al. MYH9-related disorders display heterogeneous kidney involvement and outcome. Clin Kidney J. 2019;12(4):494–502.

59. Lindheimer MD, Kanter D. Interpreting abnormal proteinuria in pregnancy: the need for a more pathophysiological approach. Obstet Gynecol. 2010;115(2 Pt 1):365–75. https://doi.org/10.1097/AOG.0b013e3181cb9644.

60. Cabarcas-Barbosa O, Capalbo O, Ferrero-Fernández A, Musso CG. Kidney-placenta crosstalk in health and disease. Clin Kidney J. 2022;15(7):1284–9. https://doi.org/10.1093/ckj/sfac060.

Chapter 15
Renal Replacement Treatment, Blood Purification, and Crosstalk in Acute Kidney Injury

Manuel Soto-Doria, Juan Pablo Cordoba, Gustavo Aroca-Martinez, and Carlos Guido Musso

15.1 Introduction

Severely ill patients in intensive care units (ICU), especially with hemodynamic instability and acute kidney injury (AKI), require replacement therapy for renal function. In hemodynamically stable patients, intermittent hemodialysis (IHD) or extended hemodialysis is indicated, in order to achieve highly efficient purifying therapies, especially in cases of hypercalcemia, severe hyperkalemia, metabolic acidosis, some acute poisonings, and tumor lysis syndrome.

In the case of hemodynamic instability, the indication is continuous renal replacement therapy (CRRT) that guarantees a very slow and sustained extraction of volume, promoting hemodynamic and cardiovascular stability, greater control of the fluid and electrolyte balance, and improvement in microcirculation due to the

M. Soto-Doria
Nephrology Division, Clínica IMAT Oncomédica Auna, Montería, Colombia

J. P. Cordoba
Internal Medicine and Nephrology, Clinica La Carolina, Bogotá, Colombia

G. Aroca-Martinez
Nephrology Division, Clínica de la Costa, Barranquilla, Colombia

Facultad de Ciencias de la Salud, Universidad Simón Bolivar, Barranquilla, Colombia

C. G. Musso (✉)
Facultad de Ciencias de la Salud, Universidad Simón Bolivar, Barranquilla, Colombia

Nephrology Division and Research Department, Hospital Italiano de Buenos Aires, Buenos Aires, Argentina
e-mail: carlos.musso@hospitalitaliano.org.ar

C. G. Musso, A. Covic (eds.), *Organ Crosstalk in Acute Kidney Injury*,
https://doi.org/10.1007/978-3-031-36789-2_15

"""

preferential elimination of interstitial fluid. In addition, it is also more useful in severe hyponatremia, given by the slow correction of sodium concentration in the blood, preventing central pontine myelinolysis. In ICU, more than 70% of renal replacement therapies (RRT) are performed with CRRT [1, 2]. The *Acute Dialysis Quality Initiative* (ADQI) group conference in 2004 and the consensus between intensivists and nephrologists of the *Acute Kidney Injury Network (AKIN) in 2007 and Kidney Disease Improving Global Outcomes (KDIGO) in 2012*. They defined and classified AKI based on criteria, this has allowed a better understanding and earlier intervention in AKI [3–5] (Table 15.1).

In patients with hemodynamic instability, the strongest evidence is to start CRRT in KDIGO stage 3 with some of the serious complications of AKI: volume overload and hypoxemia, the recommendation is to start CRRT in hypervolemia refractory to diuretics and compromise of a vital organ, patients with metabolic acidosis and electrolyte disorders: sodium bicarbonate less than 12–15 mmol/L and severe hyperkalemia (serum potassium >6.5 mmol/L), and patients with uremia, urea nitrogen >112 mg%, condition that favors platelet dysfunction, heart failure, and increased susceptibility to infection and sepsis [6].

CRRT with a high convective rate is proposed for removal of pro-inflammatory cytokines in the patient with severe sepsis, with clinical evidence of cytokine removal, but no evidence on clinical outcomes in mortality [7].

Patients with acute neurological injury (ANI), can present AKI, and a low percentage of them require RRT, IHD can aggravate cerebral edema. The usefulness of CRRT in patients with ANI and AKI is reviewed here.

Other patients with acute heart failure (AHF) or cardiorenal syndrome, as well as patients with acute liver injury (ALI), hepatorenal syndrome, or chronic liver disease exacerbated with AKI require RRT and/or extracorporeal artificial assistance of liver function. RRT modalities and liver detoxification techniques which have been evaluated are IHD, CRRT, continuous veno-venous hemofiltration (CVVHF), continuous venovenous ultrafiltration (CVVUF), plasmapheresis, albumin dialysis, and MARS systems.

Table 15.1 Acute kidney injury (AKI) stages (KDIGO 2012)

AKIN stage	Definition
1.	Increase in serum creatinine levels >0.3 mg/dL or 1.5–1.9 times the baseline creatinine value, and/or decreased urine output to 0.5 mL/kg/h for 6 h
2.	Increase in serum creatinine levels 2–2.9 times the baseline creatinine value, and/or decreased urine output to 0.5 mL/kg/h for 12 h
3.	Increase in serum creatinine levels 3 times the baseline creatinine value, increase of serum creatinine >4 mg/dL, initiation of RRT and/or decreased urine output to 0.3 mL/kg/h for 24 h or anuria for 12 h

sCr serum creatinine, *RRT* renal replacement therapy, *KDIGO* kidney disease improving global outcomes

15.2 High-Flow Kidney Replacement Therapy and Sepsis

CRRT is a treatment modality with a clear indication in the unstable patient with AKI in ICU, in addition to showing advantages in maintaining hemodynamic stability, recent studies propose its participation in immunomodulation phenomena. This property could be attributed to the removal of pro-inflammatory cytokines through convection and absorption mechanisms.

Park et al., in a study with 212 patients; 107 underwent CRRT at a conventional dose (40 mL/kg/h), and the other high-dose group with 105 patients (80 mL/kg/h), the level of cytokines (IL-6, IL-8, IL-1b and IL-10) at the entrance and exit of the dialyzer was measured at the time of starting the CRRT. In the conventional dose group, there was no difference in the level of cytokines at the entrance and exit of the dialyzer; while in the high-dose group (80 mL/kg/h), the level of cytokines was much lower at the outlet of the dialyzer compared to the inlet. On the other hand, serum cytokines were measured at the beginning and at 24 h of CRRT; in the conventional group there was no difference in the 2 moments, while in the high-volume group, the level of cytokines was lower at 24 h.

Regarding mortality, Peng Li et al., assessed high doses of CRRT vs. conventional doses; At 90 days, there was no significant difference regarding mortality in one or the other group [6, 8, 9].

The efficiency mechanism of the CRRT is based on convection and absorption. It allows the removal of substances with higher molecular weight; proinflammatory cytokines in the septic patient. High doses of CRRT achieve a greater removal of pro-inflammatory toxins, transferring a probable benefit to the critically ill patient with sepsis and AKI.

What is not clear is whether the removal of cytokines has any impact on clinical outcomes of morbidity and mortality; one explanation is that cytokine removal may have been trivial compared to the amount of toxins produced during sepsis, or that the amount of cytokines removed in 24 h have no impact on the global phenomenon of sepsis [8].

In a meta-analysis, Wang et al., reviewed 15 randomized studies where high doses of CRRT vs standard doses were evaluated in relation to mortality; no benefit was shown in relation to all-cause mortality in either group [10].

15.3 Kidney Replacement Therapy in Acute Neurological Injury (ANI) and AKI

The clinical utility of CVVHF in patients with acute ANI and AKI has been reviewed. This clinical setting can be found in patients with intracranial hematoma, cerebral infarction, meningitis, head trauma, cerebral malaria, hypoxia and ischemia in hypertensive emergencies, encephalopathy due to diabetic and hepatic coma. In the medical management of ANI, oxygenation is crucial to maintaining cerebral perfusion pressure (CPP). Intracranial pressure (ICP) secondary to bleeding or hematoma can be controlled by decreasing cerebrospinal fluid volume and cerebral blood volume. In this sense, mannitol or hypertonic saline produces a decrease in cerebral fluid due to an osmotic effect.

ANI in head trauma, and in hemorrhagic or ischemic stroke takes 10–14 days to stabilize, time in which CVVHF can be useful [11].

In patients with AKI, uremia and metabolic acidosis lead to increased plasma and brain osmolarity, an osmotic gradient is generated between the blood and the extracellular medium of the brain, leading to brain edema. IHD worsens cerebral edema since there is sodium bicarbonate entry into the extracellular environment, rapid correction of blood pH, intracellular paradoxical acidosis, intracellular osmole production, passage of water into the intracellular space, and increased cerebral edema [11, 12].

IHD can increase ICP due to cerebral edema and inflammation in chronic kidney disease (CKD) patients. In patients with ANI, there is an increase in ICP, not only due to osmotic changes and a rapid increase in blood pH, but also due to a decrease in mean arterial pressure, and consequently a decrease in CPP with aggravation of cerebral edema. Therefore, it is not a recommended therapy in this setting.

In patients with ANI and high ICP due to cerebral edema, CVVHF produces fewer changes in ICP and CPP than intermittent therapies. There are few changes in plasma osmolarity due to a slow decrease in urea and other solutes, and greater cardiovascular stability by cooling with predilution replacement fluid. The sodium balance tends to be positive, even so, a replacement fluid with sodium greater than 140 mmol/L should be used. The goal in ANI is to adjust treatment to avoid sudden drop in serum osmolarity and cardiovascular instability. Additionally, hypertonic saline or mannitol boluses can be used at the same time with extra benefits.

The advantages of CVVHF over intermittent therapy are theoretical: improved hemodynamic stability, slower and more tolerable removal of liquids and solutes. There is no evidence of a decrease in mortality from one versus the other. Numerous studies and meta-analyzes have concluded that the survival of critically ill patients with ANI and AKI is not affected by the type of therapy. Recent Kidney Disease Improving Global Outcome (KDIGO) guidelines recommend the use of slow continuous and intermittent complementary use modalities [13].

There is a single contemporary study of patients with ANI that included 4 patients: 3 treated with IHD and one with CVVHF [14]. All patients suffered from rapidly progressive edema and brain herniation and death, all related to RRT, with no other detectable causes. It is presumed that the syndrome of dialysis imbalance due to rapid reduction of urea and paradoxical acidosis was the cause of the fatal cerebral edema. All the recommendations for an adequate RRT in the patient with ANI were followed. Only one patient was treated with CVVHF, and for whom there was a need to change to IHD due to severe hyperkalemia. CVVHF was not evaluable in its entirety due to premature suspension of therapy. This result recommends abstaining from IHD.

CVVHF is recommended using a high sodium concentration in dialysate or replacement fluid with strict monitoring of serum sodium, urea nitrogen, sodium bicarbonate, neurological examination, continuous monitoring of blood pressure, and oxygenation.

15.4   Kidney Replacement Therapy in Acute Heart Failure (AHF) and AKI

Acute heart failure (AHF) is a complex syndrome with a great impact on public health. AHF problem consists of the presence of volume overload with an insufficient heart function; consequently, there is neurohormonal activation, especially of the renin-angiotensin-aldosterone system, and the sympathetic nervous system, renal cell dysregulation, and oxidative stress. Besides, glomerular filtration rate (GFR) and renal sodium excretion are decreased, while tubular sodium reabsorption is increased. The attempt to maintain an euvolemic state through prescribing water restriction and diuretics has not been able to improve survival in these patients. On the contrary, it seems to aggravate the impact on the neurohormonal system, a crucial axis in the pathophysiology of this syndrome [15].

In this condition, the central adverse effect is persistent congestion. In the ESCAPE trial [16], an elevated pulmonary pressure was the main predictor of mortality. There was increased tubular reabsorption of sodium and water with elevated central venous pressure, increased intraglomerular pressure, and further impaired GFR [17]. The high rate of hospital readmission revealed the failure of treatment to achieve sustained euvolemia. Forty percent of patients presented congestive signs at discharge, 90% of hospital admission was due to volume overload, between 20 and 30% had resistance to diuretics; 5-year survival was 50%, being the third leading cause of death from cardiovascular disease [18, 19].

Loop diuretics continue to be the first treatment option for AHF, with doubts about their safety profile and adequate dosage. Resistance to diuretics and worsening of renal function is of relevance in these patients [20].

CVVUF arises as a complementary alternative treatment in AHF patients or chronic patients who are unable to achieve euvolemia with diuretics. This procedure increasingly simple to perform, using a portable equipment with a disposable extracorporeal blood circuit. By convection, solutes and water are extracted from the plasma slowly, without further deterioration in osmolarity or neurohormonal activation.

CVVUF can achieve clinical improvement in patients with AHF by decreasing right atrial pressure, pulmonary capillary pressure, and ventricular filling pressure. It also improves ventricular function by reducing cardiac edema. The objective is to avoid the characteristic neurohormonal imbalance, and arterial underfilling of AHF, as well as diuretics treatment.

15.4.1 Cardiorenal Syndrome

Heart and kidney disorders in which the acute or chronic dysfunction of one organ causes the dysfunction of the other. Cardiorenal syndrome was previously defined as AKI secondary to acute heart disease. A new classification demonstrates the bidirectional nature of the disorder and classifies the disorder into 5 subtypes that reflect a true crosstalk in the pathophysiology of concomitant cardiac and renal dysfunction (See Chap. 10: kidney–heart crosstalk) [21].

15.4.2 Clinical Evidence

The RAPID-CHF trial [22] is the first randomized and controlled study of CVVUF with AHF. In this trial, 40 patients were studied: half of them were treated with CVVUF, and the other group was treated with usual treatment; there was no weight loss difference at 24 h; however at 24 and 48 h, the elimination of fluids and improvement of symptoms favored the CVVUF group.

Another study: UNLOAD trial, the first prospective, multicenter, randomized, large-scale study comparing isolated ultrafiltration vs diuretics treatment in patients with AHF, studied 200 patients: 100 with intravenous (IV) diuretic treatment and 100 with CVVUF for 48 h. It concluded that ultrafiltration applied early achieves a greater loss of volume than diuretics without compromising renal function. In this study was documented that after 90 days, rehospitalizations were lower (18% vs 32%), days length of stay (1.4 vs 3.8 days on average), unscheduled medical visits (21% vs 44%), adverse events were fewer; as well as need of vasoactive drugs (3.1% vs 12%) and hypokalemia cases were lower (1% vs 12%) [23].

In the CUORE trial [24], the patients treated with CVVUF presented a significant decrease in rehospitalization for AHF compared to the usual treatment group. This favorable effect was maintained up to 1 year later; and this was associated with a more stable weight, renal function preservation, and lower diuretics dose in the 6 months following discharge. It has been confirmed that congestion is the main determinant in cardiorenal prognosis. The CARRESS-HF Trial (Cardiorenal Rescue Study in Acute Decompensated Heart Failure) had the objective to compare CVVUF with pharmacological treatment in AHF patients with worsening of renal function and signs of permanent congestion. 188 hospitalized patients with AHF were evaluated, 94 patients were treated with CVVUF, while 94 patients were treated diuretics. The study concluded that drug treatment was superior to CVVUF to preserve kidney function, achieving a similar weight loss in both strategies. There was no difference in mortality at 60 days, although CVVUF was associated with more adverse events. Besides, half of the cases of therapy discontinuation were due to causes not related to congestion.

Due to lack of evidence of benefit, and a higher number of adverse events in the CVVUF group, inclusion was terminated early. It is worth mentioning that the studied groups were not totally comparable, no inotropic or vasodilator drugs were authorized in the CVVUF group, while in the diuretic group, dose adjustments of vasoactive drugs and diuretics were allowed. Ultrafiltration was uniform throughout the CVVUF group, and perhaps very excessive in some groups of patients [25].

The safety and efficacy of CVVUF depend on the ability to eliminate solutes without causing hemodynamic instability, worsening renal function, or neuroendocrine activation. CVVUF should be formulated at a rate of 100–200 mL/h, so as not to impact intravascular volume depletion. The overall results in reference to these studies lead to complex strategies in relation to fluid extraction, kidney function, and clinical outcomes. In patients with severe congestion, recent weight gain, diuretic resistance, and low cardiac output without shock, CVVUF may be beneficial.

15.5 Kidney Replacement Therapy in Acute Liver Injury (ALI) and AKI

Acute liver injury (ALI) is a serious condition that warrants management in the ICU, being its only effective treatment liver transplantation, since without transplantation ALI mortality is 80%. ALI patients usually present AKI (40–80%) requiring RRT and sometimes extracorporeal artificial assistance of liver function.

The problem is the availability of organs and how to keep the patient in ideal conditions until transplantation, or the possibility of recovery of liver function. The success achieved in artificial organ support in the last 50 years has not had the same results in liver support, perhaps because of the functional complexity of the liver that includes functions of detoxification of ammonia, alcohol or drugs metabolism, as well protein synthesis, and general metabolic functions; therefore, it is difficult to artificially supply liver function. Hepatic detoxification function can be obtained by performing extracorporeal clearance, through biocompatible membranes, and based on dialysis mechanisms: filtration, convection, and absorption. Hepatic artificial biosynthesis would be possible using isolated organs or hepatocytes of human or animal origin procedures which are currently under investigation [26].

15.5.1 Artificial Extracorporeal Hepatic Assistance Systems

Extracorporeal therapy seeks to eliminate toxic substances responsible for the clinical picture of liver failure. This therapy is not a complete liver replacement, since it does not provide the synthesis function. With IHD it is possible to eliminate small water-soluble substances (up to 2000 D), although it seems not to be useful in ALI. The IHD could be contraindicated in patients with cerebral edema. Continuous slow therapies broaden the elimination spectrum of larger toxic substances, such as ammonium, lactate, gamma aminobutyric acid (GABA), through slow convection and dialysis mechanisms. In addition, due to its greater hemodynamic tolerance, its beneficial effect on intracranial pressure and the possibility of eliminating pro-inflammatory cytokines, CRRT has become the therapy of choice for patients suffering from ALI and AKI [27].

15.5.2 Plasmapheresis

This procedure allows the elimination of substances present in plasma and others bound to proteins, which are in a different spectrum of those removed by IHD and CRRT. Performing plasmapheresis and CRRT at the same time can offer better results in neurological outcomes, and even survival. The simultaneous use of plasmapheresis and absorptive procedures has shown efficacy in septic patients with severe liver failure [28].

15.5.3 Dialysis with Albumin

Plasma albumin, due to its transport action, transports bilirubin, aromatic amino acids, copper, or bile acids. Albumin dialysis allows the elimination of toxic substances bound to albumin with positive results in clinical improvement [29]. The MARS system (Molecular Adsorbent Recirculating System) is a simple, tolerable procedure which has few complications. MARS allows achieving longer treatments by reusing albumin, and consequently lowering costs. Albumin circulates in the countercurrent of the blood through a high-flux membrane, removing dialysable substances such as urea, ammonium, creatinine, and removing substances bound to albumin such as bilirubin, and bile acids. The additional use of CRRT allows the control of AKI by eliminating water and larger dialyzable molecules [30]. From the clinical point of view, although based on a series of few cases, an improvement is shown in renal and cardiovascular parameters, encephalopathy degree, as well as a decrease in bilirubin toxicity, with indirect improvement in liver detoxification function than in hepatic biosynthetic function [31]. Regarding MARS impact on mortality, this procedure achieves an evident biochemical improvement, which leads to an improvement in encephalopathy, hemodynamics, as well as in bilirubin, creatinine, urea, albumin, ammonium, and international normalized ratio (INR) levels. However, there is very little evidence regarding MARS significant positive results in patient's mortality. Two studies with positive effects on survival have been reviewed. In a prospective study by Mitzner et al. [30], based on patients with type 1 hepatorenal syndrome, mortality was 100% in the control group, while it was 62.5% at day 7 and 75% at 30 days in patients treated with MARS ($p < 0.01$). In another study, based on 24 patients suffering from decompensated cirrhosis (bilirubin 20 mg%), Heemann et al., demonstrated clinical and biochemical improvement in liver function, and a reduction in mortality at 30 days (11/12 in MARS group vs 6/12 in control group ($p < 0.05$). It is worth mentioning that the low sample of this study was because of the early completion due to the excellent results obtained. Besides, this study documented that renal dysfunction was presented in 8% of the patients in the MARS group compared to 58% of patients in the control group [31].

15.5.4   Hemoperfusion in Sepsis and AKI

Sepsis and AKI are frequent conditions in the ICU patients. Sepsis is still one of the major causes of death among medical and surgical patients in ICU. Usually, these patients result in multiple organ dysfunction (MOD) syndromes, where the kidney is one of the most frequently affected organs. MOD has been attributed to an inflammatory response induced by pro-inflammatory cytokines and activated neutrophils [32].

Host inflammatory response can produce harm not only by cytokine-induced cytotoxic effect but also by perpetuating and expanding the immune cellular activation. This phenomenon leads to systemic inflammation and consequently to increased vascular permeability and thrombosis [33–36]. In this sense, interleukin (IL) IL-6 and IL-8, which can be produced by macrophages and lymphocytes in response to endotoxins and other cytokines, such as IL-1 or tumor necrosis factor-α (TNFα), can expand the inflammatory reaction by stimulating potent neutrophil activation [36]. Other clinical trials using polymyxin B-immobilized fiber direct hemoperfusion (PMX-DHP) have been demonstrating the safety of PMX in the treatment of septic shock and its capacity to decrease endotoxin levels [37, 38]. However, new evidence is still required to define the indications and timing of this type of therapies.

While we continue understanding the role of all inflammatory mediators and the correct timing of each one of them in controlling the septic/inflammatory process or causing more harm to the organism, it makes sense to try to mitigate the cytokines storm. Here is when the concept of blood purification procedures takes place and relevance. Thus, due to the association between high serum inflammatory cytokines levels and adverse clinical outcomes in critical patients, it has been proposed that reducing cytokines activity could improve their prognosis. Therefore, a variety of strategies have been developed to reduce inflammatory cytokine response based on pharmaceutical or extracorporeal removal approaches [39].

Regarding the pharmaceutical approach, despite anti-endotoxin monoclonal antibodies and cytokine antagonists having been unsuccessful in controlling sepsis inflammation in some clinical studies performed in animal models, they have shown some therapeutic efficacy [36].

With regard to the extracorporeal removal approach, depending on the patient's organ dysfunction and on the target substance to be removed, different extracorporeal therapies can be applied. These blood purification procedures can be based on one of the following physicochemical principles or its combination (most of them have already been discussed in this chapter): hydrostatic pressure gradient across the membrane leading to solvent drag (convection), and solute binding to sorbent material contained within a cartridge (adsorption). Hemoperfusion (HPF) is the procedure based on the principle of adsorption. HPF can remove solutes by binding them to hydrophobic sorbent-based cartridges (charcoal or non-ionic resin), or to ionic resin-based cartridges through chemical exchange. HPF based on non-ionic resin cartridge (HA) contains biocompatible neutral macroporous adsorption resin made of coated polystyrene. This sort of cartridge can remove middle-high weight molecules (5–60 kDa), depending on the subtype of cartridge used: HA130, HA230, HA330/HA380 [33, 34]. While HA130 and HA230 cartridges are effective in purifying blood from uremic toxins and drugs, respectively; HA330/HA338 cartridges are effective in purifying inflammatory cytokines [33]. Apart from its biocompatibility, other advantages of HPF are its lower risk of removing nutrients and drugs and its lower relative cost compared to convective procedures (e.g., hemofiltration) [35].

Furthermore, HPF cartridges usually have a much higher weight cut-off than conventional high-flux hemodiafilters [33, 34]. The HA330 cartridge absorbs most inflammatory cytokines, such as IL-1, IL-6, IL-8, TNFα, and many reports have documented the clinical benefit and safety of this sort of cartridge in treating patients with septic shock [34]. Besides, in sepsis-induced acute lung injury patients, HPF with HA330 cartridge significantly improved patients' hemodynamic and organ function, as well as reduced their mortality, with respect to those who did not receive it [33]. HPF with HA330 has been applied to patients suffering from different inflammatory conditions (sepsis, acute lung injury, hepatitis, pancreatitis) showing significant reduction of inflammatory cytokines with improvement in their clinical evolution. HPF treated patients had better hemodynamics, lower mechanical ventilation and RRT requirement, and shorter ICU length stay and mortality. Furthermore, HPF treated patients had no significant adverse effect, compared to the control group. Additionally, HPF with HA330 reduced circulating and alveolar levels of pro-inflammatory cytokines (IL and TNFα), improved oxygenation, and attenuated lung injury [32, 38].

15.5.5 Hemoperfusion in AKI Associated with COVID-19

COVID-19 associated inflammatory response can affect many organs, particularly the lungs, kidney, heart, digestive tract, blood, and nervous system [11, 13]. IL-6 and ferritin are among the main parameters described as characteristic of the systemic inflammatory syndrome associated with COVID-19. During systemic stress, serum ferritin comes from acute cell destruction, and it is responsible for stimulating innate immunity cells (e.g., macrophages) which induce the cytokine storm. This phenomenon induces severe multi-organ damage through the massive release of inflammatory mediators such as IL-1, IL-2, IL-6, IL-8, IL-10, TNF-α, MCP-1, and IFN-γ. Because of that it has been speculated that cytokines removal from blood could limit organ damage in this condition [33–35]. In this sense, it has been observed that HPF treated patients improved their clinical evolution, associated with persistent serum reduction over time of key inflammatory mediators such as IL-6, IL-8, and TNF-α, in comparison to those patients treated without HPF. This clinical improvement was associated with significant C-reactive protein level reduction, systemic hemodynamic and oxygenation parameters (PaO_2/FiO_2, SpO_2) improvement, peripheral lymphocytes count increase, and reduced intubation requirement [35, 36]. The prompt serum IL-6 reduction induced by HPF, points to its effective removal through the cartridge resin absorption as the mechanism causing clinical improvement, but it has also been speculated that this improvement could be also attribute to a reset of blood IL-8 and TNF-α levels due to cytokine spectrum reprogramming, due to perhaps an inhibitory effect of HA HPF on cytokines production [35, 36]. Furthermore, it has been documented that HPF was effective with sessions that lasted 4 h rather than longer since the bulk of cytokine removal occurs in the first hours of treatment. However, HPF should be applied at an adequate time of the inflammatory process since it has been demonstrated that mortality was lower in HPF treated patients compared with control patients only when their SOFA score was lower than 8 at ICU admission [36, 40–44].

15.5.6 Hemoperfusion in Cardiovascular Surgery

As it has been mentioned above, harmful inflammatory response may appear in those patients who will be submitted to cardiovascular surgery, a population with high prevalence of AKI. As it was published in June 2021 in Blood Purification journal [45], the group exposed to HPF had significantly lower levels of IL-6, IL-8, and IL-10, and significantly lower levels of creatinine (Cr), aminotransferase (AST), and total bilirubin (TBil) compared to the control group. In the same way, the group exposed to HPF had significantly less vasopressor requirement and shorter mechanical ventilation time, and ICU stay length compared to the control group. So, the authors concluded that the HA380 HPF cartridge could effectively reduce the systemic inflammatory responses and improve cardio-pulmonary bypass postoperative recovery in adult patients. This evidence shows the importance of controlling the inflammatory storm in critical ill patients, and the positive impact of HPF in other organs, which could explain the beneficial effects of HPF in avoiding multisystemic syndromes.

15.6 Conclusion

In seriously ill patients in the intensive care unit (ICU), acute kidney injury (AKI) is a component with a worse prognosis in the context of multiple organs failure. In fact, it always implies a higher rate of morbidity and mortality. In ICU patients with AKI and hemodynamic instability, and failure of other organs, the best renal supportive therapy is continuous renal replacement therapy (CRRT). In acute neurological injury (ANI) and AKI, continuous veno-venous hemofiltration (CVVHF) is preferred with a sodium concentration > 140 mmol/L in the dialysate. In acute heart failure (AHF) and AKI with failure in regular treatment with diuretics, continuous venovenous ultrafiltration (CVVUF) is the best alternative. In acute liver injury (ALI) and AKI, the best indication is CRRT together with a detoxification therapy. In severe sepsis and AKI, high-flux CRRT demonstrates effectiveness in removing proinflammatory cytokines without yet achieving positive result in survival, and the new evidence is supporting the use of hemoperfusion as an alternative to control the pro-inflammatory storm. Still, we need more robust evidence to define a critical point as is the correct "time" to start these hemo-adsorptive therapies. The earliest intervention in general, perhaps with a nephroprotective criterion, would prevent damage to other organs; so, an individualized therapy, using the best medical criteria and center expertise will always be the best approach.

References

1. Chawla LS, Bellomo R, Bihorac A, Goldstein SL, Siew ED, Bagshaw SM, Bittleman D, Cruz D, Endre Z, Fitzgerald RL, Forni L, Kane-Gill SL, Hoste E, Koyner J, Liu KD, Macedo E, Mehta R, Murray P, Nadim M, Ostermann M, Palevsky PM, Pannu N, Rosner M, Wald R, Zarbock A, Ronco C, Kellum JA. Acute kidney disease and renal recovery: consensus report of the acute disease quality initiative (ADQI) 16 workgroup. Nat Rev Nephrol. 2017;13(4):241–57.
2. Villa G, Ricci Z, Romagnoli S, Ronco C. Multidimensional approach to adequacy of renal replacement therapy in acute kidney injury. Contrib Nephrol. 2016;187:94–105.
3. KDIGO. Clinical practice guideline for acute kidney injury. Kidney Int Suppl. 2012;2(1):1–38.
4. Bellomo R, Ronco C, Kellum JA, Metha RL, Palevsky P, ADQI Workgroup. Acute renal failure-definition, outcome measure, animal models, fluid therapy and information technology needs: The Seconds International Consensus Conference of the Acute Dialysis Quality Initiative (ADQI) Group. Crit Care. 2004;8:R204. https://doi.org/10.1186/cc2872.
5. Metha RL, Kellum JA, Shah SV, Molitoris BA, Ronco C, Warnock DG, Levin A. Acute Kidney Injury Network (AKIN): report of an initiative to improve outcomes in acute kidney injury. Crit Care. 2007;11:R31. https://doi.org/10.1186/cc5713.
6. Badel JC, García LA, Soto-Doria MJ, Musso CG. Dialysis prescription in acute kidney injury: when and how much? International urology and nephrology. Int Urol Nephrol. 2021;53:489. https://doi.org/10.1007/s11255-020-02601-z. ISSN 0301-1623.
7. Payen D, Mateo J, Cavaillon JM, Fraisse F, Floriot C, Vicaut E. Hemofiltration and Sepsis Group of the Collège National de Réanimation et de Médecine d'Urgence des Hôpitaux extra-Universitaires. Impact of continuous venovenous hemofiltration on organ failure during the early phase of severe sepsis: a randomized controlled trial. Crit Care Med. 2009;37:803–10. https://doi.org/10.1097/CCM.0b013e3181962316.

8. Park JT, Lee H, Kee YK, Park S, Oh HJ, Han SH, Joo KW, Lim CS, Kim YS, Kang SW, Yoo TH, Kim DK, HICORES Investigators. High-dose versus conventional-dose continuous venovenous hemodiafiltration and patients and kidney survival and cytokine removal in sepsis-associated acute kidney injury: a randomized controlled trial. Am J Kidney Dis. 2016;68(4):599–608. https://doi.org/10.1053/j.ajkd.2016.02.049.

9. Metha RL, Pascual MT, Soroko S, Savage BR, Himmelfarb J, Ikizler TA, Paganini EP, Chertow GM. Program to improve care in acute renal disease. Spectrum of acute failure in the intensive care unit: the PICARD experience. Kidney Int. 2004;66(4):1613–21.

10. Wang Y, Gallagher M, Li Q, Lo S, Cass A, Finfer S, Myburgh J, Bouman C, Faulhaber-Walter R, Kellum JA, Palevsky PM, Ronco C, Saudan P, Tolwani A, Bellomo R. Renal replacement therapy intensity for acute kidney injury and recovery to dialysis. Nephrol Dial Transplant. 2018;33(6):1017–24. https://doi.org/10.1093/ndt/gfx308.

11. Davenport A. Continuous renal replacement therapies in patients with acute neurological injury. Semin Dial. 2009;22:165–8. https://doi.org/10.1111/j.1525139X.2008.00548.X.

12. Davenport A. Renal replacement therapy for the patient with acute traumatic brain injury and severe acute kidney injury. Contrib Nephrol. 2007;156:333–9.

13. Khwaja A. KDIGO clinical practice guideline for acute kidney injury. Nephron Clin Pract. 2012;120(4):C179–84. https://doi.org/10.1159/000339789.

14. Osgood M, Compton R, Carandang R, Hall W, Kershaw G, Muehlschlegel S. Rapid unexpected brain herniation in association with renal replacement therapy in acute brain injury: caution in the Neurocritical care unit. Neurocrit Care. 2015;22:176–83.

15. Francis G, Benedict C, Johnstone DE, Kirlin PC, Nicklas J, Liang CS, Kubo SH, Rudin-Toretsky E, Yusuf S. Comparison of neuroendocrine activation in patients with left ventricular dysfunction with and without congestive heart failure: a sub study of the studies of left ventricular dysfunction (SOLVD). Circulation. 1990;82(5):1724–9.

16. Binanay C, Califf RM, Hasselblat V, O'Connor CM, Shah MR, Sopko G, et al. Evaluation study of congestive heart failure and pulmonary artery catheterization effectiveness: the ESCAPE trial. JAMA. 2005;294:1625–33. https://doi.org/10.1001/jama.294.13.1625.

17. Mullens W, Abrahams Z, Francis GS, Sokos G, Taylor DO, Starling RC, et al. Importance of venous congestion for worsening of renal function in advanced decompensated heart failure. J Am Coll Cardiol. 2009;53:589–96. https://doi.org/10.1016/j.jacc.2008.05.068.

18. Rodriguez-Artalejo F, Banegas-Banegas JR, Guallar-Castillón P. Epidemiology of heart failure. Rev Esp Cardiol. 2004;57:163–70.

19. Ronco C, Cicoira M, McCullough PA. Cardiorenal syndrome type 1: pathophysiological crosstalk. Cardiorenal syndrome type 1: pathophysiological crosstalk leading to combined heart and kidney dysfunction in the setting of acutely decompensated heart failure. J Am Coll Cardiol. 2012;60:1031–42. https://doi.org/10.1016/j.jacc.2012.01.077.

20. Sarraf M, Masoumi A, Schrier RW. Cardiorenal syndromes in acute decompensated heart failure. Clin J Am Soc Nephrol. 2009;4:2013–26. https://doi.org/10.2215/CJN.03150509.

21. Ronco C, Bellasi A, LucaDi LL. Cardiorenal syndrome: an overview. ACKD. 2018;25(5):382–90. https://doi.org/10.1053/j.ackd.2018.08.004.

22. Bart BA, Boyle A, Bank AJ, Anand I, Olivari MT, Kraemer M, Mackedanz S, Sobotka PA, Schollmeyer M, Goldsmith SR. Ultrafiltration versus usual care for hospitalized patients with heart failure: the relief for acutely fluid-overloaded patients with decompensated congestive heart failure(rapid-CHF) trial. J Am Coll Cardiol. 2005;46:2043–6. https://doi.org/10.1016/j.jacc.2005.05.098.

23. Costanzo MR. Ultrafiltration versus intravenous diuretics for patients hospitalized for acute decompensated heart failure. Am Coll Cardiol. 2007;49(6):675–83. https://doi.org/10.1016/j.jacc.2006.07.073.

24. Marenzi M, Muratori M, Cosentino ER, Rinaldi ER, Donghi V, Milazzo V, Ferramosca E, Borghi C, Santoro A, Agostoni P. Continuous ultrafiltration for congestive heart failure: the CUORE trial. J Card Fail. 2014;20:9–17. https://doi.org/10.1016/j.cardfail.2013.11.004.

25. Bradley A, Goldsmith SR, Lee KL, Givertz MM, O'Connor CM, Bull D, Redfield MM, Deswal A, Rouleau JL, LeWinter MM, Ofili EO, Stevenson LW, et al. For the heart failure clinical research network. Ultrafiltration in decompensated heart failure with Cardiorenal syndrome. N Engl J Med. 2012;367:2296–304. https://doi.org/10.1056/NEJMoa1210357.

26. Stravitz RT, Kramer AH, Davern T, Shaikh AOPS, Caldwell SH, Metha RL, Blei A, Fontana R, Mcguire B, Rossaro L, Alastair D, Lee M. Intensive care of patients with acute liver failure: recommendations of the U.S. acute liver failure study group. Crit Care Med. 2007;35:2498–508.

27. Davenport A, Will EJ, Davison AM, Swindells S, Cohen AT, Miloszewski KJ. Changes in intracranial pressure during hemofiltration in oliguric patients with grade IV hepatic encephalopathy. Nephron. 1989;53:142–6.

28. Ronco C, Brendolan A, Lonnemann G, Bellomo R, Piccinni P, Digito A, Dan M, Irone M, La Greca G, Inguaggiato P, Maggiore U, De Nitti C, Wratten ML, Ricci Z, Tetta C. A pilot study of coupled plasma filtration with absorption in septic shock. Crit Care Med. 2002;30:1250–5.

29. Stange J, Ramlow W, Mitzner S, Schmidt R, Klinkmann H. Dialysis against a recycled albumin solution enables the removal of albumin-bound toxins. Artif Organs. 1993;17:809–13.

30. Mitzner SR, Stange J, Klammt S, Risler T, Erley CM, Bader BD, Berger ED, Lauchart W, Peszynski P, Freytag J, Hickstein H, Loock J, Löhr M, Liebe S, Emmrich J, Korten G, Schmidt R. Improvement of hepatorenal syndrome with extracorporeal albumin dialysis MARS: results of a prospective, randomized, controlled clinical trial. Liver Transpl. 2000;6(3):277–86. https://doi.org/10.1002/lt.500060326.

31. Heemann U, Treichel U, Loock J, Philipp T, Gerken G, Malago M, Klammt S, Loehr M, Liebe S, Mitzner S, Schmidt R, Stange J. Albumin dialysis in cirrhosis with superimposed acute liver injury. A prospective and controlled study. Hepatology. 2002;36(4PT1):949–58.

32. Huang Z, Wang SR, Su W, Liu JY. Removal of humoral mediators and the effect on the survival of septic patients by Hemoperfusion with neutral microporous resin column., therapeutic apheresis and dialysis. Ther Apher Dial. 2010;14(6):596–602. https://doi.org/10.1111/j.1744-9987.2010.00825.x.

33. Pomarè-Montin D, Ankawi G, Lorenzin A, Neri M, Caprara C, Ronco C. Biocompatibility and cytotoxic evaluation of new sorbent cartridges for blood hemoperfusion. Blood Purif. 2018;46(3):187–95.

34. Ankawi G, Fan W, Pomarè Montin D, Lorenzin A, Neri M, Caprara C, de Cal M, Ronco C. A new series of sorbent devices for multiple clinical purposes: current evidence and future directions. Blood Purif. 2019;47:94–100.

35. Rampino T, Gregorini M, Perotti L, Ferrari F, Pattonieri EF, Grignano MA, Valente M, Garrone A, Islam T, Libetta C, Sepe V, Albertini R, Bruno R, Belliato M. Hemoperfusion with CytoSorb as adjuvant therapy in critically ill patients with SARS-CoV2 pneumonia. Blood Purif. 2021;50:566–71.

36. Huang Z, Wang SR, Su W, Liu JY. Removal of humoral mediators and the effect on the survival of septic patients by hemoperfusion with neutral microporous resin column. Ther Apher Dial. 2010;14(6):596–602.

37. Suyama H, Kawasaki Y, Morikawa S, Kaneko K, Yamanoue T. Early induction of PMX-DHP improves oxygenation in severe sepsis patients with acute lung injury. Hiroshima J Med Sci. 2008;57:79–84.

38. Kushi H, Miki T, Nakahara J, Okamoto K, Saito T, Tanjo K. Hemoperfusion with an immobilized polymyxin B fiber column improves tissue oxygen metabolism. Ther Apher Dial. 2006;10:430–5.

39. He Z, Lu H, Jian X, Li G, Xiao D, Meng Q, Chen J, Zhou C. The efficacy of resin Hemoperfusion cartridge on inflammatory responses during adult cardiopulmonary bypass. Blood Purif. 2021;1:98. https://doi.org/10.1186/s12966-019-0860-z.

40. Wang D, Hu B, Hu C, Zhu F, Liu X, Zhang J, Wang B, Xiang H, Cheng Z, Xiong Y, Zhao Y, , Li Y, Wang X, Peng Z. Clinical characteristics of 138 hospitalized patients with 2019 novel coronavirus-infected pneumonia in Wuhan, China, JAMA 2020;323(11):1061–1069.

41. Ronco C, Bagshaw SM, Bellomo R, Clark WR, Husain-Syed F, Kellum JA, Ricci Z, Rimmelé T, Reis T, Ostermann M. Extracorporeal blood purification and organ support in the critically ill patient during COVID-19 pandemic: expert review and recommendation. Blood Purif. 2021;50(1):17–27.
42. Ronco C, Reis T. Kidney involvement in COVID-19 and rationale for extracorporeal therapies. Nat Rev Nephrol. 2020;16:308–10.
43. Musso CG, Cordoba JP, Aroca-Martinez G, Terrasa S, Barriga-Moreno A, Lozano-Sanchez M, Barón-Alvarez RA, Gonzalez-Torres H, Cantos J, Huespe I. Negative alactic base excess is reversed by hemoperfusion in septic patients. G Clin Nefrol Dial. 2022;34:122–4.
44. Barriga-Moreno A, Lozano-Sanchez M, Barón-Alvarez RA, Cordoba JP, Aroca-Martinez G, Dianda D, Gonzalez-Torres H, Musso CG. Mortality rate and acute kidney injury prevalence reduction in COVID-19 critical patients treated with hemoperfusion. Indian J Nephrol. 2023;7:S369.
45. Hea Z, Lua H, Jiana X, Xiaoa GLD, Menga Q, Chena J, Zhoua C. The efficacy of resin hemoperfusion cartridge on inflammatory responses during adult cardiopulmonary bypass. Blood Purif. 2022;51(1):31–7. https://doi.org/10.1159/000514149.

Chapter 16
Acute Kidney Injury and Organ Crosstalk in COVID-19

Camila Juana, Victoria Paula Musso-Enz, Guido Mateo Musso-Enz, Gustavo Aroca-Martinez, and Carlos Guido Musso

16.1 Acute Kidney Injury in COVID-19 (AKI-COVID-19)

In December 2019, the first cases of a lung disease of unknown etiology began to be described in the province of Wuhan (China). These were later attributed to a new variety of coronavirus, which was named as *severe acute respiratory syndrome coronavirus 2 (SARS-CoV-2)*, and the disease it causes as *COVID-19* [1, 2].

COVID-19 can affect many other organs in addition to the respiratory system, particularly the kidney, heart, digestive tract, blood, and nervous system [3]. As for the kidney alterations, they vary depending on the specific type of reported renal affectation: albuminuria (34%), proteinuria (63%), hematuria (27%), proteinuria with hematuria (44%), and/or acute kidney injury (AKI) (14%–27%) [4].

Direct deleterious action of this virus on the kidney has been demonstrated by the histopathological analysis of organ samples collected from patients who died of COVID-19. Findings include loss of the brush border and non-isometric tubular vacuolation, microvascular luminal occlusions (glomerular and peritubular)

C. Juana · V. P. Musso-Enz
Physiology Department, Instituto Universitario del Hospital Italiano de Buenos Aires, Buenos Aires, Argentina
e-mail: camila.juana@hospitalitaliano.org.ar; victoria.musso@hospitalitaliano.org.ar

G. M. Musso-Enz
Facultad de Medicina, Universidad Católica de Buenos Aires, Buenos Aires, Argentina

G. Aroca-Martinez
Facultad de Ciencias de la Salud, Universidad Simón Bolivar, Barranquilla, Colombia

C. G. Musso (✉)
Facultad de Ciencias de la Salud, Universidad Simón Bolivar, Barranquilla, Colombia

Fisiologia, Instituto Universitario del Hospital Italiano de Buenos Aires, Buenos Aires, Argentina
e-mail: carlos.musso@hospitalitaliano.org.ar

© The Author(s), under exclusive license to Springer Nature Switzerland AG 2023
C. G. Musso, A. Covic (eds.), *Organ Crosstalk in Acute Kidney Injury*, https://doi.org/10.1007/978-3-031-36789-2_16

consisting mainly of erythrocytes, endothelial damage, and pigmented casts detected in association with high serum levels of creatine phosphokinase (rhabdomyolysis) [3, 4].

Moreover, SARS-CoV-2 has been found in the urine of infected patients. In addition, electron microscopy evidenced spherical viral particles characteristic of SARS-CoV-2 in podocytes and proximal tubular epithelium. This was associated with effacement of the pedicels, occasional vacuolation, and detachment of podocytes from the glomerular basal membrane, with the viral presence being confirmed by immunofluorescence [5].

There is growing evidence that acute kidney injury (AKI) is prevalent in SARS-CoV-2 infection, with a reported incidence of 8–17%, reaching 35% in critical patients, and that this condition is considered a poor prognostic factor [6]. In this sense, the development of AKI in the context of COVID-19 (AKI-COVID-19) has an associated mortality of 91.7% [7]. SARS-CoV-2 spike (S) protein binds to the angiotensin-converting enzyme 2 (ACE2) receptor, employing cellular transmembrane serine proteases (TMPRSSs) for priming. When the SARS-CoV-2 binds to the ACE2 receptor, protein S becomes activated and cleaved by the TMPRSSs, allowing virus endocytosis [6, 7].

Among the risk factors associated with its development, the following have been identified: presence of malignant pathology, sepsis, right heart failure, and disseminated intravascular coagulation [8]. It has been proposed that the mechanism by which the virus produces renal injury has multiple causes, including direct cytopathic effects mediated by viral binding to angiotensin-converting enzyme II receptors, as well as acute tubular necrosis triggered by factors such as volume depletion, cytokine storm, hypoxia, shock or rhabdomyolysis and, finally, immune complex deposition [9].

Aroca et al., in a recent study found that the prevalence of AKI-COVID-19 was 41%, ranging from 5% to 76% of the prevalence reported by other studies. This difference possibly depends on whether all inpatients are included in the study or only those admitted to the intensive care unit [10–12]. Similar to other reports, the onset of AKI was within the first week of admission. Likewise, the finding of a predominance for this condition in older adults (61 ± 15 years), particularly males, also coincides with what observed by other authors. With respect to the AKI subtype (AKIN), based on their experience, the most common class was AKIN 3 and the least frequent was AKIN 2; proportion that matches that of most previous reports, with the exception of some authors who reported that AKIN 1 was the most common class, followed by AKIN 3 [13, 14] (Table 16.1). It could be speculated that this difference in the AKIN type prevalence could be attributed to the evolution time at which AKI was diagnosed in each study [13–16].

Renal replacement therapy (RRT) was required in 29% of the patients affected by AKI due to COVID-19, clinical picture that Meijers et al. have proposed to be designated as "COVAN" [17] (COVID-19-associated nephropathy). However, it should be taken into account that it is not yet clear if this condition is secondary to SARS-CoV-2 or just an association (AKI secondary COVID-19 disease). This

Table 16.1 Acute kidney injury (AKI) stages (KDIGO 2012)

AKIN stage	Definition
1.	Increase in serum creatinine levels >0.3 mg/dL or 1.5–1.9 times the baseline creatinine value, and/or decreased urine output to 0.5 mL/kg/h for 6 h
2.	Increase in serum creatinine levels 2–2.9 times the baseline creatinine value, and/or decreased urine output to 0.5 mL/kg/h for 12 h
3.	Increase in serum creatinine levels 3 times the baseline creatinine value, increase of serum creatinine >4 mg/dL, initiation of RRT and/or decreased urine output to 0.3 mL/kg/h for 24 h or anuria for 12 h

sCr serum creatinine, *RRT* renal replacement therapy, *KDIGO* kidney disease improving global outcomes

percentage of patients receiving RRT is in line with what has been reported in the literature, where RRT use oscillates between 14% and 38% [13, 14]. Aroca et al. found that the percentage of patients suffering from AKI-COVID-19 who recovered during admission, either totally or partially, was approximately 31% [10–12]. The percentage of recovery described by other authors oscillates between 17.4% and 50% [14].

As for the urinary manifestations of AKI-COVID-19, proteinuria was predominant (35%), followed by hematuria (31%), and, to a lesser extent, leukocyturia (4%). This order of frequency is commonly reported in scientific publications, with some variations depending on the various clinical contexts: proteinuria (44–84%), hematuria (25–81%), and leukocyturia (4–60%) [9, 14, 18]. The origin of these abnormalities has been attributed to the various mechanisms of kidney damage detailed below. However, it has been postulated that the clear preponderance of proteinuria, whose prevalence exceeds even the proportion of patients developing AKI, may be secondary to the febrile state inherent to this condition or to the activation of glomerular hyperfiltration in the context of a systemic inflammatory state [14, 18–20]. Mechanisms identified as a cause of AKI-COVID-19 include [4, 5, 9, 13, 15–26]:

- Direct cytopathic action of the virus, as detected in the urine and renal tissue (podocytes and proximal tubules), where angiotensin II-converting enzyme, considered the putative receptor of the virus mediating cell entry, is expressed in abundance. It is worth mentioning that some authors deny this mechanism.
- Acute tubular necrosis generated by various factors such as bacterial sepsis, cytokine storm, tissue hypoxia, rhabdomyolysis, mechanical ventilation induced hypoperfusion, renal microvascular thrombotic compromise, and nephrotoxic drug use (e.g., beta-lactams, remdesivir, etc.).
- Injury caused by immune complexes due to viral antigen deposition.

It should be noted that the development of AKI-COVID-19 is a risk factor for admission to the intensive care unit, RRT requirement, and death [14, 16]. CKD (6%) and end-stage kidney disease (2%) have also been reported as AKI-COVID-19 sequelae [18]. Regarding the symptomatology characteristic of COVID-19, other reports have also described fever (100%) as well as respiratory (76%) and muscle (43%) symptomatology [21]. As in other studies, among the inflammatory biochemical and systemic compromise markers (direct and indirect), C-reactive protein, ferritin, and D-dimer stood out. This reinforces the idea that the renal and systemic damage generated by COVID-19 is fundamentally reactive, induced by the patient's own immune system and by a series of mediators (cytokines) released during the so-called cytokine storm [5, 16]. When assessing the comorbidities of our patients, they coincided in type and proportion with those reported in other studies, the most significant ones being high blood pressure (60%), obesity (30%), chronic kidney disease (CKD) (34%), diabetes mellitus (30%), chronic obstructive pulmonary disease (14%), and oncological pathology [15]. Aroca et al. reported, in line with the literature, that the vast majority of critical patients required inotropic and ventilatory support (80–90%). Nevertheless, mortality was overly high (73%) when compared with previous reports, where it ranged between 16.1% and 62% [13–15, 22]. This phenomenon may be linked to the considerable proportion of frail patients reported in this population (31%). The homeostatic capacity of individuals allows them to successfully cope with clinical situations that jeopardize their body integrity. This capacity can be measured by applying a simple and validated scale: the Clinical Frailty Scale (CFS) (Table 16.2). To assess the impact of this clinical condition on the evolution of AKI-COVID-19, the degree of frailty of the study

Table 16.2 Clinical frailty scale

1. Very fit	Robust, active, energetic, and motivated persons. These persons commonly exercise regularly. They are among the most fit for their age
2. Well	Persons who have no active diseases and no symptoms, but who are less fit than those in the previous category. They often exercise or are very active from time to time
3. Managing well	Persons whose medical problems are well controlled but are not regularly active beyond routine walking
4. Vulnerable	While not dependent on others for daily help, their symptoms often limit activities. A common complaint is being "slowed up" and/or being tired during the day
5. Mildly frail	These persons often have more evident slowing and need help with more complex activities (managing their finances, medicines, transportation, and heavy housework)
6. Moderately frail	These persons need help with all outdoor activities. Indoors, they need help with cleaning and often have problems climbing stairs. They also need help bathing and may need minimal assistance to get dressed
7. Severely frail	Completely dependent for personal care either due to physical or cognitive reasons. Even so, they seem stable and not at high risk of dying
8. Very severely frail	Completely dependent, and close to the end of their life (within 6 months)
9. Terminally ill	Approaching the end of life. This category applies to anyone with a life expectancy <6 months, who is not evidently fragile

population was determined and its relationship with the evolution of the disease was analyzed by these authors. They found that 69% of the patients who developed AKI were robust (CFS: 1–3), 21% were frail (CFS: 4–5), and 10% were very frail (CFS: 6–7). The degree of frailty was significantly correlated with mortality, with a 33% increase for each rise in the degree of frailty, which is reasonable given the impact that a reduced functional reserve has on the patient's evolution.

Aroca et al. also found that viral load (3.12 ± 0.3 copies/mL) was not significantly correlated with the degree of frailty, renal replacement requirement, or mortality. Although a previous report noted that viral load (6.2 copies/mL, range: 3.0–8.0 copies/mL) showed a significant independent association with mortality, the viral loads were much higher than in the studied population [23]. The authors hypothesized that the viral load in the airway did not correlate with AKI severity, since renal damage depends on the urine (tubular) viral load or, even more likely, on the sort of the patient's immunological response [25–28].

Regarding the significant correspondence observed by Aroca et al. between the robust condition and the serum ferritin level, as well as between the frailty status and the D-dimer value, this could be interpreted as follows [28–35]:

Ferritin, transferrin, IL6, D-dimer, fibrinogen, and C-reactive protein are among the parameters described as characteristic of the systemic inflammatory syndrome associated with acute infection by COVID 19. With respect to ferritin, it is an intracellular iron storage protein. In moments of systemic stress, serum ferritin comes from the acute destruction of cells previously at rest, such as hepatocytes, macrophages, or bone marrow cells. This sudden serum ferritin increase is responsible for the systemic stimulation of cells of innate immunity such as macrophages. The macrophage response is the secretion of cytokines, generating the so-called cytokine storm, the activation of recruitment mechanisms of acute inflammatory mediators and subsequently the presentation of antigens [29–35].

Regarding serum D-dimer levels, it is a marker of fibrinolysis and, therefore, thrombus formation. During coagulation, apart from the activation of coagulation factor, another system, called the fibrinolytic system comes into place. Its aim is to maintain equilibrium between the thrombotic formation and degradation. It consists of plasmin, plasminogen, plasminogen activators, and inhibitors of plasminogen activators. Plasmin is a proteolytic enzyme whose main aim is to degrade fibrin and, in this process, it releases fibrin degradation products among them, D-dimer.

There is a constant interaction between the immune system and the coagulation system in response to infection by any microorganism to prevent its indiscriminate spread, causing the condition called disseminated intravascular coagulation (DIC). This parameter is related to the presence of previously existing acute or chronic endothelial damage or activation. Differences in the host's previous status at the time of SARS-CoV2 virus infection may be the factor that determines the degree of existing endothelial stress. The progression of the predominant biomarkers in the evolution of the systemic inflammatory syndrome would be the result of the combination of variables between the host and the virus. In a previously robust organism without apparent prior pathology, the poor evolution of COVID-19 infection would depend on the way in which the immune system orchestrates its response. In this sense, a patient which has acute serum ferritin elevation as a predominant systemic inflammation mechanism will cause cytokine storm and organ damage. In contrast, in a fragile organism, previously chronically stressed forms of severe endothelial inflammation occur. In this case, SARS-CoV-19 infection could potentiate the host frailty status, inducing an acute microthrombotic activity, evidence in significantly elevated dimer D levels in blood. This biomarker would, in turn, determine the poor clinical evolution due to microthromboembolic activity or disseminated intravascular coagulation (DIC) [32].

16.2 Crosstalk in AKI COVID-19

16.2.1 Cytokine Storm

In SARSCoV-2 infection, multiple organ failure (MOF) is more likely to be responsible for AKI than the virus itself. Cytokine profiles in AKI-COVID-19 showed interferon-gamma (IFN-γ) and interleukin (IL)-1, IL-6, and IL-12 elevation for 2 weeks after disease onset, without elevation of anti-inflammatory cytokines IL-10, IL-2, and IL-4. It is worth mentioning that acute respiratory distress syndrome induced hypoxia can increase inflammation, through hypoxia-inducible factor and nuclear factor-κB [26].

Cell apoptosis and pyroptosis can be caused by the elevation of leukocyte derived proinflammatory cytokines, such as tumor necrosis-alpha (TNF-α), interleukin (IL) 6 and IL-1β. These cellular damages cause different tissue dysfunction depending on the organ, such as tubular damage and intestinal fibrosis in kidneys and digestive system, respectively [21]. This can be demonstrated by the strong-moderate leukocyte infiltration in kidneys of patients who died of COVID-19. Apart from leukocyte infiltration, these tissues showed CD68+ macrophages in tubule-interstitium and, a lesser proportion, showed CD8+ T cells and an even lesser proportion evidenced a low number of CD56+ natural killer (NK). The above indicates that there exists a cellular recruitment in tubule-interstitium of predominantly CD68+ macrophages in SARS-CoV2 infection. Moreover, deposits of the complement membrane-attack complex (MAC), composed by C5b to C9 further damage the tubules and glomeruli [5]. Consequently, kidney damage secondary to MAC was further assessed by studying postmortem kidney tissues of patients who died of COVID-19. In all of the six tissues, an extensive deposit of MAC in tubules was observed. Conversely, glomeruli and capillaries deposits were low and observed in only two of those tissues. To contrast with the previous results, MAC tubular deposits in postmortem kidneys of trauma victims were negative, while in hepatitis B virus associated nephropathy was only slight. The previously stated suggests that SARS-CoV2 infection also induces renal damage by MAC deposition.

16.2.2 Chemokines

Chemokine type and proportions vary between patients with mild COVID-19 and patients that require admission to the Intensive Care Unit (ICU). The former, present higher levels of IL1-β, INF-γ, CXCL 10/IP-10 ,and CCL/MCP-1, while the latter presented higher levels of G-CSF, CXCL10/IP-10, CCL2/MCP-1, and CCL3/MIP-1α.

The RUBY study, a multi-center international prospective observational study, has an objective to identify molecules that could serve as biomarkers that indicate a persistent stage 3 AKI, as defined by the Kidney Disease Improving Global Outcome (KDIGO) guidelines. A large cohort of molecules were recognized, still, the most promising one was a newly identified urinary chemokine, called C-C motif ligand 14 (CCL-14). CCL14 urinary levels persistence is specific to patients who persisted with AKI. Consequently, CCL-14 could be of great relevance as a biomarker and mediator of renal tissue damage and recovery and it could serve as a novel diagnostic and prognostic factor. Therefore, it could be of great importance on a patient's clinical management, such as deciding on the initiation of renal replacement therapy. CCL1 belongs to the CC chemokine family and has been attributed to pro-inflammatory roles. The CC chemokine family has been recognized to be crucial in the recruitment of monocytes/macrophages and their role in tissue injury and repair. CCL14 not only binds to typical CC chemokine receptors 1, 5, and 3 (CCR1, CCR5, and CCR3), but also binds to the atypical chemokine receptor ACKR2. In proinflammatory environments, injured tissues release inflammatory mediators, such as TNF-α and when it binds to its receptor, the TNF receptors, it leads to the release of CCL14 from tubular epithelial cells. Then, CCL14 binds to its receptors on monocytes and T-lymphocytes, CCR1 and CC5, inducing chemotaxis to the site of injury. Then, monocytes differentiate into macrophages and naive T-lymphocytes onto proinflammatory T-lymphocytes helper 1 (Th1), this being pathogenic in the lesion and help magnify and extend tissue damage. C–C motif ligand 1 (CCL2) or Monocyte Chemotactic Protein-1 (MCP1), member of the chemokine family binds to conventional CC chemokine receptor 2 (CCR2) on monocytes. This results in the traffic of monocytes from bone marrow to tissues in response to inflammatory signals. Furthermore, similar to what happens in CCL14, the fine tuning of the bioavailability of CCL2 relies on its binding to the atypical chemokine receptor ACKR2. In this manner, the crucial role of this chemokine receptor and its proinflammatory ligands in AKI is confirmed. It has been shown that mRNA expression increases in ischemia–reperfusion injury, thus, being of value as a biomarker for mononuclear inflammatory processes that occur after ischemic AKI. Studies showed the role of CCL2, as being a potent chemokine produced by kidney cells and mediating processes of acute ischemic and toxic kidney injuries. Moreover, the use of CCL2 as a biomarker was proven by clinical assessment, as it was observed that CCL2 increases in urine in patients with AKI. Lastly the elevation of CCL2 in plasma has been associated with an increased risk of AKI and death after cardiac operations [36].

One of the pivotal inflammatory elements linked to renal tissue damage is the expression of C-X3-C motif ligand 1 (CX3CL1), also called fractalkine. Lipopolysaccharides (LPS) induce the production of CX3CL1, and its participation in inflammatory responses in various organ systems is due to its binding to the CX3CL1 receptor, the CX2CR1. The vast majority of the performed studies show its role as a promoter of nephropathies. As found in a recent study, LPS causes both in vivo and in vitro inflammatory responses on glomerular podocytes that result in decreased podocyte-specific mARNm, decreased protein production, and an involvement in the development of AKI.

Nevertheless, a number of recent studies demonstrated that its role might also be to mitigate these same damages. Therefore, to date, the CX3CL1/CX3CR1 axis is considered to be a double-edged sword that could impart novel perspectives into the pathogenesis and treatment of renal diseases and disorders [36].

16.2.3 Immune Cells Response

16.2.3.1 Innate Immune Response

An effective innate immune response to control the viral replication against viral infection depends on the Interferon-1d6fc (IFN-1d6fc) and toll-like receptor (TRL) expressions Endothelium mainly expressed IFN-1d6fc, TLR 3, and TLR 9 against viruses and bacteria. Innate immune responses during ongoing SARS-CoV2 infection, such as increased neutrophil and reduced lymphocyte, are related to the ongoing infection and severity of disease, therefore contributing to patient's death. The increased secretion of proinflammatory mediators is probably the leading cause of the life-threatening respiratory disease in COVID-19 patients. Granulocytes and proinflammatory macrophages, both cells from the innate immune system, release inflammatory mediators that damage cells and induce lung inflammation. To contrast, the involvement of the adaptive immune system in COVID-19 infections appears to be lower, as shown by the lower frequency of monocytes (CD16 + and CD14+) recruitment in the COVID-19 patient's blood. The exception is the natural killer (NK) cells count, as no difference was shown between a COVID-19 infected patient and NK physiological levels [37].

16.2.3.2 Acquired Immune Response

CD4 + T cells and CD8 + T cells play a significant role in the development of autoimmunity and anti-inflammation. CD4 + T cells stimulate the production of virus-specific antibodies and activate T-dependent B cells. The role of CD8 + T cells is to perform direct cytotoxic activity to the virally infected cells. In addition, the expression and survival of the previously mentioned CD4 + T cells and CD8 + memory T cells rely on the endothelium. In SARS-CoV-2 infected patients,

CD4 + T cells and CD8 + T cells, excessive activation can be evidenced by a substantial decrease of blood count levels of these cells and elevated levels of HLA-DR. Moreover, the increased concentration of proinflammatory substances in CD4 + T cells and the increased granules count in CD8 + T cells justify severe immune response in this patient [36, 37].

16.2.4 Other Organ Compromise in COVID-19

16.2.4.1 Lung

During acute lung injury, several processes that occur may lead to kidney injury; the release of proinflammatory cytokines leads to systemic inflammation and hemodynamic changes, such as reduced cardiac output with high intrathoracic pressure and reduction in kidney medullary perfusion due to hypoxemia [38]. In vitro studies have shown increased sensitivity of lung cells to IFN-γ. Additionally, IFN-γ causes renal cell apoptosis. IL-6 levels in AKI-COVID-19 patients are 10–40 times lower than those previously reported in acute respiratory distress syndrome (ARDS). Given that the mortality rate from COVID-19 associated ARDS is up to 50%, lower cytokine level compared with ARDS does not imply lower lung damage. Thus the inflammatory response is probably not the main cause of AKI but may contribute to it [38, 39].

A randomized study comparing ARDS patients assigned to receive either a "lung-protective" ventilation strategy (prone position) or conventional ventilation (control group), documented that the control group had significantly higher mediator concentrations in plasma and in broncho-alveolar fluids. Besides, the right ventricle badly tolerates high-positive end-expiratory pressure (PEEP) in this population, and prone positioning is an efficient means of controlling right ventricular pressure in ARDS patients [26, 39].

16.2.4.2 Heart

The proportion of lung cells expressing the ACE2 receptor is about 2%, while this proportion increases to 4% for the renal tubular cells and up to 7.5% for myocardial cells. This phenomenon could explain the possibility of the heart and kidney significant affectation by SARS-CoV2. Moreover, patients with chronic heart failure may become unstable in the presence of viral infection due to the imbalance between the patient's low myocardial reserve and the increased metabolic demand due to infection. This imbalance increases the risk of acute coronary syndrome, cardiac decompensation, and sudden death. Acute myocarditis has been reported in these patients, showing lymphocyte infiltration surrounding myocyte necrosis but with negative SARS-CoV-2 S protein.

SARS-CoV-2 AKI is consistent with type 5 cardiorenal syndrome, which is characterized by the combined presence of acute heart and AKI due to a systemic disorder [26, 40].

16.2.4.3 Muscles

Rhabdomyolysis with elevation of creatine kinase beyond 10,000 international units (IU)/L has been reported in association with SARS-CoV-2. The released myoglobin can cause intrarenal vasoconstriction, direct and ischemic tubular injury, and tubular obstruction.

Interestingly, postmortem kidney histopathologic analysis of COVID-19 patients has shown pigmented casts in the kidney tubules and increased creatine kinase; possibly representing rhabdomyolysis [26, 38].

16.2.4.4 Coagulation

COVID-19 patients have a coagulation disorder that leads to a procoagulant state. This can be shown by the documentation of an altered prothrombin time, altered activated partial thromboplastin time, D-dimer, fibrinogen, and fibrin/fibrinogen degradation products (FDPs) in COVID-19 patients. Besides, differences in terms of coagulation were found between COVID-19 patients who were survivors and patients who were non-survivors, since the latter had significantly higher D-dimer and FDP levels. In addition, 71.4% of non-survivors met the criteria of disseminated intravascular coagulation (DIC) during their hospital stay. The release of inflammatory mediators and the uninhibited effects of angiotensin II may trigger the coagulation cascade, causing hypercoagulability. A high incidence of thrombotic complications has been reported, even in those patients who were on prophylactic anticoagulation. In a postmortem kidney pathohistological analysis, fibrin thrombi were present in the absence of red blood cell fragmentation and platelet thrombi. Due to this, a hypercoagulable state is suspected. Therefore, endothelial cell dysfunction that leads to activation of the coagulation cascade and thrombosis of the microcirculation may also play a role in AKI [26, 38].

16.2.4.5 Vessels

DIC and endothelial dysfunction are conditions that can lead to thrombotic microangiopathy. Cases of thrombotic microangiopathy have been reported in association with a wide range of infections and one of the consequences is AKI. Viral elements have been found within endothelial cells, and inflammatory factors can lead to endothelial cell apoptosis [26].

16.2.4.6   Colon

Chemokine C-X-C motif ligand (CXCL) 1 has been proven to be the major mediator of colon-kidney organ crosstalk, as shown in a model of dextran sodium sulfate colitis. Furthermore, chemokine CXCL8, or IL-8, the human homolog of rodent CXCL1, is an early proinflammatory chemokine secreted by mononuclear immune cells and epithelial cells. When released, it promotes neutrophil chemotaxis and neutrophil activation by binding to conventional CXC chemokine receptors 1 and 2 (CXCR1 and CXCR2). This can be supported with the implication of CXCL8/CXCL1 in a broad range of diseases that are characterized by their polymorphonuclear neutrophils cell infiltration, including AKI. As aforementioned, CXCL8 involvement in the local immune response is by the promotion of neutrophil chemotaxis and activation by NF-kB pathway. Therefore, a persistence or upregulation of this chemokine maintains immune cell recruitment, generating constant deleterious effects on inflamed tissue. In a recent Amrouche et al. study, it has been found that miR-146a targets the NF-κB pathway in tubular cells, consequently, regulating CXCL8 secretion. Therefore, in vivo deletion of miR-146a enhances the formation of tubular lesions after unilateral AKI, immune cells infiltration, and renal fibrosis development [36, 41].

16.3   Conclusion

Acute kidney injury associated with COVID-19 induced pneumonia is a paradigmatic example of pathologic kidney–lung crosstalk.

References

1. World Health Organization. New coronavirus. China. 2020.
2. Musso-Enz GM. Why was the SARS-COV epidemic (2002–2003) so rapidly contained while SARS-COV-2 easily spread since December 2019 and gave rise to the actual pandemic? Electron J Biomed. 2021;3:34–6.
3. Wang D, Hu B, Hu C, et al. Clinical characteristics of 138 hospitalized patients with 2019 novel coronavirus-infected pneumonia in Wuhan, China. JAMA. 2020;323(11):1061–9.
4. Naicker S, Yang CW, Hwang SJ, Liu BC, Chen JH, Jha V. The novel coronavirus 2019 epidemic and kidneys. Kidney Int. 2020;97(5):824–8. https://doi.org/10.1016/j.kint.2020.03.001.
5. Su H, Yang M, Wan C, et al. Renal histopathological analysis of 26 postmortem findings of patients with COVID-19 in China. Kidney Int. 2020;98(1):219–27. https://doi.org/10.1016/j.kint.2020.04.003.
6. Gabarre P, Dumas G, Dupont T, Darmon M, Azoulay E, Zafrani L. Acute kidney injury in critically ill patients with COVID-19. Intensive Care Med. 2020;46(7):1339–48. https://doi.org/10.1007/s00134-020-06153-9.
7. Cheng Y, Luo R, Wang K, et al. Kidney impairment is associated with in-hospital death of COVID-19 patients. medRxiv. 2020:1–21. https://doi.org/10.1101/2020.02.18.20023242.

8. Sang L, Chen S, Zheng X, et al. The incidence, risk factors and prognosis of acute kidney injury in severe and critically ill patients with COVID-19 in mainland China: a retrospective study. BMC pulmonary Med. 2020;20:1–10.
9. Shafi ST. Covid-19 and acute kidney injury: recent updates. Pak J Kidney Dis. 2020;4(2):225–7.
10. Aroca-Martínez G, Musso CG, Avendaño-Echavez L, González-Torres H, Vélez-Verbel M, Chartouni-Narvaez S, Peña-Vargas W, Acosta-Hoyos A, Ferreyra L, Cadena-Bonfanti A. Impact of frailty and viral load on acute kidney injury evolution in patients affected by COVID-19. Saudi J Kidney Dis Transpl. 2021;32(5):1356–64.
11. Aroca-Martínez G, Musso CG, Avendaño-Echavez L, Vélez-Verbel M, Chartouni-Narvaez S, Hernandez S, Hinojosa-Vidal MA, Espitaleta Z, Cadena-Bonfanti A. Differences between COVID-19-induced acute kidney injury and chronic kidney disease patients. J Bras Nefrol. 2022;44(2):155–63.
12. Avendaño-Echavez L, Musso CG. COVID-19 and acute kidney injury: current knowledge. Rev Colomb Nefrol. 2020;7(Supl 2):168–9.
13. Gondo-an K, Temel S, Baran Ketencio-lu B, Rabah B, Tutar N, Sungur M. Acute kidney injury in SARS-CoV-2 infected critically ill Patients Turkish. J Nephrol. 2020;29:185–9.
14. Chan L, Chaudhary K, Saha A, et al. On behalf of the Mount Sinai COVID informatics center (MSCIC). AKI in hospitalized patients with COVID-19. J Am Soc Nephrol. 2020;32:151. https://doi.org/10.1681/ASN.2020050615.
15. King-Vela E, Muñoz J, Rico-Fontalvo J, et al. Acute kidney injury in Colombian patients with COVID-19 who received kidney support therapy with genius® 90 technology. J Clin Nephrol. 2020;4(3):056–60.
16. Cheng Y, Luo R, Wang K, et al. Kidney disease is associated with in-hospital death of patients with COVID-19. Kidney Int. 2020;97(5):829–38.
17. Meijers B, Hilbrands LB. The clinical characteristics of coronavirus-associated nephropathy. Nephrol Dial Transplant. 2020;35(8):1279–81.
18. Molina-Barragan AM, Pardo E, Galichon P, et al. SARS-COV2 renal impairment in critical care: A retrospective study of 42 cases—Kid COVID Study. J Clin Med. 2021;10(8):1571. https://doi.org/10.21203/rs.3.rs-64088/v1.
19. Golmai P, Larsen DVM, et al. Histopathologic and ultrastructural findings in postmortem kidney biopsy material in 12 patients with AKI and COVID-19. J Am Soc Nephrol. 2020;31:1944–7. https://doi.org/10.1681/ASN.2020050683.
20. Batlle D, Soler MJ, Sparks MA, et al. Acute kidney injury in COVID-19: emerging evidence of a distinct pathophysiology. J Am Soc Nephrol. 2020;31(7):1380–3. https://doi.org/10.1681/ASN.2020040419.
21. Sise ME, Baggett MV, Shepard JO, Stevens JS, Rhee EP. Case 17-2020: a 68-year-old man with Covid-19 and kidney acute injury. N Engl J Med. 2020;382(22):2147–56.
22. Hernandez-Arroyo CF, Varghese V, Mohamed MMB, Velez JCQ. Urinary sediment microscopy in acute kidney injury associated with COVID-19. Kidney360. 2020;1(8):819–23. https://doi.org/10.34067/KID.0003352020.
23. Pujadas E, Chaudhry F, McBride R, et al. SARS-CoV-2 viral load predicts COVID-19 mortality. Lancet. 2020;8(9):e70.
24. Khan S, Chen L, Yang CR, et al. Does SARS-CoV-2 Infect the Kidney? J Am Soc Nephrol. 2020;31:1–3. https://doi.org/10.1681/ASN.2020081229.
25. Braun F, Huber T, Puelles V. Proximal tubular dysfunction in patients with COVID-19: what have we learnt so far? Kidney Int. 2020;98(5):1092–4. https://doi.org/10.1016/j.kint.2020.09.002.
26. Redant S, De Bels D, Honoré PM. Severe acute respiratory syndrome coronavirus-2-associated acute kidney injury: a narrative review focused upon pathophysiology. Crit Care Med. 2021;49(5):e533–40.
27. González C, Yama E, Yomayusa N, et al. Colombian consensus of experts on evidence-informed recommendations for the prevention, diagnosis and management of sars-cov-2/covid-19 acute kidney injury. Rev Colomb Nefrol. 2020;7(Supl.2):50–69. https://revistanefrologia.org/index.php/rcn/article/view/473.

28. Lee J, Silberzweig J, Akchurin O, et al. Characteristics of acute kidney injury in hospitalized COVID-19 patients in an urban Academic Medical Center. Clin J Am Soc Nephrol. 2021;16:1–3. https://doi.org/10.2215/CJN.07440520.
29. Zhou F, Ting Y, Ronghui D, et al. Clinical course and risk factors for mortality of adult inpatients with COVID-19 in Wuhan, China: a retrospective cohort study. Lancet. 2020;395:1054–62.
30. Ruan Q, Yang K, Wang W, et al. Clinical predictors of mortality due to COVID-19 based on an analysis of data of 150 patients from Wuhan, China. Intensive Care Med. 2020;46:846–8. https://doi.org/10.1007/s00134-020-05991-x.
31. Páramo Fernández J. Coagulación, Dímero D y COVID-19. Sociedad Española de Trombosis y Hemostasia (SETH). https://www.seth.es/index.php/noticias/noticias/noticias-de-la-seth/1588-coagulacion-dimero-d-y-covid-19.html.
32. Pérez G. Coronavirus. Impacto cardiovascular Sociedad Interamericana de Cardiología http://www.siacardio.com/novedades/covid-19/coronavirus-y-su-impacto-cardiovascular/.
33. Driggin E, Madhavan MV, Bikdeli B, Chuich T, Laracy J, Bondi-Zoccai G, Brown TS, Nigoghossian CD, Zidar DA, Haythe J, Brodie D, Beckman JA, Kirtane AJ, Stone GW, Krumholz HM, Parikh SA. Cardiovascular considerations for patients, health care workers, and health systems during the coronavirus disease 2019 (COVID-19) pandemic. J Am Coll Cardiol. 2020;75:2352. https://doi.org/10.1016/j.jacc.2020.03.031.
34. Qin C, Zhou L, Hu Z, et al. Dysregulation of immune response in patients with COVID-19 in Wuhan, China. Clin Infect Dis. 2020;71:762. https://doi.org/10.1093/cid/ciaa248.
35. Mehta P, McAuley DF, Brown M, Sanchez E, Tattersall RS, Manson JJ. COVID-19: consider cytokine storm syndromes and immunosuppression. Lancet. 2020;395:1033. https://doi.org/10.1016/S0140-6736(20)30628-0.
36. Taverna G, Di Francesco S, Borroni EM, Yiu D, Toniato E, Milanesi S, Chiriva-Internati M, Bresalier RS, Zanoni M, Vota P, Maffei D, Justich M, Grizzi F. The kidney, COVID-19, and the chemokine network: an intriguing trio. Int Urol Nephrol. 2021;53(1):97–104. https://doi.org/10.1007/s11255-020-02579-8.
37. Loganathan S, Kuppusamy M, Wankhar W, Gurugubelli KR, Mahadevappa VH, Lepcha L, Choudhary AK. Angiotensin-converting enzyme 2 (ACE2): COVID 19 gate way to multiple organ failure syndromes. Respir Physiol Neurobiol. 2021;283:103548. https://doi.org/10.1016/j.resp.2020.103548.
38. Hassanein M, Radhakrishnan Y, Sedor J, Vachharajani T, Vachharajani VT, Augustine J, Demirjian S, Thomas G. COVID-19 and the kidney. Cleve Clin J Med. 2020;87(10):619–31.
39. Saeedi Saravi SS, Barbagallo M, Reiner MF, Schmid HR, Rutishauser J, Beer JH. Acute kidney injury associated with COVID-19: a prognostic factor for pulmonary embolism or coincidence? Eur Heart J. 2020;41(48):4601. https://doi.org/10.1093/eurheartj/ehaa637.
40. Vakili K, Fathi M, Pezeshgi A, Mohamadkhani A, Hajiesmaeili M, Rezaei-Tavirani M, Sayehmiri F. Critical complications of COVID-19: a descriptive meta-analysis study. Rev Cardiovasc Med. 2020;21(3):433–42. https://doi.org/10.31083/j.rcm.2020.03.129.
41. Sam Kant S, Menez SP, Hanouneh M, Fine DM, Crews DC, Brennan DC, Sperati CJ, Jaar BG. The COVID-19 nephrology compendium: AKI, CKD, ESKD and transplantation. BMC Nephrol. 2020;21:449. https://doi.org/10.1186/s12882-020-02112-0.

Index